Clinical Trials in Rheumatoid Arthritis and Osteoarthritis

Series Editors

Derek Pearson, BSc, PhD
Joint Service Manager
Medical Physics & Clinical Engineering
Department
Nottingham University Hospitals NHS
Trust
City Hospitals Campus
Hucknall NG5 1PB
UK

Colin G. Miller, PhD, FICR
Senior Vice President
Medical Affairs
Bio-Imaging Technologies Inc.
826 Newtown-Yardley Road
Newtown, PA 18940
USA

Other Titles in This Series

Clinical Trials in Osteoporosis (2nd Edition)
Derek Pearson and Colin G. Miller

Clinical Trials in Rheumatoid Arthritis and Osteoarthritis
David M. Reid and Colin G. Miller

David M. Reid • Colin G. Miller

Editors

Clinical Trials in Rheumatoid Arthritis and Osteoarthritis

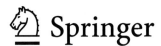 Springer

Editors

David M. Reid, MBChB, MD, FRCP
Department of Medicine and Therapeutics
University of Aberdeen
Aberdeen, UK

Colin G. Miller, BSc, PhD, FICR
Bio-Imaging Technologies Inc.
Newtown, PA, USA

ISBN: 978-1-85233-874-9   e-ISBN: 978-1-84628-742-8
DOI: 10.1007/978-1-84628-742-8

British Library Cataloguing in Publication Data
Clinical trials in rheumatoid arthritis and osteoarthritis
    1. Rheumatoid arthritis - Treatment 2. Osteoarthritis -
    Treatment 3. Clinical trials
    I. Reid, David, 1951- II. Miller, Colin G., 1960-
    616.7'22060724
ISBN-13: 9781852338749

Library of Congress Control Number: 2007937490

Printed on acid-free paper

9 8 7 6 5 4 3 2 1

Springer Science+Business Media
springer.com

Contents

Contributors

Adewale O. Adebajo, MBBS, MSc, FRCP
Honorary Senior Lecturer, Academic Rheumatology Group, University of Sheffield, Sheffield UK

François Abram, PhD
ArthroVision Inc., Montreal, Canada

Nigel Arden, MBBS, MSc, MD
Senior Lecturer in Rheumatology, MRC Unit, Southampton General Hospital, Southampton, UK

Anna M. Baratelle, ASRT, (R)(MR)
Clinical Imaging Lead, Centocor, Malvern, Pennsylvania, USA. Previously, Director, Business Development and Clinical Education, Bio-Imaging Technologies, Inc., Newtown, Pennsylvania, USA

Neil Basu, MBChB (Hons), MRCP(UK)
Specialist Registrar, NHS Grampian, Aberdeen Royal Infirmary, Aberdeen, UK

Yolanda Bravo Vergel, BA, MA, MSc
Research Fellow, Centre for Health Economics, University of York, York, UK

Shirish Dubey, MB, BS, MRCP (Ireland), DMedEd
Previously Clinical Lecturer in Rheumatology and Medical Education, Academic Unit of Medical Education, University of Sheffield, Sheffield, UK

Mario R. Ehlers, MD, PhD
Chief Medical Officer, Pacific Biometrics, Inc., Seattle, Washington, USA

Mark D. Endres, BS, CNMT
Vice President, Global Business Development, Bio-Imaging Technologies, Inc., Newtown, Pennsylvania, USA

David R. Eyre, BS, PhD
Department of Orthopaedics and Sports Medicine, University of Washington, Seattle, Washington, USA

Pieter Geusens, MD, PhD
Department of Rheumatology, University Hospital, Maastricht, The Netherlands *and* Biomedical Research Institute, University Hasselt, Diepenbeek, Belgium

Elizabeth T. Leary, PhD
Chief Scientific Officer, Pacific Biometrics, Inc., Seattle, Washington, USA

L. Stefan Lohmander, MD, PhD
Institute of Clinical Sciences, Department of Orthopaedics, Lund University
Hospital, Lund, Sweden

Johanne Martel-Pelletier, PhD
Osteoarthritis Research Unit, Notre-Dame Hospital, University of Montreal
Hospital Centre (CHUM), Montreal, Canada

Colin G. Miller, BSc, PhD, FICR
Senior Vice President, Medical Affairs, Bio-Imaging Technologies Inc., Newtown,
Pennsylvania, USA

Derek Pearson, BSc, PhD
Clinical Director, Medical Physics, City Hospital, Nottingham, UK

Jean-Pierre Pelletier, MD
Osteoarthritis Research Unit, Notre-Dame Hospital, University of Montreal
Hospital Centre (CHUM), Montreal, Canada

Stuart H. Ralston, MD, FRCP, FMedSci, FRSE
Head of School of Molecular and Clinical Medicine & Professor of Rheumatology,
Molecular Medicine Centre, University of Edinburgh, Edinburgh, UK

Jean-Pierre Raynauld, MD, FRCPC
Osteoarthritis Research Unit, Notre-Dame Hospital, University of Montreal
Hospital Centre (CHUM), Montreal, Canada

David M. Reid, MBChB, MD, FRCP edin, FRCP lon
Professor of Rheumatology, Head of Department of Medicine & Therapeutics,
University of Aberdeen, Aberdeen, UK

Julie Shotton, BSc
Previously Senior Research Nurse, Osteoporosis Research Unit, Department of
Medicine & Therapeutics, University of Aberdeen, Aberdeen, UK

David Torgerson, MSc, PhD
Director of York Trials Unit, Department of Health Sciences, University of York,
York, UK

Désirée van der Heijde, MD, PhD
Professor of Rheumatology, Leiden University Medical Center, Department
of Rheumatology, Leiden, The Netherlands

Cornelis van Kuijk, MD, PhD
Department of Radiology, VU University Medical Center, Amsterdam,
The Netherlands

Chapter 1
Introduction

David M. Reid and Colin G. Miller

Why a Book About Clinical Trials in Rheumatoid Arthritis and Osteoarthritis?

From an etiology of disease perspective, a book on rheumatoid arthritis (RA) and osteoarthritis (OA) is a strange combination; however, from a clinical trial perspective, the primary end points are very similar. The primary end points in both disease states are imaging and serum or urine biomarkers as recognized by the U.S. Food and Drug Administration (FDA) The FDA guidance documents for OA [1] refer to the RA guidance documents for the imaging end points [2]. During the writing of this book, the Osteoarthritis Research Society International (OARSI) has teamed up with the Outcomes Measures and Evaluation in Rheumatoid Arthritis Clinical Trials (OMERACT) to create the OMERACT-OARSI working group. This is an obvious recognition of similar end points of the disease states.

The evolution of the trials in RA and OA is at an interesting point in time. There have been a number of successful therapeutic disease-modifying agents that have been developed and are now on the market for RA. The same is not true for OA, where at the time of writing there have been no successful FDA submissions for a disease modifying osteoarthritis anti-rheumatic drug (DMOARD), partly due to a lack of compounds and partly due to the challenges of running the trials. With RA, there is now a standard pattern and expectation for performing these trials with three anti-TNF-α and one anti-B-cell monoclonal antibody products on the market in a number of indications and many more to follow. For OA, the one large trial testing a potential DMOAD, using the bisphosphonate risedronate [3], sadly missed its primary end point. There are now a handful of studies evaluating glucosamine and chondroitin sulfate in both the United States and Europe [4, 5]. The first results are not only suggestive of a potential positive outcome but also more importantly demonstrate that with careful controls, a study in OA looking at joint space narrowing can be achieved (see Chapter 14).

D.M. Reid
Professor of Rheumatology, Head of Department of Medicine & Therapeutics, University of Aberdeen, Aberdeen, UK

D.M. Reid, C.G. Miller (eds.), *Clinical Trials in Rheumatoid Arthritis and Osteoarthritis*,
© Springer-Verlag London Limited 2008

OA is a crippling disease that has approximately 10 times the prevalence of RA, and there is a huge unmet medical need for good drugs to halt disease progression. This is not to minimize the pain of RA; rather, the lessons learned from the RA field can be applied to OA.

Clinical trials are requiring more and more rigor, and the specific end points are becoming more complex, with an increasing and bewildering number of regulatory hurdles. This is the case with trials in RA and OA. The similarity of design makes the therapeutic combination come together. This book is intended for those new to conducting clinical trials in these areas: a handbook or a "how to." It is not intended as an all-encompassing text on the results of those studies that have gone before or a thorough in-depth analysis of how to get through the regulations like the Code of Federal Regulations (CFR 21 Part 11, Electronic Records and Use of Electronic Signatures) [6]. This is the second book in the series (the first one being *Clinical Trials on Osteoporosis*) and it follows a similar format, allowing the reader to be able to read each chapter in isolation or to put the pieces together to obtain an overall picture. As with the book on osteoporosis, this book is also unique in that it brings together both the clinical trial aspect and the therapeutic aspect into one volume.

How This Book Works

The aim of this book is to lead the research through all the stages of a clinical trial. The first part covers background to current and some future therapies for RA and OA (Chapters and 3), and the second part examines study design (Chapters 4 to 7) and the pretrial phase including ethical considerations specific to trials in RA and OA (Chapter 7).

The third part (Chapters 8 to 11) looks at the day-to-day running of the trial from the four main constituents involved in patient collection and data management: the sponsor, the site, the central blood or biomarker lab, and the central imaging core lab. It is interesting to note that the primary end points of biomarkers, be they serologic or imaging, are all now processed through independent third-party groups as a *de facto* standard. This would not have been the case 15 years ago.

The fourth part (Chapter 12) covers data analysis and presentation and includes a guide to writing a paper for a peer-reviewed journal to a standard that will ensure that readers will gain full benefit from one's trial and the results will be easily included into subsequent meta-analyses.

The final part examines imaging end points and biochemical markers for both RA and OA (Chapters 13 to 16) and describes new possible end points of pharmacogenomics (Chaper 17) and pharmacoeconomics (Chapter 18).

We have attempted to use standard terminology throughout the book. This includes the sponsor (usually a pharmaceutical company who is funding the research), the contract research organization (or CRO), which is a company responsible for administering the trial, assuring the quality of the data, analyzing the data, and producing the final report. A clinical research associate (CRA) is the representative of the sponsor or CRO who liaises between the CRO and each site participating in the trial. The investigator is the researcher at the local site who has responsibility for recruiting research subjects and running the study locally. We have chosen to refer to those taking part in clinical trials as *subjects* rather than *patients* for the very reason that many of them are not ill but are normal women and men. The drug under investigation is usually under development by the sponsor and is known throughout the book as the new molecular entity (NME).

Most chapters contain many references to other source material. These allow the reader to take any of the issues covered in the book to greater depth. As always, there are many abbreviations in the book, thus a glossary is given as an appendix.

References

1. FDA. Osteoarthritis guidance documents. Available at http://www.fda.gov/cder/guidance/2199dft.pdf.
2. FDA. RA guidance documents. Available at http://www.fda.gov/cder/guidance/raguide.pdf.
3. Spector TD, Conaghan PG, Buckland-Wright JC, et al. Effect of risedronate on joint structure and symptoms of knee osteoarthritis: results of the BRISK randomized, controlled trial. Arthritis Res Ther 2005;7(3):625–633.
4. Clegg DO, Reda DJ, Harris CL, et al. Glucosamine, chondroitin sulfate, and the two in combination for painful knee osteoarthritis. N Engl J Med 2006;354(8):795–808.
5. Herrero-Beaumont G, Román Ivorra RA, del Carmen Trabado M, et al. Glucosamine sulfate in the treatment of knee osteoarthritis symptoms: a randomized, double-blind, placebo-controlled study using acetaminophen as a side comparator. Arthritis Rheum 2007;56(2):555–567.
6. U.S. Code of Federal Regulations. CFR 21 Part 11. Available at http://www.fda.gov/ora/compliance_ref/part11/.

Chapter 2
Historical and Current Perspectives on Management of Osteoarthritis and Rheumatoid Arthritis

Shirish Dubey and Adewale O. Adebajo

Historical and Current Perspectives on Management of Osteoarthritis

Osteoarthritis (OA) is a slowly evolving but active disease of degeneration of the articular cartilage associated with symptoms of joint pain, stiffness, and limitation of movement. Typically, these symptoms tend to be worse with weight bearing and activity and improve with rest. Physical examination often reveals tenderness on palpation, bony enlargement, crepitus on movements, and limitation of joint movement. OA can occur in any joint but is most common in the hip, knee, and the joints of the hand, foot, and spine. OA is the most prevalent disease in our society and the second most common cause of disability in the elderly in the Western world, second only to cardiovascular disease [1]. In fact, more than 75% of persons above 70 years of age show some radiographic evidence of OA [2]. The World Health Organization (WHO) figures of worldwide estimates are that 9.6% of men and 18% of women aged more than 60 years have symptomatic OA [3]. The prevalence of OA increases with age because the condition is not reversible. Men are affected more often than women among those aged less than 45 years, whereas women are affected more frequently among those aged more than 55 years [4]. The prevalence of OA is only likely to rise further, due to a variety of reasons. Life expectancy has steadily increased over the years and continues to do so. The triad of increasing numbers of elderly people, obesity, and lack of exercise plaguing Western society at the moment is likely to have a significant effect on the burden of OA facing people and society in the next few decades.

S. Dubey
Previously Clinical Lecturer in Rheumatology and Medical Education, Academic Unit of Medical Education, University of Sheffield, Sheffield, UK

D.M. Reid, C.G. Miller (eds.), *Clinical Trials in Rheumatoid Arthritis and Osteoarthritis*,   5
© Springer-Verlag London Limited 2008

Historical Aspects

Perhaps the earliest descriptions of OA were provided by Heberden and Haygarth in the 19th century [5, 6]. In the 1930s and 1940s, Stecher showed that there were two forms of this disease, idiopathic and posttraumatic [7]. It was in the 1950s that the link between Heberden's nodes and large joint OA was established with the publication of a paper by Kellgren and Moore [8]. The first x-ray grading system was developed in the 1950s by Jonas Kellgren and John Lawrence [9]. Lawrence led the application of this to epidemiology leading to the observation of discordance between radiographic and symptomatic OA [10]. Surgical options were pioneered as early as the 1950s and 1960s. John Charnley [11] and George McKee [12] both published their landmark papers during the 1960s, which transformed the surgical management of these patients.

Predisposing Factors

A variety of factors are recognized as predisposing factors for individuals with OA. These are summarized in Table 2.1.

Pathogenesis

OA is a dynamic process with intermittent progression characterized by an adaptive response of synovial joints to a variety of stresses. One of the first changes in OA appears to be cartilage loss. The cartilage normally consists of proteoglycans and glycosaminoglycans in the framework of type 2 collagen. There is a progressive depletion of the cartilage proteoglycan in the early stages of OA, leading to a net loss of matrix from the cartilage [13]. This in turn leads to a cascade of events including decrease in hyaluronic acid content, changes in the enzymatic cleavage of

Table 2.1 Predisposing factors for OA

Age
Female gender
Genetic predisposition of the individual
Previous trauma
Mechanical factors like malalignment
Previous or current occupation (e.g. farming, miners, jackhammer operators, etc)
Previous inflammatory arthritis
Biochemical and metabolic abnormalities (e.g., pyrophosphate arthropathy)
Exercise, particularly for professional sports persons
Obesity
Nutritional (low Vitamin C and Vitamin D levels)

Source: Adapted from Felson DT. Epidemiology of osteoarthritis, pages 9–14; in Osteoarthritis. Eds Brandt KD, Doherty M, Lowmander LS; Oxford University Press, 2003, 2nd ed.

proteoglycans, and increase in minor collagen types leading to structural and functional deterioration of the cartilage. Certain enzymes play a vital role in this process of breakdown of cartilage [14, 15], and these include the matrix metalloproteinase enzymes (MMPs). Collagenase (MMP-1) appears to have a significant role in this, as there is a correlation between the levels of collagenase and the severity of cartilage lesions in OA [16, 17]. A number of inhibitors of MMPs have also been identified with tissue inhibitors of metalloproteinase-1 (TIMP-1) and TIMP-2 being the most common in humans [18, 19]. This disease process that begins in the articular cartilage eventually involves the surrounding bone, the synovium, and the surrounding soft tissues. Often, there is evidence of bony sclerosis that is seen on radiographs [20], but after the initial stages of cartilage degeneration, there may be a delay of many years before any symptoms appear or there is radiologic evidence of OA. At least in part, this is due to lack of innervation of the cartilage whereas the surrounding structures, which include the periosteum, subchondral bone, and the joint capsule, appear to be richly innervated.

Treatment of OA

The goals of contemporary management of a patient with OA include control of pain and improvement in function as well as quality of life [21]. A number of issues need to be considered to decide the optimum management of a patient with OA, including level of pain and discomfort, level of disability, comorbidity, the joint involved, and the degree of radiologic damage [22].

A suggested protocol for managing OA is shown in Figure 2.1.

Nonpharmacological Therapies

A number of nonpharmacologic interventions are available for patients with OA and form an integral part of the treatment plan for these patients. Some of these include patient education therapies that are available for these patients include patient education, self-management programs, weight loss (if overweight), aerobic exercise programs, muscle strengthening exercises, medial taping of the patella, appropriate footwear, occupational therapy, joint protection and energy conservation, and assistive devices for ambulation or activities of daily living [21]. There is considerable evidence to suggest that nonpharmacological options are useful not only early but also later on in the course of the disease and help to reduce disability [23–25].

Pharmacological Therapy

Analgesics

Generally, pharmacological options should be used in addition to nonpharmacological measures [26]. For many patients, simple painkillers like paracetamol or

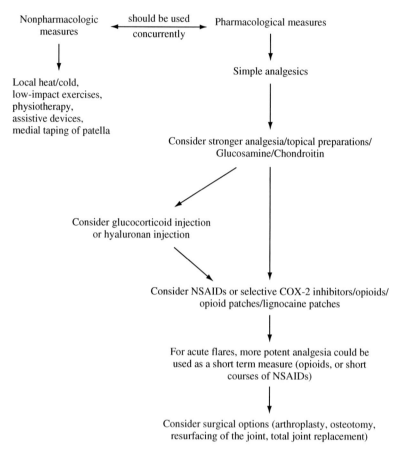

Fig. 2.1 Suggested protocol for managing osteoarthritis

acetaminophen are enough to provide significant symptom relief. Quite often for mild to moderate pain, the benefit to patients from simple analgesics is comparable with that from nonsteroidal anti-inflammatory drugs (NSAIDs) [27–29]. A meta-analysis of trials comparing simple analgesics with NSAIDs in patients with knee OA did find that NSAID-treated patients had significantly greater improvement in both pain on rest and pain on motion [30]. For moderate to severe pain, simple analgesics might not be sufficient and these patients would benefit from combination of simple analgesics with low-dose opioids, semi-synthetic opioids, transdermal opioids, or NSAIDs. There is some evidence to support the use of Buprenorphine patches and Lignocaine patches in these patients [31, 32].

Paracetamol and acetaminophen should be used with caution in patients with existing liver disease and avoided in patients with chronic alcohol abuse. These drugs can also prolong the half-life of warfarin, and careful monitoring of the INR is necessary in these patients.

NSAIDs

In some patients, the combination of nonpharmacological interventions and simple analgesics will not be enough to optimally control symptoms. In this group of patients, additional pharmacological agents should be considered; most commonly this will be in the form of a NSAID. The choice of the NSAID agent depends on a number of factors including the age of the person, comorbid medical conditions, history of upper gastrointestinal (GI) bleeding or ulcers, and anticoagulant and steroid use. In these cases, it might be safer to use selective cyclooxygenase (COX)-2 inhibitors rather than nonselective NSAIDs. The National Institute of Clinical Excellence in the United Kingdom has issued guidelines for the use of selective COX-2 agents [33]. Selective COX-2 inhibitors have the advantage of reduced risk of GI side effects alongside comparable efficacy compared with the traditional NSAIDs [34–38]. Another advantage of the selective COX-2 inhibitors is that they have no effect on platelet function, which is a major advantage during the perioperative period, as well as for patients on warfarin [39]. The common traditional NSAIDs include ibuprofen, diclofenac, naproxen, indomethacin, piroxicam, and so forth. The common selective COX-2 inhibitors include celecoxib, etoricoxib, meloxicam, parecoxib, and etodolac. NSAIDs, both selective and nonselective, have to be used with caution because of certain common side effects in patients with hypertension, congestive heart failure, or renal impairment. Severe renal impairment is a contraindication for use of NSAIDs.

Recently, the cardiovascular safety of the selective COX-2 inhibitors has received a lot of attention. Various studies involving rofecoxib and valdecoxib (which were consequently withdrawn from the market), celecoxib, and parecoxib have shown an increased vascular risk mainly in the form of myocardial infarctions and strokes. Consequently, these drugs are now used more cautiously. The cardiovascular safety of standard NSAIDs has also received some attention recently, and there is now considerable evidence to suggest that standard NSAIDs share the vascular risk with selective COX-2 inhibitors [40]. Hence the Medicine and Healthcare Products Regulatory Agency (MHRA) recommends that 'the lowest effective dose of the NSAID should be used for the shortest period of time' [41].

Other Conservative Treatments

In patients with OA of the knee, topical analgesia is also an option. This could be in the form of a nonsteroidal gel, for example piroxicam gel, or in the form of capsaicin cream [41]. In some patients, this combination will still not be enough to provide adequate pain relief. In such patients, alternative analgesics could be used, including opioid analgesics like codeine phosphate [28] or synthetic opioids like tramadol. Tramadol, a synthetic opioid that inhibits reuptake of noradrenaline and serotonin, is a centrally acting analgesic used for treating moderate to severe pain. It tends to have fewer side effects than would normally be associated with opioids, such as drowsiness, constipation, and respiratory depression. Its efficacy has found to be similar to ibuprofen in OA and is a useful adjunct [42, 43].

Intra-articular Injections

An alternative approach in the management of joint pain would be the use of intra-articular therapy. This could be in the form of glucocorticoid injections (particularly if there is evidence of joint effusion) or in the form of hyaluronic acid injections. The mechanism of action of hyaluronic acid appears to be unclear as the duration of benefit exceeds its synovial half-life. Proposed mechanisms include inhibition of inflammatory mediators such as cytokines and prostaglandins, and stimulation of cartilage matrix synthesis. In clinical trials, patients receiving intra-articular hyaluronic acid preparations had significantly greater pain relief than that seen with intra-articular injection of placebo and comparable with that seen with oral NSAIDs [44–46]. The extent of pain relief was similar to that experienced by patients treated with intra-articular glucocorticoid [46]. Intra-articular hyaluronic acid therapy is indicated for use in patients who have not responded to a program of nonpharmacological therapy and simple analgesics and could also be used in patients in whom nonsteroidals are contraindicated. However, real-life experience from use of hyaluronic acid therapy is not as positive as would be indicated from the trials alone.

Intra-articular glucocorticoids can be extremely useful in the treatment of patients with OA, particularly in the presence of a joint effusion [47]. In animal experiments, intra-articular glucocorticoids have demonstrated a protective effect with reduction of cartilage erosions and osteophyte size [48, 49]. There is, however, very little data from randomized, double-blind, placebo-controlled clinical trials in humans. Despite this, most clinicians have had experience of some benefit in patients with OA with the local administration of glucocorticoids. The difficulty lies in accurately predicting which patients will benefit with this form of therapy. Furthermore, repeated injections into the same joint tend to show diminishing response, although the reasons for this clinical phenomenon are unknown. The usual recommended dose of triamcinolone is 5 to 10 mg for a small joint such as the finger or thumb, 10 to 20 mg for joints like the ankle, wrist, and elbow, and 30 to 40 mg in a large joint like the shoulder or knee.

Glucosamine and Chondroitin

A meta-analysis of the evidence for use of glucosamine and chondroitin performed by McAlindon et al. [50] revealed moderate to large effects for these drugs in the treatment of hip or knee OA. Both glucosamine and chondroitin are derivatives of glycosaminoglycans found in the articular cartilage. However, their mechanism of action is unclear as they cannot be absorbed from the gut intact [1]. One clinical trial demonstrated some efficacy in not only reduction of symptoms but also reduction in knee medial compartment changes over 3 years [51]. A Cochrane review of glucosamine and chondroitin as well as a review of knee OA by the European League Against Rheumatism (EULAR) have both recommended that there is reasonable evidence to support the use of these agents in the management of patients with OA [52, 53].

Experimental Treatments

Cod liver oil in the dose of 1000 mg daily has been found to have an effect on reducing the levels of enzymes responsible for degradation of the cartilage in patients undergoing knee replacement (data unpublished as yet). It is possible that in the future, cod liver oil may have a role to play in reducing the symptoms of OA or reducing progression. Other forms of treatment using delivery of anti-inflammatory cytokines or gene induction using gene transfer [54] may provide novel approaches to treatment of OA. It is possible that these therapies may provide the crucial breakthrough in terms of reducing the progression of disease, which has not been clearly established with any other form of treatment yet.

Surgical Treatments

Surgery of the joints in the form of joint replacement has been available for more than 40 years for the hip and 30 years for the knee. The numbers of knee prostheses are increasing more than the number of hip prostheses, such that the demand for both is now about equal. Joint replacement, however, is not the only surgical option available to patients with OA. A number of other options are available, particularly for the younger patients; these include surgical repair and cell and tissue transplantation. In the hip, surface replacement has been introduced [55], and in the knee, arthroscopic osteotomy [56], interpositional spacers [57], and unicompartmental knee arthroplasty [58] are all options.

The primary purpose of joint surgery is to relieve pain and restore function. Two surgeons in the 1960s, John Charley and George McKee, pioneered hip replacements. The former introduced metal-on-polyethylene hip prostheses fixed with cement [59], and this was the mainstay of hip replacements for about 3 decades, and the latter was responsible for metal-on-metal hip prostheses [12], which did not gain popularity until recently due to poor fixation. The Charnley approach was adopted as the standard approach for hips [60–63] and was applied to the knees as well. However, with time, the limitations of this started to become apparent, mainly the problems relating to cement and localized bone resorption [64–67] and fracture of femoral stems [68]. The risk of fracture was reduced by changes in the metal alloys and changes in the geometric design. However, the risk of localized bone resorption persisted despite the advent of cementless prostheses. This was later recognized to be due to polyethylene wear debris [69–74]. Research into polyethylene stability revealed that the gamma irradiation in the presence of air was responsible for causing the compound to become unstable [75]. In addition, it gave rise to an increase in the wear rate as well as contributing to the osteolytic potential [76–78]. This has led to a new generation of designs and bearing materials for hip prostheses. Metal-on-polyethylene prostheses were developed for the knee and were commonly used for a number of years, with similar results.

All the above prostheses have a limited life span (of about 15 to 20 years), due to the inherent problems with them. However, for older patients with life expectancy of less than 20 years, these would still be perfectly acceptable options. For younger patients, there have been new developments including the use of ceramic femoral heads, ceramic-on-ceramic bearings, and metal-on-metal bearings that have led to alternative bearing options with better long-term results and less long-term risk of osteolysis [69,79–82]. For the knee, the major advance has been the introduction of a stable and oxidization-resistant polyethylene, which reduces the risk of delamination failure [82] and osteolysis [83–85]. Improved designs have also led to reduced wear and tear of these prostheses. Unicompartmental knee replacements have been shown to have some success in reducing the bone loss [58, 86], though long-term data are awaited. Recently, hip resurfacing has also been tried with some success [55]. Experimental work on cartilage culture and transplantation has shown some promise but is still more than a few years away from routine clinical use.

Summary

OA is primarily a disease of the cartilage later leading to ligament damage and instability of the joint. Management of this, the most common form of arthritis, involves a combination of nonpharmacological, pharmacological, and, in advanced cases, surgical options with early involvement of the multidisciplinary team. None of the therapeutic options are curative, but the aim of treatment is to reduce symptoms and improve quality of life. OA remains a significant health burden at the moment and is likely to remain so for the foreseeable future.

Historical and Current Perspectives on Management of Rheumatoid Arthritis

Rheumatoid arthritis (RA) is an autoimmune disorder of unknown etiology characterized by symmetric polyarthritis that affects the small and large joints. The cardinal features of active RA include pain, swelling, morning stiffness (commonly more than an hour), warmth, redness, and limitation of function. Additional features present include malaise, tiredness, morning stiffness, and night pains. As RA progresses, additional features of chronic synovitis are superimposed. Chronic synovitis with its attendant synovial proliferation and joint effusion can lead to instability of the joint. At the same time, destructive pannus destroys cartilage and subchondral bone. Joint deformities result and contribute to joint instability and malfunction, alongside distended joint capsule and torn ligaments and tendons. This leads to considerable disability among this group of patients, along with major economic loss. Consequently, RA can have a profound impact on patients, families, and society in general.

In about 20% of patients, the onset of RA is acute. Frequently, disease activity is at first intermittent, becoming more sustained over time. Some patients may have no more than a few months of discomfort, while others may become severely disabled. Spontaneous remission can occur, but is unlikely if the disease has been continuous for 2 or more years.

Medical management has most to offer in the early stages of the disease, when the aim is to prevent or control joint damage, prevent loss of function, and halt the systemic features of the disease. Various types of medication are used to achieve this aim. Simple analgesics are used for pain control, alongside anti-inflammatory drugs (NSAIDs). Other drugs used for control of systemic inflammation are labeled under the group called disease-modifying antirheumatic drugs (DMARDs). These drugs have also been known in the past as second-line drugs, remission-inducing drugs, and slow-acting antirheumatic drugs (SAARDs). Some of these drugs have been available for more than 50 years (e.g., gold, antimalarials, and corticosteroids), whereas others are relatively new, particularly the biologics, which will be discussed in greater detail in Chapter 12.

Evolutional History of Pharmacotherapeutics in RA

The past century saw considerable development in the pharmacological therapy of RA. This progress has been continued in this century with the increased usage and advent of the biologic agents. The 20th century began with the synthesis of salicylic acid, which was the first NSAID and led later to the discovery of other NSAIDs, including more recently the selective COX-2 inhibitors (discussed earlier). In the early part of the past century, salicylates were used extensively for pain relief and as antipyretics. This was subsequently studied in clinical trials in the 1960s [87] and the association with significant side effects led to the development of indomethacin, phenylbutazone, and other NSAIDs, which later became the mainstay of pain relief and anti-inflammatory activity. Along with this, other forms of treatment for RA were also studied, with reports suggesting good efficacy with intramuscular Gold in 1945 [88] and substance E (hydrocortisone) in 1949 [89]. At the same time, other drugs were being experimented with. These included sulfasalazine, which was first tried in 1948 [90], and antimalarials that were tried in the 1950s and 1960s, although there had been some history of use of chloroquine for joint problems from the 19th century [91]. D-Penicillamine was studied in some controlled studies in the 1970s [92–94], and methotrexate was added to the armory of RA drugs, along with cyclophosphamide, azathioprine, and later ciclosporin (previously named cyclosporine). More recently, leflunomide has become available. Along with these developments, there have also been developments in the newer NSAIDs, particularly in the past decade with the advent of the selective COX-2 inhibitors. The selective COX-2 inhibitors are generally regarded as being safer than the traditional NSAIDs mainly because of a reduced rate of ulceration and bleeding from the gastrointestinal tract, although recent data has raised some concerns relating to the cardiovascular and cerebrovascular safety of these drugs, more so for selective COX-2 inhibitors, but also for the traditional NSAIDs.

Perhaps the biggest change in the treatment of RA lies not in the increased choice available to the doctors and the patients but in the manner in which these drugs are used. Traditionally, the treatment of RA revolved around control of symptoms with painkillers and NSAIDs, with the more "toxic" agents being limited to use after the former drugs had failed to control the arthritis (hence, the concept of second-line agents). With the increase in the knowledge about RA, availability of better instruments for measuring disease activity, better assessments for determining long-term prognosis, and the devastating effects of progressive disease on joint and general health, there is a marked change in the use of these drugs. Rheumatologists now use DMARDs early in the natural history of the disease and are less inclined to await untoward events before resorting to more powerful agents [95]. Perhaps the best indicator of current perceptions for treatment are the guidelines for management of RA published by the American College of Rheumatology Subcommittee on Rheumatoid Arthritis Guidelines (2002 update). These guidelines state very clearly that "the majority of patients with newly diagnosed RA should be started on a disease-modifying antirheumatic drug within 3 months of the diagnosis" [96]. Experience from the Early Arthritis Clinics across the world suggests that there is a therapeutic "window of opportunity" that exists before the inflammatory load becomes significant. Evidence would suggest a better prognosis for initiation of DMARDs in very early RA (within 3 months of onset of symptoms) compared with later early RA (up to 12 months from onset of symptoms) [97]. When early RA is treated aggressively, there appears to be a reduction in degree of joint damage, long-term disability and improves the chances of remission [98, 99].

Once a diagnosis of RA has been made, treatment begins by educating the patient about the disease and the risks of joint damage and disability, as well as discussion of the available forms of treatment and the risks and benefits of these. Patients should be referred to physiotherapists, occupational therapists, and social workers as part of a multidisciplinary approach. As it is quite difficult for patients to grasp all of these issues in one visit, it is preferable to give patients sufficient time to understand and reflect on the significance of the discussion, without delaying the initiation of treatment. Patient education is a continuous process based on patient and physician partnership. NSAIDs and glucocorticoids (intra-articular or low-dose oral) can be used in the meantime for symptom control. The majority of patients with newly diagnosed RA should be started on DMARD therapy within 3 months of diagnosis, and the trend is to start therapy even sooner in a bid to improved overall long-term prognosis. Treatment of RA is an iterative process, and continuous reassessment of patients is extremely important.

Initial Assessment of Patients with RA

Any patient suspected of having RA should undergo a baseline assessment that should include symptoms of active disease (history of joint pain and swelling, duration of morning stiffness, diurnal variation of symptoms), functional status, clinical evidence of synovitis, presence of extra-articular disease, radiographic damage, and baseline laboratory investigations. The baseline laboratory investigations include full blood count (FBC), erythrocyte sedimentation rate (ESR), C-reactive protein (CRP), rheumatoid factor, renal function tests, liver function tests (including hepatic enzymes, alkaline phosphatase, and albumin), and urinalysis. In certain instances, a synovial fluid analysis may be deemed necessary to rule out other differential diagnoses like septic arthritis or crystal arthritis. The assessment of renal and hepatic function tests is necessary as a number of antirheumatic drugs (including NSAIDs) can cause renal and/or hepatic damage and may be contraindicated in the presence of impairment of these organs.

Along with these baseline laboratory investigations, the patient should be assessed for comorbid conditions, and a validated tool should be used for assessment of pain, disease activity, and quality of life [100, 101]. Poor prognostic markers should be identified. These include early age of disease onset, high titer of rheumatoid factor, elevated ESR, and swelling of more than 20 joints [102]. Extra-articular manifestations of RA include rheumatoid nodules, sicca syndrome, interstitial lung disease, eye involvement (episcleritis, scleritis, and, in later stages, scleromalacia perforans), pericardial involvement, and systemic vasculitis. These may indicate a worse prognosis. Antibodies to citrullinated peptides have recently been shown to have significant association with erosive disease [103]. Aggressive treatment with DMARDs should be initiated in patients with RA as soon as the diagnosis has been made to reduce the incidence and severity of joint damage.

Further Management of RA Patients

Once the diagnosis of RA has been made and the treatment commenced, the focus of the consultation shifts to determining whether there has been an improvement in the patient's condition and whether there is any continuing evidence of disease activity. Various assessments are useful in this regard. It is important to document duration of morning stiffness, severity of joint pain, presence of swollen and tender joints, as well as limitation of function. It is also worthwhile repeating at intervals the tools used for making the initial assessment of disease activity, pain and quality of life measures. Other indicators of progression or improvement include ESR, CRP, and repeat radiographs (not normally repeated at intervals of less than 12 months). It can sometimes be difficult to determine whether a decline in function is the result of inflammation, mechanical damage, or a combination of both. These distinctions are important, as treatment strategies will differ accordingly.

Although there are a number of markers of disease activity, one that has gained substantial acceptance in clinical practice appears to be the Disease Activity Score (DAS). The DAS-28 score forms the basis for defining disease activity in the UK,

Table 2.2 Criteria to define complete remission

1. Absence of symptoms of active inflammatory joint pain
2. No morning stiffness
3. No fatigue
4. No synovitis on joint examination
5. No progression of damage on sequential radiographs
6. Normal erythrocyte sedimentation rate (ESR) and C-reactive protein (CRP)

Source: From Pinals RS, Masi AT, Larsen RA, and the subcommittee for criteria of remission in RA of the American Rheumatology Association Diagnostic and Therapeutic Criteria Committee. Preliminary criteria for clinical remission in rheumatoid arthritis. Arthritis Rheum 1981;24:1308–15.

with regards to decisions about initiation of biologic agents. This is calculated on the basis of number of swollen and tender joints, ESR (or CRP), and global health assessment on the basis of a 100 mm visual analogue scale. Other measures that can be used to determine the functional status include Arthritis Impact Measurement Scales [104] and Health Assessment Questionnaire [105]. The American College of Rheumatology (ACR) has developed criteria for defining improvement [98] and clinical remission [106] in RA (see Table 2.2). Whereas these criteria have gained considerable acceptance for outcome assessment in clinical trials, they have not had the same degree of success in terms of their adoption in clinical practice. The ACR criteria for 20% clinical improvement (the ACR20) require a 20% improvement in the tender and swollen joint count, as well as a 20% improvement in three of the following five parameters: patient's global assessment, physician's global assessment, patient's assessment of pain, degree of disability, and level of acute-phase reactant (CRP). These criteria have been expanded to include criteria for 50% and 70% improvement measures (i.e., ACR50, ACR70). Other criteria, such as the Paulus criteria [105], have also been employed. Radiographic progression using the Sharp or the modified Sharp score [107–110] have been used as an outcome measure of joint damage. Another concept that has gained considerable ground recently is use of quality of life measures. Perhaps the best of these is the Quality Adjusted Life Years (QALY), which has been used by the National Institute for Clinical Excellence in the United Kingdom to evaluate the use of biologic agents.

Nonpharmacological Treatment of RA

There are a number of nonpharmacological options that play an important role in the treatment of patients with RA. Patient education is an extremely important aspect of management. Not only the patient but also the patient's family needs to understand the condition and become involved in the process of making decisions about treatment. If treatment does not fully control the disease, the patient may struggle emotionally as well as physically in adjusting to this chronic disease, its flares, and the concomitant loss of function. Rheumatologists, other physicians, and support staff (nurses, physiotherapists, occupational therapists, social workers, etc.) play important roles in educating the patient and the patient's family about the disease and providing ongoing supportive care. Organizations like the Arthritis Foundation in the United States and the Arthritis Research Campaign in the United Kingdom are an important source of educational material and/or programs. A range of health professionals including nurses, physical therapists, occupational therapists, social workers, health educators, health psychologists, and orthopedic surgeons may also be involved in a multidisciplinary team approach to the comprehensive management of RA. For example, participation in dynamic and aerobic conditioning exercise programs in patients with RA improves joint mobility, muscle strength, aerobic fitness and function, and psychological well-being without increasing fatigue or joint symptoms [110–113].

Short periods for rest can form part of management, particularly in the presence of a flare. Interestingly, whole-body rest can decrease the general systemic inflammatory response and was one of the forms of therapy that was used relatively commonly until the past decade. A judicious use of exercise and rest is recommended so as to maintain full range of motion of joints.

Pharmacological Treatment of RA

Pharmacological therapy for RA often consists of combinations of NSAIDs, DMARDs, and/or glucocorticoids. The common DMARDs used are described in Table 2.3 along with their dosing schedules and efficacy.

Table 2.3 Dosages, approximate time to benefit and comparative efficacy of some common DMARDS

Drug	Approximate time to benefit	Efficacy	Usual maintenance dose
Abatacept	2–12 weeks	+ + +	10mg/kg intravenous infusion every 4 weeks
Adalimumab	Few days to 12 weeks	+ + + +	40mg subcutaneous every fortnight
Anakinra	2–12 weeks	+ +	30-150mg subcutaneous daily
Azathioprine	8–16 weeks	+ +	50-150mg/day
Ciclosporin	8–16 weeks	+ +	2.5-4mg/kg/day
D-penicillamine	12–24 weeks	+ +	250-750mg/day
Etanercept	Few days to 12 weeks	+ + + +	25mg subcutaneous twice a week
Hydroxychloroquine	8–24 weeks	+ +	200mg twice a day
Gold, oral	16–24 weeks	+	3mg twice a day
Gold, intramuscular	12–24 weeks	+ + +	50mg every 4 weeks
Infliximab (plus methotrexate)	Few days to 16 weeks	+ + + +	3-10mg/kg IV every 8 weeks;
Leflunomide	4–12 weeks	+ + +	10-20mg/day
Methotrexate	6–12 weeks	+ + +	Oral: 7.5-25mg once a week; Injectable: 7.5-20mg/week
Minocycline	4–12 weeks	+ +	100mg twice a day
Rituximab	12 weeks	+ + +	2 infusions of 1000mg each 2 weeks apart, repeated approx. every 40-60 weeks
Sulphasalazine	6–12 weeks	+ + +	1 gm two to three times a day

NSAIDs

The historical treatment of RA usually involved the use of NSAIDs to reduce joint pain, joint swelling, and morning stiffness. These drugs were used before the decision to start a DMARD was taken, however, now these agents are used much less commonly as an adjunct to DMARD therapy. These agents help to reduce pain and have anti-inflammatory properties but do not alter the course of the disease or prevent joint destruction. Furthermore, the use of this group of drugs is limited by their side effects, particularly GI toxicity, though the newer selective COX-2 inhibitors are thought to be less toxic to the GI tract. NSAIDs should not be used as the sole treatment for RA. A number of agents are available and the choice of which drug to use is probably dictated by a combination of factors including efficacy, safety, convenience, incidence of GI side effects, comorbidity, and cost. NSAIDs act by inhibiting one or both of the cyclooxygenase enzyme isoforms, COX-1 and COX-2, which are responsible for the production of prostaglandins. COX-1 is present in many cells, including platelets, cells of the gastric and intestinal mucosa, and endothelial cells. COX-2 is the enzyme that specifically appears to be involved in inflammation. COX-2 also appears to be produced in the kidneys; hence selective COX-2 inhibitors may not necessarily be safe from nephropathy. However, selective COX-2 inhibitors do tend not to have an effect on platelet function [114], which may be of benefit when considering GI bleeding but may be a drawback when looking at the vascular complications of RA. Studies comparing nonselective NSAIDs to selective NSAIDs suggest that selective COX-2 inhibitors have a significantly lower risk of serious adverse GI effects than do nonselective NSAIDs [114, 115]. However, cost constraints may limit the use of selective COX-2 inhibitors as first-line NSAIDs in other than high-risk patients. These risk factors include advanced age (65 years or more), history of ulcer, concomitant use of corticosteroids or anticoagulants, higher dosage of NSAID, use of multiple NSAIDs, or a serious comorbid illness [116]. Evidence would also suggest that the combination of a nonselective NSAID with a proton pump inhibitor can provide the same level of protection from GI bleeds as a selective NSAID, though there is very little difference in the cost [117, 118]. As selective COX-2 inhibitors do not have any effect on platelet function [114], in patients with a vascular risk, low-dose aspirin should be used, which unfortunately may reduce the gastroprotective benefit of using selective COX-2 inhibitors. Some studies have suggested that use of selective COX-2 inhibitors is associated with the increased incidence of thrombotic events such as myocardial infarction compared with traditional NSAIDs. Quite a few selective COX-2 inhibitors have now been shown to have adverse vascular complications when used in high doses for long periods, and the use of these drugs in the presence of established cardiovascular and cerebrovascular disease is not recommended. Recent MHRA guidelines state that 'NSAIDs should be used in the lowest effective dose for the shortest duration' in view of recent evidence of vascular complications with traditional NSAIDs (see section on NSAIDs in management of OA).

DMARDs

DMARDs should be considered in every patient with RA, either alone or in combination with NSAIDs and/or glucocorticoids. Although NSAIDs and glucocorticoids may alleviate symptoms, joint damage may continue to occur and to progress, though there is now some evidence to support the use of glucocorticoids in reducing radiographic progression of RA [119]. DMARDs have the advantage of reducing or preventing joint damage and preserving joint integrity and function. Ultimately, this leads to better quality of life and may even result in economic benefit by keeping patients working for longer and reducing the need for joint surgery. DMARDs have traditionally been used when the disease is not responding to conservative treatment with NSAIDs. This is no longer best practice. The commoner DMARDs include methotrexate, gold, leflunomide, D-penicillamine, cyclosporine, sulfasalazine, hydroxychloroquine, azathioprine, and the new biologic agents (Table 2.3). DMARDs differ from NSAIDs in that the onset of effect is usually delayed for at least a few weeks, and they have no analgesic effect. They appear to act on various molecules at different levels of the inflammatory cascade, but are generally not curative.

Considerable evidence exists to support the efficacy of DMARDs in the treatment of RA. Recently, emphasis has focused on the best combination of DMARDs and on retardation of joint erosions based on radiographic evidence. DMARDs generally are effective at reducing the rate of progression of joint erosions or destruction and can sometimes even cause remission of the disease (Table 2.2). This, however, is likely to be short-lived when these drugs are discontinued.

From time to time, RA patients will experience a flare in their disease despite the patient being on DMARDs. This should prompt a careful consideration of further options including increase of dose, addition of another DMARD, or even changing to another DMARD. In instances where the active disease is limited to a few joints, intra-articular injections of corticosteroids may have an important role. For patients with severe symptoms, systemic corticosteroid therapy may be indicated, either oral (low-dose oral prednisolone) or in the form of methylprednisolone intramuscularly or intravenously (pulses).

Methotrexate

Methotrexate (MTX) has become one of the most widely used DMARDs in the treatmentof RA. Antifolates (aminopterin) have been tried as early as 1951 for nonmalignant disease [120], but the introduction of steroids took attention away from this group of drugs, which included the less toxic methotrexate. This was still used for psoriasis and an improvement in psoriatic arthritis was noticed as well, but it was not until the 1980s that MTX gained acceptance as a good option for treatment of RA. During the 1990s, the popularity of MTX appeared to grow further, and it gradually became the drug of choice for most patients with RA. Recent trends would indicate that methotrexate is rapidly becoming the most common initial DMARD, especially for patients whose RA is more active. There are a number of reasons for this. MTX has an established track record in the treatment of RA but also has the advantage of being cheap, easy to administer, having one of the best efficacy-toxicity ratios, and appears to be the best drug from the point of view of long-term patient compliance [121, 122]. RA patients taking MTX are more likely to discontinue treatment because of adverse reactions than because of lack of efficacy [123]. As a result, MTX has become the standard by which new DMARDs are evaluated. Randomized clinical trials have not only established the efficacy of MTX in RA but also provided evidence to support the view that MTX retards radiographic progression. It is usually administered once a week with doses ranging from 7.5 mg to 25 mg, and the anti-inflammatory effect may be obvious within 3 to 4 weeks, though in some instances, it does take considerably longer. In some patients, absorption of MTX from the GI tract can be patchy and erratic, and these patients may benefit from parenteral administration of MTX.

Despite extensive research, the precise mechanism of action of MTX remains unclear. MTX does inhibit the enzyme dihydrofolate reductase and causes reduced leukotriene production and interleukin-1 expression. The efficacy of MTX does not appear to be affected by the administration of folic acid, which is used frequently to reduce the incidence of side effects associated with MTX. Patients with RA are considered to be at higher risk of vascular events [124], and MTX therapy is associated with an elevation of serum homocysteine levels [125]. Elevation of serum homocysteine can cause increased predisposition to vascular injury [126, 127]. Folic acid or folinic acid administration can reduce the elevation of serum homocysteine seen in these patients [128]. Both these effects (increase of homocysteine and response to folic/folinic acid) appear to be independent of the C677T mutation in the methyltetrahydrofolate reductase (MTHFR) gene [129]. Hence, folate supplementation is increasingly becoming considered a standard part of therapy for patients on MTX.

Adverse effects of MTX include stomatitis, nausea, diarrhea, and alopecia, all of which may decrease with concomitant folic acid or folinic acid [130–132]. Other side effects of MTX therapy include leukopenia, bone marrow suppression (both usually reversible on stopping the drug), pulmonary symptoms, including MTX pneumonitis and pulmonary fibrosis, and rarely liver fibrosis and cirrhosis. Though the risk of liver cirrhosis is low, the most frequent side effect of MTX is deranged liver enzymes, and these do need to be monitored closely. A liver biopsy is indicated when there is persistent derangement of liver enzymes despite discontinuation of treatment [133].

Relative contraindications for MTX therapy include preexisting liver disease, renal impairment, significant lung disease, or alcohol abuse. Serious or life-threatening pulmonary toxicity is rare but can occur at any time. MTX is potentially teratogenic and should be discontinued 3 to 6 months before attempting conception.

Hydroxychloroquine

Antimalarials have been used for the treatment of rheumatic diseases as far back as the early 19th century [91], but it was not until the 1950s and 1960s that they were evaluated as part of controlled studies. The general consensus on the use of these drugs would be that this group of drugs is at best moderately effective for control of RA [134–138]. It does, however, have a better risk/benefit ratio than azathioprine or auranofin.

Hydroxychloroquine (HCQ) is the least toxic of the quinolones, and perhaps the least toxic of the DMARDs. Its therapeutic action can be delayed; response is seen in the majority within 3 to 6 months, though optimal benefit can take 9 to 12 months [139]. HCQ alone does not appear to slow radiographic damage to joints, despite the significant impact of HCQ on long-term patient outcome when initiated early. Patients given HCQ do not need any specific laboratory monitoring but do need periodic ophthalmic checks for early signs of reversible retinal toxicity. Other side effects include dermatitis, nausea, epigastric pain, myopathy, and hemolytic anaemia. HCQ is normally used in doses of 400 mg daily (up to 6.5mg/kg/day), and its role in RA appears to be in early/mild disease and/or as background treatment in combination with other DMARDs. Particularly common combinations appear to be combinations of MTX, sulfasalazine, and HCQ [140–143]; MTX and HCQ [142]; and cyclosporine and HCQ [143]. HCQ is relatively safe during pregnancy and can be continued through pregnancy, although breast-feeding should be avoided.

Sulfasalazine

Sulfasalazine (SASZ) is one of the few drugs originally developed for treatment of RA and is another antifolate drug (though weaker than MTX). Several studies have demonstrated good benefit with SASZ in patients with RA [144–146], though the evidence on the efficacy of SASZ in retarding radiographic progression is conflicting. Clinical response with SASZ is usually apparent within 2 to 4 months. This drug also appears to have a better long-term tolerance than some other drugs used for treatment of RA (particularly gold), with 22% of patients continuing the drug after 5 years in one study [147].

SASZ appears to be generally well tolerated, though some patients develop unacceptable side effects mainly in the form of nausea and abdominal discomfort within the first few weeks of initiation of the drug. Traditionally, SASZ has been started off at 500 mg once daily with weekly increments of 500 mg until the full dose of 2 to 3 g daily has been reached. It is, however, debatable whether this schedule is necessary and in particular whether it reduces the risk of GI side effects. SASZ however, can cause leukopenia, particularly in the first year of treatment, and derangement of liver enzymes, and laboratory monitoring is essential. SASZ appears to be more popular in Europe, where it tends to be used more commonly both alone and in combination therapy with MTX and HCQ. SASZ can cause neonatal hemolysis, although according to the *British National Formulary*, it could be continued in pregnancy with adequate folate supplementation.

Leflunomide

Several randomized controlled clinical trials have established leflunomide as an effective agent for control of RA, either as monotherapy or in combination with other agents [144, 148–153]. It tends to be particularly useful in patients who cannot tolerate MTX or cannot be given MTX because of chest problems. The benefit with leflunomide appears to be similar to that with MTX, both in terms of reducing disease activity and slowing radiographic progression. It can also be used in combination with MTX in the event of suboptimal disease control with MTX alone. However, in patients where the combination is being used, careful monitoring of liver function tests is essential, as both drugs are potentially hepatotoxic and do frequently cause derangement of liver enzymes [149, 151].

Leflunomide has a long half-life, and although loading dose was previously recommended, is rarely used now due to increased frequency of side-effects. The usual dose for leflunomide is 20 mg daily (10 mg daily for elderly patients). In addition, the drug tends to accumulate in the body, and in cases of toxicity or unacceptable side effects, leflunomide would need to be washed out with cholestyramine or activated charcoal. The common side effects of leflunomide include weight loss, hypertension, deranged liver function tests, and altered taste. Leflunomide is potentially teratogenic, and women taking leflunomide who wish to conceive must discontinue leflunomide and undergo cholestyramine or activated charcoal washout before attempting conception. Leflunomide should not be used in patients with obstructive biliary disease, liver disease, viral hepatitis, severe immunodeficiency, inadequate birth control, and rifampin therapy (which raises leflunomide levels).

Gold Salts

Gold compounds were first used in the 1920s to treat arthritis, and Forestrier's report in 1935 furthered this [154]. In 1960, the Empire Rheumatism Council published their double-blind trial, which suggested that gold salts were beneficial in about 60% to 80% of patients with RA. Gold compounds diminish the acute and chronic inflammatory response at a number of points in the inflammatory cascade. Several other studies have also proved the efficacy of gold salts [155–157]. Despite this, gold salts are not first-choice DMARDs, mainly due to the fact that oral gold is less effective [155, 156] and parenteral gold ideally needs to be administered on a weekly basis for the first 6 months. After this, the gold injection schedule can be reduced to fortnightly or monthly. Gold salts require regular monitoring, as risk of hematologic side effects is relatively high. Gold salts can also give rise to renal complications like nephrotic syndrome, and urine monitoring for proteinuria is essential. Rash is common with an incidence of 15 to 30%, and can be so severe that gold salts may need to be permanently discontinued.

Ciclosporin (Previously Named Cyclosporine)

Ciclosporin is an immunosuppressant that can be used in RA both as monotherapy [158, 159] and in combination with other drugs [160]. Despite its undoubted efficacy, its use has been limited by its side-effect profile, which includes hypertension and renal impairment [161, 162]. Several drugs interact with ciclosporin and thus increase the risk of nephrotoxicity. Furthermore, ciclosporin is relatively expensive, and hence ciclosporin treatment is primarily confined to patients with refractory RA.

Other DMARDs

Azathioprine, a purine analogue myelosuppressant, has demonstrated benefits in RA but has limited effectiveness [156, 157, 163–165]. Recent data suggests that it is worth measuring serum thiopurine methyltransferase levels to assess the risk of developing bone marrow toxicity with azathioprine [166]. D-Penicillamine is also effective [92, 93, 156, 157], but its use is limited, in part, by an inconvenient dosing schedule (i.e., slow increases in the dosage) and rare but potentially serious complications, including autoimmune diseases, such as Goodpasture's syndrome and myasthenia gravis. Minocycline has recently been found to be effective in controlling RA in some randomized, double-blind, placebo-controlled trials [167–170]. Importantly, one trial showed long-term benefit of minocycline and a decrease in radiographic progression in a subset of patients who were positive for the human leucocyte antigen-DR4 shared epitope [171]. Further research is necessary before the role of minocycline in the treatment of RA is clearly defined.

Glucocorticoids

Glucocorticoids were used for arthritis as far back as the early 1950s (substance E; 1949) [89], and since then this group of drugs has always had a role to play in control of RA. A patient disabled by active polyarthritis may experience marked and rapid improvement in functional status within a matter of days after initiation of low-dose glucocorticoids (up to 10 mg of prednisolone daily). Indeed, in terms of its short-term efficacy, very few drugs can match the response obtained with glucocorticoids. Frequently, disabling synovitis recurs when glucocorticoids are discontinued, even in patients who are receiving combination therapy with one or more DMARDs. As a result, patients with RA may become functionally dependent on glucocorticoids and continue them long-term. There is some recent evidence to support the role of

Table 2.4 Common glucocorticoid preparations, equivalent dosing, and half-lives

Drug	Anti-inflammatory potency	Equivalent dose (mg)	Biologic half-life (h)
Hydrocortisone	1	20	8–12
Cortisone	0.8	25	8–12
Prednisone	4	5	12–36
Prednisolone	5	4	12–36
Methylprednisolone	5	4	12–36
Triamcinolone	5	4	12–36
Dexamethasone	20–30	0.75	36–54

glucocorticoids in slowing the rate of joint damage and hence their consideration as having DMARD properties [119]. Joint damage may increase on discontinuation of glucocorticoids [172]. The common glucocorticoid preparations with their equivalent dosing and half-lives are shown in Table 2.4.

Glucocorticoid doses given several times a day are more potent than once-a-day dosing, however, the risk of adrenal suppression is highest with the multiple-times-a-day dosing. The benefits of low-dose systemic glucocorticoids should always be weighed against their adverse effects. The adverse effects of long-term oral glucocorticoids (even at low doses) include osteoporosis, hypertension, weight gain, fluid retention, hyperglycemia, cataracts, skin fragility, hirsutism, and premature atherosclerosis. These adverse effects need to be considered and discussed in detail before the decision to initiate steroids is taken. Almost all patients starting on long-term glucocorticoids will need bone protection for osteoporosis, probably in the form of a bisphosphonate at the time of commencing glucocorticoids [173, 174]. Patients taking glucocorticoids at dosages of less than 5 mg/day may also have an increased risk of osteoporosis, and densitometry to assess bone loss should be performed at regular intervals for the duration of glucocorticoid treatment [175]. Glucocorticoid-treated patients should receive 1500 mg elemental calcium per day (including diet and supplements) and 400 to 800 IU of vitamin D per day [174–176].

Glucocorticoid injection of joints is a safe and effective way of managing single-joint flare-ups of the disease in patients with RA. It is, however, extremely important to rule out infections before undertaking this. Local glucocorticoid injections may also allow the patient to participate more fully in rehabilitation programs to restore lost joint function. As a general rule, the same joint should not be injected more than three times a year. The need for repeated injections in the same joint or for injections in multiple joints reiterates the need for reassessment of DMARD therapy or for other forms of management such as surgery.

In the situation where rapid amelioration of symptoms is needed, treatment can be initiated with a short course of , or even a single dose of, high-dose glucocorticoid. Intramuscular injection of methylprednisolone up to 120 mg or pulsed methylprednisolone in a dose of 500 mg to 1 g for 1 to 3 infusions (daily or alternate days) can be extremely efficacious in the rapid improvement of symptoms of RA with benefit lasting up to 12 weeks [177]. This should, however, be accompanied with a reassessment of the overall management strategy.

Combination DMARD Therapy

Rheumatologists all over the world now tend to use a combination of DMARDs when a single agent alone provides insufficient benefit [142, 178]. However, the issue of whether to start off with a combination of DMARDs early in the natural history of the disease is a vexed one and needs careful consideration. The question of whether to "step-up" the treatment or to "step-down" has generated considerable debate among rheumatologists. Although there are no easy answers to this question, there do appear to be some combination therapies that appear to be safe and well tolerated. The major worry with combination DMARD therapy is that of increased toxicity, without increased benefit. Some studies do support this argument [179–181], but this is counterbalanced by other studies that have shown certain combinations of DMARDs achieving a substantial increase in efficacy without an increase in toxicity. The combination of MTX, SASZ, and HCQ has now gained some acceptance even for early arthritis [140, 141] with or without steroids. Evidence would suggest that patients on this triple therapy appear to have less radiographic progression, fewer problems with toxicity or lack of efficacy, and better disease control. The combination of MTX and leflunomide has also undergone successful trials [182–184], though this combination would need careful monitoring particularly because of the risk of hepatotoxicity. Other combinations that have shown improved efficacy include the combination of MTX and ciclosporin [185, 186], though this benefit is augmented by increased side effects (hypertension, renal impairment). The role of combination therapy in the long-term management of patients with RA is now well established, though its role in early arthritis is undergoing an evolutionary process. With more long-term data, it is likely that combinations of DMARDs will be increasingly used in the early treatment of RA.

Surgical Treatment of RA

Some patients will continue to have problems despite pharmacotherapy and other interventions. In these patients, surgery of an individual joint may be an option. The indications for surgery in patients with chronic RA are shown in Table 2.5.

Surgical procedures for RA include carpal tunnel release, synovectomy, resection of the metatarsal heads, total joint arthroplasty, and joint fusion. New prosthetic materials and cements for fixing joint prostheses have contributed to significant increases in the longevity of total joint prostheses in patients with RA [187–191]. Preoperative functional status is an important determinant of the rate of recovery of functional independence after surgery. Several strategies have been tried for optimizing the functional status of this high-risk group of patients. Strategies that

Table 2.5 Common indications and surgical options in patients with RA

Symptoms	Surgical option
Unacceptable levels of pain	Joint replacement, arthrodesis
Structural damage leading to limitation of function	Joint replacement
Joint instability/mechanical imbalance	Joint replacement/arthrodesis
Resistant monoarticular active synovitis	Synovectomy
Paresthesia of lateral three fingers (carpal tunnel syndrome)	Carpal tunnel release

have yielded some success include early surgical intervention, intensive physiotherapy prior to surgery, and even electrical muscle stimulation to improve muscle strength [192].

Summary

RA is a chronic, symmetric polyarthritis that frequently causes substantial disability. The optimal management of these patients involves a multidisciplinary approach with physiotherapists, occupational therapists, nurses, and other health professionals working alongside doctors to reduce the substantial morbidity and disability. The ideal goal of treatment is to achieve remission, and to achieve this, a variety of non-pharmacological, pharmacological, and surgical interventions might be necessary. Long-term planning, early intervention, and aggressive treatment in a multidisciplinary setting are essential to maximize function and achieve a good long-term outcome.

References

1. Haq I, Murphy E, Dacre J. Osteoarthritis. Postgrad Med J 2003;79:377–383.
2. National Center for Health Statistics. Prevalence of osteoarthrits in adults by age, sex, race and geographic area: United States 1960–62. Vital Health Stat 11(15).
3. Murray CJL, Lopez Ad, eds. The global burden of disease. A comprehensive assessment of mortality and disability from diseases, injuries, and risk factors in 1990 and projected to 2020. Cambridge, MA: Harvard School of Public Health on behalf of the World Health Organisation and the World Bank; 1996.
4. Silman AJ, Hochberg MC. Epidemiology of the rheumatic diseases. Oxford: Oxford University Press; 1993.
5. Heberden W. Commentaries on the history and causes of disease. London: Payne; 1802.
6. Haygarth J. A clinical history of diseases. II. Nodosity of the joints. London: Gadell and Davies; 1805.
7. Stecher RM. Heberden's nodes: heredity in hypertrophic arthritis of the finger joints. Am J Med Sci 1941:201;801–809.
8. Kellgren JH, Moore R. Generalised osteoarthritis and Heberden's nodes. Br Med J 1952;1:181–187.
9. Kellgren JH, Lawrence JS. Radiological assessment of osteo-arthrosis. Ann Rheum Dis 1957;16(4):494–502.

10. Lawrence JS, Bremmer JM, Bier F. Osteoarthrosis: prevalence in the population and relationships between symptoms and X-ray changes. Ann Rheum Dis 1966;25:1–24.
11. Charnley J. Arthroplasty of the hip: a new operation. Lancet 1961;1:1129–1132.
12. McKee GK, Watson-Farrar J. Replacement of arthritic hips by the McKee-Farrar prosthesis. J Bone Joint Surg Br 1966;48(2):245–259.
13. Mankin H. The reaction of articular cartilage to injury and osteoarthritis. N Engl J Med 1990;291:1285.
14. Dean D. Proteinase-mediated cartilage damage in osteoarthritis. Semin Arthritis Rheum 1991;20(Suppl):2.
15. Pelletier J, Roughley P, Dibattista JA, et al. Are cytokines involved in osteoarthritic pathology? Semin Arthritis Rheum 1991;20(Suppl):63.
16. Martel-Pelletier J, Pelletier JP, Cloutier JM, et al. Neutral protease capable of proteoglycan digesting activity in osteoarthritic and normal human cartilage. Arthritis Rheum 1984;27:305.
17. Pelletier JP, Martel-Pelletier J, Cloutier JM, et al. Proteoglycan-degrading acid metalloproteinase activity in human osteoarthritic cartilage, and the effect of intraarticular steroid injections. Arthritis Rheum 1987;19:541.
18. Dean D, Woessner J Jr. Extracts of human articular cartilage contain an inhibitor of tissue metalloproteinases. Biochem J 1984;218:277.
19. Dean D, Martel-Pelletier J, Pelletier JP, et al. Evidence of metalloproteinase and metalloproteinase inhibitor (TIMP) imbalance in human osteoarthritic cartilage. J Clin Inv 1989;84:678.
20. Wolff J. The law of bone remodelling. New York: Springer-Verlag; 1986.
21. American College of Rheumatology Subcomitteee on Osteoarthritis Guidelines. Recommendations for the medical management of osteoarthritis of the hip and knee. Arthrits Rheum 2000;43(9):1905–1915.
22. Ettinger WH Jr, Bums R, Messier SP, et al. A randomized trial comparing aerobic exercise and resistance exercise with a health education program in older adults with knee osteoarthritis: the Fitness Arthritis and Seniors Trial (FAST). JAMA 1997;277:25–31.
23. Van Baar ME, Dekker J, Oostendorp RAB, et al. The effectiveness of exercise therapy in patients with osteoarthritis of the hip or knee: a randomized clinical trial. J Rheumatol 1998;25:2432–2439.
24. Hurley MV, Scott DL, Rees J, et al. Sensorimotor changes and functional performance in patients with knee osteoarthritis. Ann Rheum Dis 1997;56:641–648.
25. American Geriatrics Society Panel on Chronic Pain in Older Persons. The management of chronic pain in older persons. J Am Geriatric Soc 1998;46:635–651.
26. Bradley JD, Brandt KD, Katz BP, et al. Comparison of an anti-inflammatory dose of ibuprofen, an analgesic dose of ibuprofen, and acetaminophen in the treatment of patients with osteoarthritis of the knee. N Engl J Med 1991;325:87–91.
27. Williams HJ, Ward JR, Egger MJ, et al. Comparison of naproxen and acetaminophen in a two-year study of treatment of osteoarthritis of the knee. Arthritis Rheum 1993;36:1196–206.
28. Towheed TE, Hochberg MC. A systematic review of randomized controlled trials of pharmacological therapy in patients with osteoarthritis of the knee. Semin Arthritis Rheum 1997;27:755–770.
29. Eccles M, Freemantle N, Mason J, for the North of England Non-Steroidal Anti-Inflammatory Drug Guideline Development Group. North of England Evidence Based Guideline Development Project: summary guideline for non-steroidal antiinflammatory drugs versus basic analgesia in treating the pain of degenerative arthritis. BMJ 1998;317:526–30.

30. Guidance on the use of cyclo-oxygenase (Cox) II selective inhibitors,celecoxib, rofecoxib, meloxicam and etodolac for osteoarthritis and rheumatoid arthritis. Available at http://www.nice.org.uk/pdf/coxiifullguidance.pdf. Accessed 14 April 2005.

31. Griessinger N, Sittl R, Likar R. Transdermal buprenorphime in clinical practice – a post-marketing surveillance study in 13,179 patients. Curr Med Res Opin 2005;21(8): 1147–1156.

32. Gammaitoni AR, Galer BS, Onawola R, Jensen MP, Argoff CE. Lignocaine patch 5 % and its positive impact on pain qualities in osteoarthritis: results of a pilot, open-label study using the Neuropathic Pain Scale. Curr Med Res Opin. 2004;20(suppl2):S13–S19.

33. Hawkey CJ. COX-2 inhibitors. Lancet 1999;353:307–314.

34. Crofford LJ, Lipsky PE, Brooks P, et al. Basic biology and clinical application of specific cyclooxygenase-2 inhibitors. Arthritis Rheum 2000;43:4–13.

35. Simon LS, Lanza FL, Lipsky PE, et al. Preliminary study of the safety and efficacy of SC-58365, a novel cyclooxygenase 2 inhibitor: efficacy and safety in two placebo-controlled trials in osteoarthritis and rheumatoid arthritis, and studies of gastrointestinal and platelet effects. Arthritis Rheum 1998;41:1591–1602.

36. Simon LS, Weaver AL, Graham DY, et al. Anti-inflammatory and upper gastrointestinal effects of celecoxib in rheumatoid arthritis: a randomized controlled trial. JAMA 1999;282:1921–1928.

37. Laine L, Harper S, Simon T, et al. A randomized trial comparing the effect of rofecoxib, a cyclooxygenase 2-specific inhibitor, with that of ibuprofen on the gastroduodenal mucosa of patients with osteoarthritis. Gastroenterology 1999;117:776–783.

38. Hawkey C, Laine L, Simon T, et al. Comparison of the effect of rofecoxib (a cyclooxygenase 2 inhibitor), ibuprofen, and placebo on the gastroduodenal mucosa of patients with osteoarthritis: a randomized, double-blind, placebo-controlled trial. Arthritis Rheum 2000;43:370–377.

39. Karim A, Tolbert D, Piergies A, et al. Celecoxib, a specific COX-2 inhibitor, lacks significant drug-drug interactions with methotrexate or warfarin. Arthritis Rheum 1998;41,9(Suppl):S315.

40. Kearney PM, Baigent C, Godwin J, Halls H, Emberson JR, Patrono C. Do selective cyclo-oxygenase-2 inhibitors and traditional non-steroidal anti-inflammatory drugs increase the risk of atherothrombosis? Meta-analysis of randomised trials. BMJ 2006;332: 1302–1308.

41. Medicines and Healthcare Products Regulatory Agency. Cardiovascular safety of COX-2 inhibitors and non-selective NSAIDs. Available at http://www.mhra.gov.uk/home/ideplg?ldcService=SS_GET_PAGE&nodeld=227. Last accessed 1st January 2008.

42. Dalgin P, and the TPS-OA Study Group. Comparison of tramadol and ibuprofen for the chronic pain of osteoarthritis [abstract]. Arthritis Rheum 1997;40(Suppl 9):S86.

43. Roth SH. Efficacy and safety of tramadol HCI in breakthrough musculoskeletal pain attributed to osteoarthritis. J Rheumatol 1998;25:1358–1363.

44. Altman RD, Moskowitz RW, and the Hyalgan Study Group. Intra-articular sodium hyaluronate (Hyalgan) in the treatment of patients with osteoarthritis of the knee: a randomized clinical trial. J Rheumatol 1998;25:2203–2212.

45. Adams ME, Atkinson MH, Lussier AJ, et al. The role of viscosupplementation with hylan G-F 20 (Synvisc) in the treatment of osteoarthritis of the knee: a Canadian multicenter trial comparing hylan G-F 20 alone, hylan G-F 20 with non-steroidal anti-inflammatory drugs (NSAIDs) and NSAIDs alone. Osteoarthritis Cartilage 1995;3:213–225.

46. Kirwan JR, Rankin E. Intra-articular therapy in osteoarthritis. Baillieres Clin Rheumatol 1997;11:769–794.

47. Ayral X. Injections in the treatment of osteoarthritis. Best Pract Res Clin Rheumatol 2001;15:609–626.

48. Williams JM, Brandt KD. Triamcinolone hexacetonite protects against fibrillation and osteophyte formation following chemically induced cartilage damage. Arthritis Rheum 1985;28(11):1267–1274.

49. Pelletier JP, Martel-Pelletier J. Protective effects of corticosteroids on cartilage lesions and osteophyte formation in the Pond-Nuki dog model of osteoarthritis. Arthritis Rheum 1989;32(2):181–193.

50. McAlindon TE, LaValley MP, Gulin JP, et al. Glucosamine and chondroitin for treatment of osteoarthritis: a systematic quality assessment and meta-analysis. JAMA 2000;283(11):1469–1475.

51. Reginster JY, Deroisy R, Rovati LC, et al. Long-term effects of glucosamine sulphate on osteoarthritis progression: a randomised, placebo-controlled clinical trial. Lancet. 2001;357(9252):251–256.

52. Jordan KM, Arden NK, Docherty M, et al. EULAR Recommendations 2003: an evidence based approach to the management of knee osteoarthritis: Report of a Task Force of the Standing Committee for International Clinical Studies Including Therapeutic Trials (ESCISIT). Ann Rheum Dis 2003;62:1145–1155.

53. Towheed TE, Anastassiades TP, Shea B, Houpt J, Welch V, Hochberg MC. Glucosamine therapy for treating osteoarthritis. Cochrane Database Syst Rev 2001;(1):CD002946.

54. Fernandes JC, Martel-Pelletier J, Pelletier J-P. Gene therapy for osteoarthritis. Clin Orthop 2000;379(Suppl):S262–272.

55. McMinn D, Treacy R, Lin K, Pynsent P. Metal on metal surface replacement of the hip: experience of the McMinn prosthesis. Clin Orthop 1996;329(Suppl):89–98.

56. Iorio R, Healy WL. Unicompartmental arthritis of the knee. J Bone Joint Surg Am 2003;85(7):1351–1364.

57. McKeever DC. Tibial plateau prosthesis. Clin Orthop 1960;18:86–95.

58. Murray DW, Goodfellow JW, O'Connor JJ. The Oxford medial unicompartmental arthroplasty: a ten-year survival study. J Bone Joint Surg Br 1998;80(6):983–991.

59. Charnley J. The long-term results of low-friction arthroplasty of the hip performed as a primary intervention. J Bone Joint Surg Br 1972;54(1):61–76.

60. Wroblewski BM. 15-21-year results of the Charnley low-friction arthroplasty. Clin Orthop 1986;211:30–35.

61. Callaghan JJ, Forest EE, Olejniczak JP, et al. Charnley total hip arthroplasty in patients less than fifty years old: a twenty to twenty-five-year follow-up note. J Bone Joint Surg Am 1998;80(5):704–714.

62. Charnley J, Cupic Z. The nine and ten year results of the low-friction arthroplasty of the hip. Clin Orthop Relat Res 1973;95:9–25.

63. Charnley J, Halley DK. Rate of wear in total hip replacement. Clin Orthop 1955;Oct 170–179.

64. Harris WH, Schiller AL, Scholler JM, et al. Extensive localized bone resorption in the femur following total hip replacement. J Bone Joint Surg Am 1976;58(5):612–618.

65. Charnley J, Follacci FM, Hammond BT. The long-term reaction of bone to self-curing acrylic cement. J Bone Joint Surg Br 1968;50(4):822–929.

66. Jones LC, Hungerford DS. Cement disease. Clin Orthop 1987;225:192–206.

67. Willert HG. Reactions of the articular capsule to wear products of artificial joint prostheses. J Biomed Mater Res 1977;11(2):157–164.

68. Charnley J. Fracture of femoral prostheses in total hip replacement: a clinical study. Clin Orthop 1975;111:105–120.

69. Ingham E, Fisher J. Biological reactions to wear debris in total joint replacement. Proc Inst Mech Eng [H] 2000;214(1):21–37.

70. Amstutz HC, Campbell P, Kossovsky N, Clarke IC. Mechanism and clinical significance of wear debris-induced osteolysis. Clin Orthop 1992;276:7–18.

71. Howie DW, Haynes DR, Rogers SD, McGee MA, Pearcy MJ. The response to particulate debris. Orthop Clin North Am 1993;244:571–581.

72. Goodman SB, Fornasier VL, Lee J, Kei J. The histological effects of the implantation of different sizes of polyethylene particles in the rabbit tibia. J Biomed Mater Res 1990;24(4): 517–524.

73. Murray DW, Rushton N. Macrophages stimulate bone resorption when they phagocytose particles. J Bone Joint Surg Br 1990;72(6):988–992.

74. Santavirta S, Hoikka V, Eskola A, et al. Aggressive granulomatous lesions in cementless total hip arthroplasty. J Bone Joint Surg Br 1990;72(6):980–984.

75. Kurtz SM, Rimnac C, Bartel D. Degradation rate of ultra-high molecular weight polyethylene. J Orthop Res 1997;15(1):57–61.

76. Eyerer P, Ke YC. Property of UHMW polyethylene hip cup endoprostheses during implantation. J Biomed Mater Res 1984;18(9):1137–1151.

77. Fisher J, Chan KL, Hailey JL, et al. Preliminary study of the effect of ageing following irradiation on the wear of ultrahigh-molecular-weight polyethylene. J Arthroplasty 1995;10(5):689–692.

78. Besong AA, Tipper JL, Ingham E, et al. Quantitative comparison of wear debris from UHMWPE that has and has not been sterilised by gamma irradiation. J Bone Joint Surg Br 1998;80(2):340–344.

79. Heisel C, Silva M, Schmalzried TP. Bearing surface options for total hip replacement in young patients. J Bone Joint Surg Am 2003;85(7):1366–1379.

80. Berry D. Editorial. Bearing surface options in total hip replacement. Semin Arthroplasty 2003;14:55–60.

81. Tipper JL, Firkins PJ, Besong AA et al. Characterisation of wear debris from UHMWPE on zirconia ceramic, metal-on-metal and alumina ceramic-on-ceramic hip prostheses generated in a physiological anatomical hip joint simulator. Wear 2001;250:120–128.

82. Fisher J. Biomedical applications. In: Bhushan B, ed. Modern tribology handbook. Volume 2: materials, coatings and industrial applications. Boca Raton: CRC Press; 2001:1593–1609.

83. Fisher J, McEwen HMJ, Barnett PI et al. Mini-Symposium: Total knee replacement – practical considerations. (i) Wear of polyethylene in artificial knee joints. Curr Orthop 2001;15:399–405.

84. Barnett PI, Fisher J, Auger DD, et al. Comparison of wear in a total knee replacement under different kinematic conditions. J Mater Sci Mater Med 2001;12(10–12):1039–1042.

85. McEwen HMJ, Fisher J, Goldsmith AAJ, et al. Wear of fixed bearing and rotating platform mobile bearing knees subjected to high levels of internal and external tibial rotation. J Mater Sci Mater Med 2001;12(10–12):1049–1052.

86. Emerton ME, Burton D. Mini-Symposium: Total knee replacement – practical considerations. (ii) The role of unicompartmental knee replacement. Curr Orthop 2001;15: 406–412.

87. Boardman PL, Hart FD. Clinical measurement of the anti-inflammatory effects of salicylates in rheumatoid arthritis. Br Med J 1967;4:264–268.

88. Fraser TN. Gold treatment in rheumatoid arthritis. Br Med J 1945;50:471–475.

89. Hench PS, Kendall EC, Slocumb CH, Polley HF. The effect of a hormone of the adrenal cortex (17-hydroxy-11-dehydrocortisone-compound E) and of the pituitary adrenocorticotrophic hormone on rheumatoid arthritis – preliminary report. Proc Staff Meetings Mayo Clinic 1949;24:181–197.

90. Sinclair RJG, Duffy JJR. Salazopyrin in the treatment of rheumatoid arthritis. Ann Rheum Dis 1948;8:226–231.

91. Wickens S, Paulus HE. Antimalarial drugs. In: Paulus HE, Furst DE, Dromgoole SH, eds. Drugs for rheumatic disease. New York: Churchill Livingstone; 1987:113.

92. Multi-Centre Trial Group. Controlled trial of D-penicillamine in rheumatoid arthritis. Lancet 1973;1:275–285.

93. Dixon AStJ, Davies J, Dormandy TL, et al. Synthetic D-penicillamine in rheumatoid arthritis – double-blind controlled study of a high and low-dose regimen. Ann Rheum Dis 1975;34:416–421.

94. Davies J, Dormandy TL, et al. Synthetic D-penicillamine in rheumatoid arthritis – double-blind controlled study of a high and low-dose regimen. Ann Rheum Dis 1975;34:416–421.
95. Girgis L, Conaghan PG, Brooks P. Disease-modifying antirheumatic drugs, including methotrexate, sulfasalazine, gold, antimalarials, and penicillamine. Curr Opin Rheumatol. 1994;6(3):252–261.
96. American College of Rheumatology Subcommittee on Rheumatoid Arthritis guidelines. Guidelines for the management of Rheumatoid Arthritis. Arthritis Rheum 2002;46(2): 328–346.
97. Nell VPK, Machold KP, Eberl G, et al. Benefit of very early referral and very early therapy with disease-modifying anti-rheumatic drugs in patients with early rheumatoid arthritis. Rheumatology 2004;43:906–914.
98. Albers JM, Paimela L, Kurki P, et al. Treatment strategy, disease activity and outcome in four cohorts of patients with early rheumatoid arthritis. Ann Rheum Dis 2001;60:453–458.
99. Breedveld FC, Kalden JR. Appropriate and effective management of rheumatoid arthritis. Ann Rheum Dis 2004;63:627–633.
100. Felson DT, Anderson JJ, Boers M, et al. The American College of Rheumatology preliminary core set of disease activity measures for rheumatoid arthritis clinical trials. Arthritis Rheum 1993;36:729–740.
101. Goldsmith CH, Boers M, Bombardier C, Tugwell P, for the OMERACT Committee. Criteria for clinically important changes in outcomes: development, scoring, and evaluation of the rheumatoid arthritis patient and trial profiles. J Rheumatol 1993;20:561–565.
102. Scott DL. Prognostic factors in early rheumatoid arthritis. Rheumatology 2000;39 (Suppl 1):24–29.
103. Kroot EJ, deBong JA, van Leeuwen MA, et al. The prognostic value of anticyclic citrullinated peptide antibody in patients with recent-onset rheumatoid arthritis. Arthritis Rheum 2000;43(8):1831–1835.
104. Meenan RF, Gertman PM, Mason JH. Measuring health status in arthritis: the Arthritis Impact Measurement Scales. Arthritis Rheum 1980;23:146–152.
105. Paulus HE, Egger MJ, Ward JR, et al., and the Cooperative Systematic Studies of Rheumatic Diseases Group. Analysis of improvement in individual rheumatoid arthritis patients treated with disease-modifying antirheumatic drugs, based on the findings in patients treated with placebo. Arthritis Rheum 1990;33:477–484.
106. Pinals RS, Masi AT, Larsen RA, and the Subcommittee for Criteria of Remission in Rheumatoid Arthritis of the American Rheumatism Association Diagnostic and Therapeutic Criteria Committee. Preliminary criteria for clinical remission in rheumatoid arthritis. Arthritis Rheum 1981;24:1308–1315.
107. Sharp JT, Lidsky MD, Collins LC, et al. Methods of scoring the progression of radiologic changes in rheumatoid arthritis: correlation of radiologic, clinical, and laboratory abnormalities. Arthritis Rheum 1971;14:706–720.
108. Sharp JT, Young DY, Bluhm GB, et al. How many joints in the hands and wrists should be included in a score of radiologic abnormalities used to assess rheumatoid arthritis? Arthritis Rheum 1985;28:1326–1335.
109. Van der Heijde DMFM, van Leeuwen MA, van Riel PLCM, et al. Biannual radiographic assessments of hands and feet in a three-year prospective follow up of patients with early rheumatoid arthritis. Arthritis Rheum 1992;35:26–34.
110. Bell MJ, Lineker SC, Wilkens AL, et al. A randomized controlled trial to evaluate the efficacy of community based physical therapy in treatment of people with rheumatoid arthritis. J Rheumatol 1998;25:231–237.
111. Komatireddy GR, Leitch RW, Cella K, et al. Efficacy of low resistance muscle training in patients with rheumatoid arthritis functional class II and III. J Rheumatol 1997;24: 1531–1539.
112. Neuberger GB, Press AN, Lindsey HB, et al. Effects of exercise on fatigue, aerobic fitness, and disease activity measures with rheumatoid arthritis. Res Nurs Health 1997;20: 195–204.

113. Van den Ende CH, Vliet Vlieland TP, Munneke M, et al. Dynamic exercise therapy in rheumatoid arthritis: a systematic review. Br J Rheumatol 1998;37:677–687.

114. Bombardier C, Laine L, Reicin A, et al., for the VIGOR Study Group. Comparison of upper gastrointestinal toxicity of rofecoxib and naproxen in patients with rheumatoid arthritis. N Engl J Med 2000;343:1520–1528.

115. Silverstein FE, Faich G, Goldstein JL, et al. Gastrointestinal toxicity with celecoxib vs non-steroidal anti-inflammatory drugs for osteoarthritis and rheumatoid arthritis: the CLASS Study: a randomized controlled trial. JAMA 2000;284:1247–1255.

116. Wolfe MM, Lichtenstein DR, Singh G. Gastrointestinal toxicity of nonsteroidal antiinflammatory drugs. N Engl J Med 1999;340:1888–1899.

117. Yeomans ND, Tulassay Z, Juhasz L, et al, for the Acid Suppression Trial: Ranitidine versus Omeprazole for NSAID-Associated Ulcer Treatment (ASTRONAUT) Study Group. A comparison of omeprazole with ranitidine for ulcers associated with nonsteroidal anti-inflammatory drugs. N Engl J Med 1998;338:719–726.

118. Hawkey CJ, Karrasch JA, Szczepanski L, et al., for the Omeprazole versus Misoprostol for NSAID-Induced Ulcer Management (OMNIUM) Study Group. Omeprazole compared with misoprostol for ulcers associated with nonsteroidal antiinflammatory drugs. N Engl J Med 1998;338:727–734.

119. Kirwan JR, and the Arthritis and Rheumatism Council Low-Dose Glucocorticoid Study Group. The effect of glucocorticoids on joint destruction in rheumatoid arthritis. N Engl J Med 1995;333:142–46.

120. Gubner R, August S, Ginsburg V. Therapeutic suppression of tissue reactivity:II. Effect of aminopterin in rheumatoid arthritis and psoriatic arthritis. Am J Med Sci 1951; 221:176.

121. Fehlauer SC, Carson CW, Cannon GW. Two year follow up of treatment of rheumatoid arthritis with methotrexate: clinical experience in 124 patients. J Rheumatol 1989;16: 307–312.

122. Weinblatt ME, Kaplan H, Germain BF, et al. Methotrexate in rheumatoid arthritis: a five-year prospective multicenter study. Arthritis Rheum 1994;37:1492–1498.

123. Suarez-Almazor ME, Belseck E, Shea B, et al. Methotrexate for treating rheumatoid arthritis (Cochrane Review). In: The Cochrane Library, Issue 4, 2001 Oxford: Update Software.

124. Boushey CJ, Beresford SAA, Omenn GS, et al. A quantitative assessment of plasma homocysteine as a risk factor for vascular disease. Probable benefits for increasing folic acid intakes. JAMA 1995;274:1040–1057.

125. Landewe RBM, van der Borne BEEM, Breedveld FC, et al. Methotrexate effects in patients with Rheumatoid arthritis with cardiovascular comorbidity. Lancet 2000;355: 1616–1617.

126. Wald DS, Law M, Morris JK. Homocysteine and cardiovascular disease: evidence on causality from a meta-analysis. BMJ 2002;325:1202–1208.

127. Arnesen E, Refsum H, Bonna KH, et al. Serum total homocysteine and coronary heart disease. Int J Epidemiol 1995;24:704–709.

128. Morgan SL, Baggott JE, Lee JY, et al. Folic acid supplementation prevents deficient blood folate levels and hyperhomocysteinaemia during longterm low dose methotrexate therapy for rheumatoid arthritis: implications for cardiovascular disease prevention. J Rheumatol 1998;25:441–446.

129. Van Ede AE, Laan RFJM, Blom HJ, et al. Homocysteine and folate status in methotrexate treated patients with Rheumatoid arthritis. Rheumatology 2002;41:658–665.

130. Morand EF, McCloud PI, Littlejohn GO. Life table analysis of 879 treatment episodes with slow acting antirheumatic drugs in community rheumatology practice. J Rheumatol 1992;19:704–708.

131. Morgan SL, Baggott JE, Vaughan WH, et al. Supplementation with folic acid during methotrexate therapy for rheumatoid arthritis: a double-blind, placebo controlled trial. Ann Intern Med 1994;121:833–841.

132. Shiroky JB, Neville C, Esdaile JM, et al. Low-dose methotrexate with leucovorin (folinic acid) in the management of rheumatoid arthritis: results of a multicenter randomized, double-blind, placebo-controlled trial. Arthritis Rheum 1993;36:795–803.

133. Kremer JM, Alarco'n GS, Lightfoot RW Jr, et al. Methotrexate for rheumatoid arthritis: suggested guidelines for monitoring liver toxicity. Arthritis Rheum 1994;37:316–328.

134. Van der Heijde DM, van Riel PL, Nuver-Zwart IH, et al. Effects of hydroxychloroquine and sulphasalazine on progression of joint damage in rheumatoid arthritis. Lancet 1989;1: 1036–1038.

135. Van der Heide A, Jacobs JW, Bijlsma JW, et al. The effectiveness of early treatment with "second-line" antirheumatic drugs: a randomized, controlled trial. Ann Intern Med 1996;124:699–707.

136. Tsakonas E, Fitzgerald AA, Fitzcharles MA, et al. Consequences of delayed therapy with second-line agents in rheumatoid arthritis: a 3-year follow-up on the Hydroxychloroquine in Early Rheumatoid Arthritis (HERA) study. J Rheumatol 2000;27:623–629.

137. Clark P, Casas E, Tugwell P, et al. Hydroxychloroquine compared with placebo in rheumatoid arthritis: a randomized controlled trial. Ann Intern Med 1993;119:1067–1071.

138. Blackburn WDJr, Prupas HM, Silverfield JC, et al. Tenidap in rheumatoid arthritis: a 24-week double-blind comparison with hydroxychloroquine-plus-piroxicam, and piroxicam alone. Arthritis Rheum 1995;38:1447–1456.

139. Runge LA. Risk/benefit analysis of hydroxychloroquine sulphate treatment in rheumatoid arthritis. Am J Med 1983;75(1A):52.

140. O'Dell JR, Haire CE, Erikson N, et al. Treatment of rheumatoid arthritis with methotrexate alone, sulfasalazine and hydroxychloroquine, or a combination of all three medications. N Engl J Med 1996;334:1287–1291.

141. Möttönen T, Hannonen P, Leirisalo-Repo M, et al. Comparison of combination therapy with single-drug therapy in early rheumatoid arthritis: a randomized trial. Lancet 1999;353: 1568–1573.

142. O'Dell J, Leff R, Paulsen G, et al. Methotrexate (M)-hydroxychloroquine (H)-sulfasalazine (S) versus M-H or M-S for rheumatoid arthritis (RA): results of a double-blind study [abstract]. Arthritis Rheum 1999;42(Suppl 9):S117.

143. Landewe' RB, Goei The' HS, van Rijthoven AWAM, et al. A randomized, double- blind, 24-week controlled study of low-dose cyclosporine versus chloroquine for early rheumatoid arthritis. Arthritis Rheum 1994;37:637–643.

144. Smolen JS, Kalden JR, Scott DL, et al. Efficacy and safety of leflunomide compared with placebo and sulphasalazine in active rheumatoid arthritis: a double-blind, randomised, multicentre trial. Lancet 1999;353:259–266.

145. Williams HJ, Ward JR, Dahl SL, et al. A controlled trial comparing sulfasalazine, gold sodium thiomalate, and placebo in rheumatoid arthritis. Arthritis Rheum 1988;31:702–713.

146. Ebringer R, Ahern M, Thomas D, et al, for the Australian Multicentre Clinical Trial Group. Sulfasalazine in early rheumatoid arthritis. J Rheumatol 1992;19:1672–1677.

147. Skosey JL. Comparison of responses to and adverse effects of graded doses of sulfasalazine in the treatment of rheumatoid arthritis. J Rheumatol Suppl 1998;16:5–8.

148. Sharp JT, Strand V, Leung H, et al., on behalf of the Leflunomide Rheumatoid Arthritis Investigators Group. Treatment with leflunomide slows radiographic progression of rheumatoid arthritis: results from three randomized controlled trials of leflunomide in patients with active rheumatoid arthritis. Arthritis Rheum 2000;43:495–505.

149. Strand V, Cohen S, Schiff M, et al. Treatment of active rheumatoid arthritis with leflunomide compared with placebo and methotrexate. Arch Intern Med 1999;159:2542–2550.

150. Mladenovic V, Domljan Z, Rozman B, et al. Safety and effectiveness of leflunomide in the treatment of patients with active rheumatoid arthritis: results of a randomized, placebo-controlled, phase II study. Arthritis Rheum 1995;38:1595–1603.

151. Emery P, Breedveld FC, Lemmel EM, et al. A comparison of the efficacy and safety of leflunomide and methotrexate for the treatment of rheumatoid arthritis. J Rheumatol 2000;39:655–665.

152. Strand V, Tugwell P, Bombardier C, et al. Function and health-related quality of life: results from a randomised controlled trial of leflunomide versus methotrexate or placebo in patients with active rheumatoid arthritis. Arthritis Rheum 1999;42:1870–1878.

153. Tugwell P, Wells G, Strand V, et al. Clinical improvement as reflected in measures of function and health-related quality of life following treatment with leflunomide compared with methotrexate in patients with rheumatoid arthritis: sensitivity and relative efficiency to detect a treatment effect in a twelve-month, placebo-controlled trial. Arthritis Rheum 2000;43:506–514.

154. Forestier J. Rheumatoid arthritis and its treatment with gold salts. J Lab Clin Med 1935;20:827.

155. Cash JM, Klippel JH. Second-line drug therapy for rheumatoid arthritis. N Engl J Med 1994;330:1368–1375.

156. Felson DT, Anderson JJ, Meenan RF. The comparative efficacy and toxicity of second-line drugs in rheumatoid arthritis: results of two meta-analyses. Arthritis Rheum 190;33: 1449–1461.

157. Ward JR, Williams HJ, Egger MJ, et al. Comparison of auranofin, gold sodium thiomalate, and placebo in the treatment of rheumatoid arthritis: a controlled clinical trial. Arthritis Rheum 1983;26:1303–1315.

158. Van Rijthoven AW, Dijkmans BA, Goei The' HS, et al. Cyclosporin treatment for rheumatoid arthritis: a placebo controlled, double blind, multicentre study. Ann Rheum 1986;45: 726–731.

159. Wells G, Haguenauer D, Shea B, et al. Cyclosporine for treating rheumatoid arthritis (Cochrane Review). In: The Cochrane Library, Issue 4, 2001 Oxford: Update Software.

160. Van den Borne BEEM, Landewe' RBM, Goei The' HS, et al. Combination therapy in recent onset rheumatoid arthritis: a randomized double blind trial of the addition of low dose cyclosporine to patients treated with low dose chloroquine. J Rheumatol 1998;25:1493–1498.

161. Altman RD, Perez GO, Sfakianakis GN. Interaction of cyclosporine A and nonsteroidal anti-inflammatory drugs on renal function in patients with rheumatoid arthritis. Am J Med 1992;93:396–402.

162. Boers M, Dijkmans BA, van Rijthoven AW, et al. Reversible nephrotoxicity of cyclosporine in rheumatoid arthritis. J Rheumatol 1990;17:38–42.

163. Levy J, Paulus HE, Barnett EV, et al. A double-blind controlled evaluation of azathioprine treatment in rheumatoid arthritis and psoriatic arthritis [abstract]. Arthritis Rheum 1972;15:116–117.

164. Urowitz MB, Gordon DA, Smythe HA, et al. Azathioprine in rheumatoid arthritis: a double-blind, crossover study. Arthritis Rheum 1973;16:411–418.

165. Woodland J, Chaput de Saintonge DM, et al. Azathioprine in rheumatoid arthritis: double-blind study of full versus half doses verses placebo. Ann Rheum Dis 1981;40:355–359.

166. Clunie GPR, Lennard L. Relevance of thiopurine methyltransferase status in rheumatology patients receiving Azathioprine. Rheumatology 2004;43:13–18.

167. Kloppenburg M, Breedveld FC, Terwiel JP, et al. Minocycline in active rheumatoid arthritis: a double-blind, placebo-controlled trial. Arthritis Rheum 1994;37:629–636.

168. Tilley BC, Alarco'n GS, Heyse SP, et al. Minocycline in rheumatoid arthritis: a 48-week, double-blind, placebo-controlled trial. Ann Intern Med 1995;122:81–88.

169. O'Dell JR, Haire CE, Palmer W, et al. Treatment of early rheumatoid arthritis with minocycline or placebo: results of a randomized double-blind, placebo controlled trial. Arthritis Rheum 1997;40:842–848.

170. O'Dell JR, Paulsen G, Haire CE, et al. Treatment of early seropositive rheumatoid arthritis with minocycline: four-year follow up of a double-blind, placebo controlled trial. Arthritis Rheum 1999;42:1691–1695.

171. Alarco'n GS, Bartolucci AA. Radiographic assessment of disease progression in rheumatoid arthritis patients treated with methotrexate or minocycline. J Rheumatol 2000;27: 530–534.
172. Hickling P, Jacoby RK, Kirwan JR, and the Arthritis and Rheumatism Council Low-Dose Glucocorticoid Study Group. Joint destruction after glucocorticoids are withdrawn in early rheumatoid arthritis. Br J Rheumatol 1998;37:930–936.
173. American College of Rheumatology Task Force on Osteoporosis Guidelines. Recommendations for the prevention and treatment of glucocorticoid-induced osteoporosis. Arthritis Rheum 1996;39:1791–801.
174. Royal College of Physicians (UK). Osteoporosis: clinical guidelines for prevention and management. London: RCP; 1999.
175. Buckley LM, Leib ES, Cartularo KS, et al. Effects of low dose corticosteroids on the bone mineral density of patients with rheumatoid arthritis. J Rheumatol 1995;22: 1055–1059.
176. Amin S, LaValley MP, Simms RW, et al. The role of vitamin D in corticosteroid-induced osteoporosis: a meta-analytic approach. Arthritis Rheum 1999;42:1740–1751.
177. Garber EK, Targoff C, Paulus HE. Corticosteroids in the rheumatic diseases: Chronic low doses, chronic high doses, "pulses", intra-articular. In: Paulus HE, Furst DE, Dromgoole SH, eds. Drugs for rheumatic disease. New York: Churchill Livingstone; 1987: 443.
178. Pincus T, O'Dell JR, Kremer JM. Combination therapy with multiple disease-modifying antirheumatic drugs in rheumatoid arthritis: a preventive strategy. Ann Intern Med 1999; 131:768–774.
179. Williams HJ, Ward JR, Reading JC, et al. Comparison of auranofin, methotrexate, and the combination of both in the treatment of rheumatoid arthritis: a controlled clinical trial. Arthritis Rheum 1992;35:259–269.
180. Haagsma CJ, van Reil PL, de Jong AJ, et al. Combination of sulfasalazine and methotrexate versus the single components in early rheumatoid arthritis: a randomized, controlled, double-blind, 52 week clinical trial. Br J Rheumatol 1997;36:1082–1088.
181. Dougados M, Combe B, Cantagrel A, et al. Combination therapy in early rheumatoid arthritis: a randomized, controlled, double blind 52 week clinical trial of sulfasalazine and methotrexate compared with the single components. Ann Rheum Dis 1999;58: 220–225.
182. Weinblatt ME, Kremer JM, Coblyn JS, et al. Pharmacokinetics, safety, and efficacy of combination treatment with methotrexate and leflunomide in patients with active rheumatoid arthritis. Arthritis Rheum 1999;42:1322–1328.
183. Kremer JM, Caldwell JR, Cannon GW, et al. The combination of leflunomide and methotrexate in patients with active rheumatoid arthritis who are failing on methotrexate treatment alone: a double-blind placebo controlled study [abstract]. Arthritis Rheum 2000;43(Suppl 9):S224.
184. Furst DE, Luggen ME, Thompson AK, et al. Adding leflunomide to patients with active rheumatoid arthritis while receiving methotrexate improves physical function and healthrelated quality of life [abstract]. Arthritis Rheum 2000;43(Suppl 9):S344.
185. Salaffi F, Carotti M, Cervini C. Combination therapy of cyclosporine A with methotrexate or hydroxychloroquine in refractory rheumatoid arthritis. Scand J Rheumatol 1996;25:16–23.
186. Tugwell P, Pincus T, Yocum D, et al. Combination therapy with cyclosporine and methotrexate in severe rheumatoid arthritis. N Engl J Med 1995;333:137–141.
187. Cook SD, Beckenbaugh RD, Redondo J, et al. Long-term follow-up of pyrolytic carbon metacarpophalangeal implants. J Bone Joint Surg Am 1999;81:635–648.
188. Creighton MG, Callaghan JJ, Olejniczak JP, et al. Total hip arthroplasty with cement in patients who have rheumatoid arthritis: a minimum ten-year follow-up study. J Bone Joint Surg Am 1998;80:1439–1446.
189. Mont MA, Yoon TR, Krackow KA, et al. Eliminating patellofemoral complications in total knee arthroplasty: clinical and radiographic results of 121 consecutive cases using the Duracon system. J Arthroplasty 1999;14:446–455.

190. Ranawat CS. Surgical management of the rheumatoid hip. Rheum Dis Clin North Am 1998;24:129–141.
191. Wolfe F, Zwillich SH. The long-term outcomes of rheumatoid arthritis: a 23-year prospective, longitudinal study of total joint replacement and its predictors in 1,600 patients with rheumatoid arthritis. Arthritis Rheum 1998;41:1072–1082.
192. Escalante A, Beardmore TD. Predicting length of stay after hip or knee replacement for rheumatoid arthritis. J Rheumatol 1997;24:146–152.

Chapter 3
Development of Biological Therapies for Inflammatory Arthritis

Neil Basu

Biological response modifiers have revolutionized the practice of rheumatology in the past few years. These potent therapeutic tools are derived from the fundamental translational concept of deciphering distinct immunopathologic mechanisms. Substances that mimic natural antagonists to these mechanisms were subsequently developed through genetic engineering.

Tumor Necrosis Factor-α for Rheumatoid Arthritis

The first class of biologics licensed were directed toward the cytokine tumor necrosis factor-α (TNF-α). Substantial evidence exists implicating the role of this mediator in several proinflammatory functions ranging from neutrophil activation to matrix metalloproteinase induction. Furthermore, the relative importance of TNF-α to other cytokines is suggested by *in vitro* experiments in which dramatic falls in interleukin (IL)-1, IL-6, IL-8, and granulocyte-macrophage colony-stimulating factor (GM-CSF) levels in response to TNF blockade were observed [1].

Within the synovial fluid of patients with rheumatoid arthritis (RA), not only is TNF-α found in high concentrations, but also its levels can be correlated with bony erosions [2]. Equally, high levels have been established in the joint fluid of psoriatic arthritis (PsA) [3], juvenile idiopathic arthritis (JIA) [4], and in the sacro-iliac joint in ankylosing spondylitis (AS) [3].

The concept of TNF-α blockade as a therapy for inflammatory arthritis has developed into a clinically efficacious therapy consuming a significant proportion of a typical rheumatology service budget.

There are currently three agents licensed for use in RA: etanercept, infliximab, and adalimumab.

N. Basu
Grampian, Aberdeen Royal Infirmary, Aberdeen, UK

D.M. Reid, C.G. Miller (eds.), *Clinical Trials in Rheumatoid Arthritis and Osteoarthritis*,   37
© Springer-Verlag London Limited 2008

Etanercept

A humanized TNF-receptor fusion protein, etanercept binds to both soluble TNF-α and TNF-β preventing interaction with their respective receptors. Administration is subcutaneous and a 25 mg twice-a-week regimen is thought to be optimal and unrelated to weight. Efficacy has been suitably demonstrated for monotherapy [5] and for combination therapy with methotrexate [6]. However, comparison between the regimens did not come until recently [7].

The TEMPO study group randomly assigned 686 patients to a treatment regimen. Significantly, patients selected had not received methotrexate (MTX) in the preceding 6 months. In addition, patients who were previously intolerant to MTX or who experienced a poor response were excluded from the trial. This allowed for a fairer comparison of the agents. Primary end points included radiographic assessment in terms of the Sharp score [8] as well as clinical response in terms of American College of Rheumatology (ACR) response 20, 50, and 70 [9].

Table 3.1 illustrates that combination therapy was particularly significant in producing ACR50 and ACR70 outcomes and suggests that joint damage can be repaired in part as indicated by a negative mean Sharp score. These results were found to be statistically significant. It is therefore recommended that etanercept be prescribed with MTX wherever possible.

Infliximab

Infliximab is a chimeric antibody that neutralizes both soluble and membrane-bound TNF-α. It not only prevents receptor interaction but also induces antibody- and complement-dependent cytotoxicity on those cells expressing TNF-α. Murine monoclonal antibodies, such as infliximab, have the propensity to become immunogenic after repeated exposures. Maini et al. [10] reported the presence of anti-infliximab antibodies in 53% and 21% of patients receiving 1 mg/kg and 3 mg/kg infusions, respectively, after 12 weeks. MTX reduces immunogenicity, so when given in combination, the levels of antiglobulin antibodies were reduced to 15% and 7% for 1 mg/kg and 3 mg/kg infusions over the same period of time. Immunogenicity leads to loss of long-term efficacy and infusion reactions, therefore infliximab is only licensed for use in combination with MTX in RA.

Table 3.1 TEMPO: ACR response (%) and change in mean Sharp score after 52 weeks

	MTX	ETA	MTX + ETA
ACR20	75	76	85
ACR50	43	48	69
ACR70	19	24	43
Sharp score	+2.8	+0.5	−0.5

MTX, methotrexate escalated from 7.5 mg to 20 mg as tolerated; ETA, etanercept 25 mg subcutaneous twice weekly.

Table 3.2 ATTRACT: ACR response (%) at 30 weeks

	MTX	MTX + INF 3 mg/kg every 8 weeks	MTX + INF 3 mg/kg every 4 weeks	MTX + INF 10 mg/kg every 8 weeks	MTX + INF 10 mg/kg every 4 weeks
ACR20	20	53	50	58	52
ACR50	5	29	27	26	31
ACR70	0	8	11	18	11

MTX, methotrexate maximum tolerated licensed dose; INF, infliximab.

Efficacy of this combination was verified in phase III trials by the ATTRACT study group [11], as shown in Table 3.2.

Follow-through studies confirmed persisting efficacy at 102 weeks and exemplified significant retardation in radiologic progression [12].

The recommended dosing for RA is the intravenous administration of 3 mg/kg at 0, 2, and 6 weeks and every 8 weeks thereafter.

Adalimumab

Another example of a monoclonal antibody is adalimumab. It is completely humanized and binds soluble and membrane-bound TNF-α, as well as mediating the death of cells expressing TNF-α. In contrast with the chimeric infliximab, formation of antiglobulin antibodies is not a significant issue and therefore the therapy can be prescribed as monotherapy, although combination with MTX is still preferred.

Efficacy and the subcutaneous dosage of 40 mg fortnightly, regardless of weight, is largely based on two randomized controlled trials (RCTs) that looked at the addition of adalimumab to patients with active RA already established on MTX, as summarised in Table 3.3.

The Keystone study also supported the radiologic benefits described in previous anti-TNF-α studies.

Ankylosing Spondylitis

Therapeutic options have been particularly limited in patients with ankylosing spondylitis, particularly in regard to axial disease. There is, however, ever increasing evidence that anti-TNF-α agents can provide clinical improvement comparable with

Table 3.3 RCTs on adalimumab efficacy

	ARMADA [13] 24 weeks		Keystone et al. [14] 52 weeks	
	MTX	ADA + MTX	MTX	ADA + MTX
% ACR20	9	45	24	59
% ACR50	5	37	9.5	41.5
% ACR70	3	18	9	23.2

MTX, methotrexate maximum tolerated licensed dose; ADA, adalimumab subcutaneous 40 mg/fortnight.

that found in RA [3]. Early magnetic resonance imaging (MRI) studies also suggest a slowing of radiographic progression. Etanercept and infliximab are currently licensed in the United States, the European Union, and the United Kingdom, the former at its usual RA dose and the latter at an increased dose of 5 mg/kg every 6 to 8 weeks. There are no data relating to combination therapy with other disease-modifying antirheumatic drugs (DMARDs) at this time.

Psoriatic Arthritis

All three anti-TNF-α agents are licensed for use in the United States, the European Union, and the United Kingdom for the treatment of psoriatic arthritis. Not only do peripheral and axial arthritic symptoms respond, but a clear benefit to the skin condition has also been demonstrated [3].

Juvenile Idiopathic Arthritis

Significantly active JIA disease, after an adequate trial of MTX, is a licensed indication to treat children/adolescents with etanercept. TNF-β is thought to play a greater role in this disease process in comparison with adult RA, and therefore there is a theoretical reason why etanercept may be particularly efficacious, being the only available biologic known to antagonize this mediator. Nonetheless, infliximab has been used successfully, and trials leading to license submission are in the pipeline [15].

Safety Considerations

When assessing any new class of drug, safety is paramount. Fear of the unknown should not preclude progress, but caution is essential. The majority of RCTs involving these exciting therapies are industry funded with a tendency to select favorable populations with minimal comorbidity. Nevertheless, the safety data from such trials have been reassuring. Commonly reported side effects are minor and include injection site reactions, headache, and nausea. However, a wide range of more severe adverse events are coming to light, and it is vital that vigilant surveillance continues. For example, in the United Kingdom, all patients commenced on anti-TNF-α therapy are submitted to the British Society for Rheumatology (BSR) biologics register [16]. Any adverse events arising while on anti-TNF therapy are immediately reported.

Serious infections have been recorded and include fatalities. It is recommended that anti-TNF-α not be started or continued during such events, however it may be initiated once successful treatment is complete. Pathogenic organisms include opportunistic infections such as histoplasmosis, *Pneumocystis carinii,* and aspergillosis as well as the more typical bacterial infections. Reactivation of latent tuberculosis has been a particular problem, especially within the first 12 months of treatment. Guidelines by the BSR call for appropriate TB screening for all patients prior to therapy. If there is a suspicion of latent disease, then review by a local TB specialist is advised and consideration given to prophylactic antituberculous therapy.

There is theoretical evidence implicating TNF-α with neoplastic suppression. Blockade may, therefore, lead to malignancy. There is no evidence thus far confirming any association clinically. There are worries regarding lymphoma with rates of between 2.3 to 6.4 times the normal population being reported [17]. However, the RA population in general is known to have an increased lymphoproliferative risk.

As mentioned, infliximab readily induces antichimeric antibodies, yet all agents have been associated with raised antinuclear titers. Drug-induced lupus is rare, but if clinical evidence is present, cessation of the biological agent is recommended.

TNF-α is abundant in the context of cardiac failure, however a trial into the therapeutic use of infliximab in congestive cardiac failure (CCF) actually reported an increase in mortality. Consequently, anti-TNF therapies should not be initiated in patients with New York Heart Association grade III/IV CCF, and consideration should be given to discontinuing treatment if CCF develops while on therapy.

Demyelination has been reported after anti-TNF therapy and is a contraindication to continued therapy. A history of demyelinating illness, such as multiple sclerosis, is also a reason to exclude potential patients.

On a final cautious note, the British registry has uncovered a potential association with pulmonary fibrosis and severe lower respiratory tract infections. Whether this is the first warning of many to be produced by this facility, only time will tell.

Economic Considerations

Evidence indicates that continuous treatment is required if efficacy is to be maintained. Economically, this adds up to approximately £ 8000 per year per patient [18]. A previous economic analysis suggested that the combination of etanercept and MTX therapy was approximately 36 times more expensive than a triple therapy regime of sulfasalazine, MTX, and hydroxychloroquine [19]. Despite there being good evidence of biological efficacy in early RA [20–22], whether they offer significant cost-benefit over traditional DMARD options remains to be seen. It would seem both economically and medically imprudent to offer anti-TNF therapy to all; indeed within the United Kingdom, a strict eligibility criteria exists [16]. Patients must:

1. Fulfil the 1987 criteria of the American College of Rheumatology classification criteria for a diagnosis of RA.
2. Have active RA (have a DAS28 score >5.1).
3. Have failed standard therapy as defined by failure to respond to or tolerate adequate therapeutic trials of at least two standard DMARDs.

The Future

There is hope that the development of oral TNF inhibitors will reduce costs in the future. AGIX4207 is an example currently undergoing phase II trials. Further TNF antagonism modalities look hopeful such as pegsunercept, a pegylated soluble TNF receptor type 1, and ISIS-104838, a TNF-α antisense inhibitor [23]. Finally, in the more immediate future, golimumab, another humanized monoclonal antibody to TNF-α, is to be marketed and will offer patients a monthly subcutaneous dosing schedule [24].

Other Biological Agents

Approximately 25% of patients prescribed anti-TNF do not gain significant benefit. For those that do respond to these agents, cure is not guaranteed and the durability of effectiveness is still in question. It is therefore important to explore further potential therapeutic routes.

Anakinra

The proinflammatory cytokine IL-1 is thought to play a key role in the pathogenesis of RA. It orchestrates several aspects of the immune and inflammatory processes. Fundamental functions include neutrophil recruitment, macrophage activation, and lymphocyte stimulation. More specifically, it induces matrix metalloproteinases and osteoclasts, both of which are inherently linked with cartilage destruction and bone erosion [25].

In vitro evidence linking RA to IL-1 is strong. Several animal models have demonstrated the development of inflammatory arthritis after the administration of IL-1. Human studies have not only confirmed the presence of high IL-1 titers in the synovial fluid of RA patients but also shown correlation with disease activity [26].

Given the evidence, it would seem reasonable to postulate that IL-1 antagonism may provide therapeutic benefit in the context of RA.

Anakinra is the first clinically available agent to specifically target IL-1. The product of recombinant human DNA technology, it mimics interleukin receptor antagonist (IL-1Ra), a naturally occurring inhibitor. IL-1Ra plays a pivotal role in balancing the proinflammatory effects of IL-1 as studies have shown its levels to be deficient in RA patents [27].

Initial U.S. licensing in November 2001 and later in the United Kingdom in April 2002 was predominately based on three large controlled efficacy studies (Table 3.4).

Safety data thus far has been favorable for both monotherapy and MTX combination therapy. Injection site reactions have been the most commonly reported

Table 3.4 Anakinra efficacy studies

	ACR20 response at 24 weeks							
	European monotherapy [28]				MTX combination [29]			Confirmatory efficacy [30]
Daily regimen	P	30 mg	75 mg	150 mg	MTX	MTX + 1 mg/kg	MTX + 2 mg/kg	MTX MTX + 100 mg
% ACR20	27	39	34	43	23	42	35	22 38

MTX, methotrexate maximum tolerated licensed dose; P, placebo.

adverse event. These tend to be dose dependent, mild, and self-resolving. There is a suggestion of a slight increase in infection rates although the evidence is conflicting. Susceptibility to lower respiratory tract infections has been noted particularly in asthmatics and elderly males. However, there have been no reports of an increase in opportunistic infections, particularly TB, or neoplasia although it will be several years before adverse long-term sequelae can be truly excluded. Finally, leukopenia is a rare potential complication, and therefore blood counts should be monitored during treatment [26].

Administration is subcutaneous, and the licensed dosage is 100 mg once a day. Monotherapy is approved in the United States, however prescription is restricted to MTX combination use in Europe.

As Table 3.4 outlines, efficacy is significant but modest. Clinicians would argue that ACR50 and ACR70 measures have more practical relevance and data to fulfill these criteria are less convincing. For example, participants of the European monotherapy trial [28] demonstrated only an 18% and 2% ACR50 and ACR70 response, respectively, after 48 weeks. Indeed, evaluation of the therapy by the National Institute of Excellence (NICE) in the United Kingdom concluded that the benefits gained were not substantial enough to merit its significant economic costs [31].

Evidence supporting the drug's role in prevention of structural damage is more impressive. An extension of the European Monotherapy study [32] showed up to a 58% reduction in radiologic progression compared with placebo after 24 weeks. Further studies confirm this effect to be sustained [26] corroborating *in vitro* evidence that IL-1 antagonism offers a protective effect to bone and cartilage. It is hypothesized that IL-1's influence predominates over pathways involving structural damage such as proteoglycan breakdown as opposed to those concerned with joint inflammation. This would explain anakinra's relatively modest showing in disease activity scores. Whether these scores are a comprehensive representation of therapeutic goals is an entirely different debate. Further explanations for its incomplete performance include its short half-life and imperfect drug delivery system. Slow-release formulations are being studied, as are alternative mechanisms of IL-1 inhibition such as the development of monoclonal antibodies against IL-1 and inhibitors of IL-1 converting enzymes.

Table 3.5 Clinical efficacy

	MTX alone		Rituximab alone		Rituximab + cyclo		Rituximab + MTX	
Week	24	48	24	84	24	48	24	48
% ACR20	38	20	65	33	76	49	73	65
% ACR50	13	5	33	15	41	27	43	35
% ACR70	5	0	15	10	15	10	23	15

Source: From Reference 34.
Cyclo, cyclophosphamide; MTX, methotrexate.

Rituximab

The role of B cells in the immunopathogenesis of RA is far from clear and is likely to involve a number of intricate mechanisms. Its importance is exemplified by the abundance of B cells producing Rh factor, proinflammatory cytokines, and TNF-α in rheumatoid synovial membrane [33]. Clinically, its significance was first considered after anecdotal case reports describing the remission of RA in patients being treated for coexisting lymphoma. The treatment in question was the genetically engineered chimeric anti-CD20 monoclonal antibody, rituximab. CD20 is an antigen specific to all B cells except stem and plasma cells. Rituximab results in a transient depletion of $CD20^+$ B-cell populations by way of several mechanisms including complement activation and antibody-dependent cell-mediated cytotoxicity.

After a number of encouraging small, open-label trials, a double-blinded, controlled study was performed randomizing 161 active RA patients resistant to previous DMARD therapy to one of oral MTX; rituximab (1 g days 1 and 15); rituximab (750 mg days 3 and 17) and cyclophosphamide; or rituximab (1 g days 1 and 15) and MTX summarised in Table 3.5 [34].

The data clearly supports a role for B-cell depletion therapy with significant improvements in disease activity for as long as 48 weeks when combination therapy is used. More recently, preliminary data from the phase III REFLEX trial was presented at the annual ACR meeting. This long-term efficacy trial observed the response of a single dose of rituximab on DMARD-resistant RA patients, and initial findings are encouraging [35].

Table 3.6 Clinical efficacy of abatacept

	ATTAIN [38] 6 months		AIM [39] 12 months	
	MTX	ABA + MTX	MTX	ABA + MTX
% ACR20	19.5	50.4	36.1	62.6
% ACR50	30.8	20.3	20.2	41.7
% ACR70	1.5	10.2	7.6	20.9

ABA, abatacept 10 mg/kg; MTX, methotrexate.

Almost complete peripheral B-cell depletion is observed and can last between 3 to 12 months [36]. The spectre of serious infection is an obvious worry over this period, and although no significant difference in adverse events was noted between the treatment groups in the mentioned study, this safety issue needs to be addressed further in larger and longer-term trials. Observed adverse events included frequent but mild infusion reactions and are not considered significant enough to lead to therapy cessation. Theoretical immune reactions against chimeric antibodies exist, and fully humanized agents such as ocrelizumab are currently undergoing phase II trials.

Available evidence is certainly supportive of this therapeutic modality, and licensing for resistant active RA has now occurred in the United States, the European Union, and the United Kingdom. It should, however, be noted that most data relate to rheumatoid factor–positive patients, and it is certainly a matter for debate whether the same response would be expected from seronegative patients.

Abatacept

Substantial evidence exists that T lymphocytes are central to the pathogenesis of RA. Not only are T cells found to significantly accumulate in joints of RA patients, but also evidence exists to show that transfer of such cells from RA synovium to immunodeficient mice results in the development of an inflammatory arthritis in the recipient organisms [37].

The activation of T cells requires dual interaction with an antigen-presenting cell (APC). Signaling between the major histocompatibility complex peptide on the APC and T-cell receptor is antigen specific. Costimulation of CD antigens on respective cells leads to cytokine production and augmentation of the T-cell population. Downstream consequences of T-cell activation include induction of IL-1, IL-6, TNF-α, matrix metalloproteinases, osteoclasts, and many more mediators involved in the erosive joint disease of RA.

The CD antigens typically involved in the activation of T cells in RA are CD80/CD86 on APCs. These combine with CD28 on T-cells. Cytotoxic T lymphocyte–associated antigen 4 (CTLA4) is a protein that binds to CD80/CD86 and thus impedes interaction with CD28. This in turn inhibits T-cell activation. Abatacept is a chimeric fusion protein with an extracellular domain that mimics CTLA4. Its consequent ability to bind to CD80/CD86 blocks the ability of APCs to stimulate T cells and their known role in the pathogenesis of RA.

Translation into clinical medicine has recently led to the U.S. Food and Drug Administration (FDA) licensing of the agent. Approval was based on three large clinical controlled trials, two looking at efficacy [38, 39] (Table 3.6) and one at safety [40].

Early evidence is certainly encouraging regarding the efficacy of monthly intravenous infusions of abatacept in combination with MTX. ACR data appear to improve with time, and longer-term outcome studies may show even greater efficacy. On the other hand, initial suggestions from AIM [39] indicate a 50% reduction in radiographic erosive rates in comparison with anti-TNF-α therapies, which regularly show improvements of 80% to 90%.

ASSURE [40] was positive concerning the therapy's safety profile. As with all biologics, infection is a worry; however, theoretically, abatacept only knocks out one costimulation pathway thus leaving numerous other T-cell avenues to provide a normal immune response against infective agents. Furthermore, memory T-cells are less dependent on CD28 costimulation and therefore should not be significantly influenced.

Thus far, only a marginal increase in infection rates has been noted apart from two subgroups of patients, those on combination therapy with anti-TNF-α products and those with a history of chronic obstructive airways disease (COAD). It is recommended that anti-TNF-α combinations no longer be used and that abatacept be used cautiously in patients with COAD. The most common adverse events to be noted were minor and included headaches, dizziness, and dyspepsia.

Modulation of T-cell activity is certainly a promising therapeutic option; current research includes the production of a CD2 antagonist, alfacept, which is in phase II development.

Tocilizumab

Developed in Japan, tocilizumab is a humanized antibody to the IL-6 receptor. The IL-6 cytokine participates in several immune stimulatory pathways including immunoglobulin production, T-cell activation, platelet production, and the promotion of acute-phase protein hepatic synthesis. The interference of IL-6 induction by tocilizumab theoretically should modulate inflammatory diseases such as RA.

Phase II trials suggest significant ACR responses, at least in the short-term, for RA [41] and particularly when used in combination with MTX. Its role in limiting acute-phase protein responses looks promising in severe systemic JIA [42], a condition where extreme levels of IL-6 are observed. Adverse events documented thus far have included reactivation of Epstein-Barr virus (EBV), a case of allergic pneumonitis, and increased lipid levels [43]. Most commonly, nasopharyngitis, skin rash, and abdominal pain have been noted. Phase III trials are progressing with a view to license submission in 2006 in Japan and 2007 elsewhere.

Clinical trials of monoclonal antibodies to IL-15 (HuMAX) and IL-12 (ABT-874) have reached phase II; IL-12 and IL-17 have also been investigated as potential therapeutic targets [43].

Others

Several other novel agents and targets have been and are being investigated.

Belimumab is a monoclonal antibody that modulates B-cell function by knocking out B-lymphocyte stimulator. It showed a significant but modest ACR20 response at 24 weeks of 35% versus 16% for placebo in a phase II trial of active rheumatoid patients who had previously failed to respond to DMARDs. Seronegative patients and those with previous exposure to anti-TNF-α did not gain benefit. Its safety profile was also considered reasonable [44].

Eculizumab, a humanized antibody directed against complement, has shown benefit when administered monthly, and trials are ongoing [45].

Natalizumab is yet another humanized monoclonal antibody. Its specific effects are antagonist toward the selective adhesion molecule (SAM) alpha 4 integrin. SAMs play specific roles in aiding migration of lymphocytes from plasma to tissue. Although at the phase II trial stage for RA [46], it has reached further development in the fields of multiple sclerosis and Crohn's disease where recently the association with progressive multiple leukoencephalopathy has led to its withdrawal from all trials [47].

CAMPATH-1H [43] antibodies, a T-cell depleter, and *NGD-200-1*, an oral C5a antagonist [48], are examples of failures in this field. More recently, the catastrophic cytokine storms that were observed in six healthy volunteers receiving the anti-CD28 antibody *TGN1412* have been widely publicized [49]. Such experiences serve to dampen excessive optimism in this indisputably exciting biological age.

References

1. Feldmann M, Brennan F, Williams RO, et al. The transfer of a laboratory based hypothesis to a clinically useful therapy: the development of anti-TNF therapy of rheumatoid arthritis. Best Pract Res Clin Rheumatol 2004;18(1):59–80.
2. Neidel J, Schulze M, Lindschau J. Association between degree of bone-erosion and synovial fluid-levels of tumor necrosis factor alpha in the knee-joints of patients with rheumatoid arthritis. Inflamm Res 1995;44:217–221.
3. Braun J, Sieper J. Biological therapies in the spondylarthritides—the current state. Rheumatology 2004;43(9):1072–1084.
4. Grom AA, Murray KJ, Luyrink L, et al. Patterns of expression of tumor necrosis factor alpha, tumor necrosis factor beta, and their receptors in synovia of patients with juvenile rheumatoid arthritis and juvenile spondylarthopathy. Arthritis Rheum 1996;39:1703–1710.
5. Moreland LW, Schiff MH, Baumgartner SE, et al. Etanercept therapy in rheumatoid arthritis: a randomised controlled trial. Ann Intern Med 1999;130:478–486.
6. Weinblatt ME, Kremer JM, Bankhurst AD, et al. A trial of etanercept, a recombinant tumour necrosis factor receptor: Fc fusion protein, in patients with rheumatoid arthritis receiving methotrexate. N Engl J Med 1999;340:253–259.
7. Klareskog L, van der Heijde D, de Jager JP, et al., for the TEMPO (Trial of Etanercept and Methotrexate with Radiographic Patient Outcome) study investigators. Therapeutic effect of the combination of etanercept and methotrexate compared with each treatment alone in patients with rheumatoid arthritis: double-blind randomised controlled trial. Lancet 2004;363:675–681.
8. van der Heijde DM, van Riel PL, Nuver-Zwart IH, Gribnau FW, van de Putte LB. Effects of hydroxychloroquine and sulphasalazine on progression of joint damage in rheumatoid arthritis. Lancet 1989;1:1036–1038.
9. Felson DT, Anderson JJ, Boers M, et al. American College of Rheumatology:preliminary definition of improvement in rheumatoid arthritis. Arthritis Rheum 1995;38:727–735.
10. Maini RN, Breedveld FC, Kalden JR, et al. Therapeutic efficacy of multiple intravenous

infusions of anti-tumor necrosis factor alpha monoclonal antibody combined with low-dose weekly methotrexate in rheumatoid arthritis. Arthritis Rheum 1998;41:1552–1563.

11. Maini R, St Clair EW, Breedveld F, et al. Infliximab (chimeric anti-tumour necrosis factor alpha monoclonal antibody) versus placebo in rheumatoid arthritis patients receiving concomitant methotrexate: a randomised phase III trial. ATTRACT Study Group. Lancet 1999;354:1932–1939.

12. Lipsky PE, van der Heijde DM, St Clair EW, et al. Infliximab and methotrexate in the treatment of rheumatoid arthritis. Anti-Tumor Necrosis Factor Trial in Rheumatoid Arthritis with Concomitant Therapy Study Group. N Engl J Med 2000;343:1594–1602.

13. Weinblatt ME, Keystone EC, Furst DE, et al. Adalimumab fully human anti-tumor necrosis factor alpha monoclonal antibody, for the treatment of rheumatoid arthritis in patients taking concomitant methotrexate: the ARMADA trial. Arthritis Rheum 2003;48:35–45.

14. Keystone EC, Kavanaugh AF, Sharp JT, et al. Radiographic, clinical and functional outcomes of treatment with adalimumab (a human anti-tumor necrosis factor monoclonal antibody) in patients with active rheumatoid arthritis receiving concomitant methotrexate therapy: a randomised, placebo-controlled, 52 week trial. Arthritis Rheum 2004;50:1400–1411.

15. Wilkins N, Jackson G, Gardner J. Biologic therapies for juvenile arthritis. Ann Dis Childhood 2003;88(3):186–191.

16. Ledingham J, Deighton C. Update on the British Society for Rheumatology guidelines for prescribing TNFα blockers in adults with rheumatoid arthritis (update of previous guidelines of April 2001). Rheumatology 2005;44:157–163.

17. Brown SL, Greene MH, Gershon SK, Edwards ET, Braun MM. Tumour necrosis factor antagonist therapy and lymphoma development. 26 cases reported to the Food and Drug Administration. Arthritis Rheum 2002;46:3151–3158.

18. NICE. The clinical effectiveness and cost effectiveness of etanercept and infliximab for rheumatoid arthritis and juvenile poly-articular idiopathic arthritis. Available at www.nice.org.uk/pdf/RAAssessmentReport.pdf. Accessed February 10, 2006.

19. Choi HK, Seeger JD, Kuntz KM. A cost effectiveness analysis of treatment options for patients with methotrexate resistant rheumatoid arthritis. Arthritis Rheum 2000;43(10):2316–2327.

20. Banthon JM, Martin RW, Fleischmann RM, et al. A comparison of etanercept and methotrexate in patients with early rheumatoid arthritis. N Engl J Med 2000;343:1586–1593.

21. St Clair EW, van der Heijde DM, Smolen JS, et al. Combination of infliximab and methotrexate therapy for early rheumatoid arthritis: a randomized, controlled trial. Arthritis Rheum. 2004;50:3432–3443.

22. Breedveld FC, Weisman MH, Kavanaugh AF, et al. The PREMIER study: a multicenter, randomized, double-blind clinical trial of combination therapy with adalimumab plus methotrexate versus methotrexate alone or adalimumab alone in patients with early, aggressive rheumatoid arthritis who had not had previous methotrexate treatment. Arthritis Rheum 2006;54:26–37.

23. Goldblatt F, Isenberg D. New therapies for rheumatoid arthritis, Clin Exp Immunol 2005;140(2):195–204.

24. Kay J, Matteson EL, Dasgupta B, et al. Subcutaneous injection of CNTO 148 compared with placebo in patients with active rheumatoid arthritis despite treatment with methotrexate: a randomized, double-blind, dose-ranging trial. 2005 ACR/ARHP Annual Scientific Meeting, November 12–17, 2005, San Diego, CA. Presentation 1921.

25. Dinarello CA. Biologic basis for interleukin-1 in disease. Blood 1996;87(6):2095–2147.

26. Cohen SB. The use of anakinra, an interleukin-1 receptor antagonist, in the treatment of rheumatoid arthritis. Rheum Dis Clin North Am 2004;2(30):365–380.

27. Firestein GS, Boyle DL, Yu C, et al. Synovial interleukin-1 receptor antagonist and interleukin-1 balance in rheumatoid arthritis. Arthritis Rheum 1994;37(5):644–6650.

28. Bresnihan B, Alvaro-Gracia J-M, Cobby M, et al. Treatment of rheumatoid arthritis with recombinant human interleukin-1 receptor antagonist. Arthritis Rheum 1998;41:2196–2204.

29. Cohen S, Hurd E, Cush J, et al. Treatment of rheumatoid arthritis with recombinant human interleukin-1 receptor antagonist, in combination with methotrexate. Results of a twenty-four week, multicenter, randomised, double-blind, placebo-controlled trial. Arthritis Rheum 2002;46:614–624.

30. Cohen SB, Moreland LW, Cush JJ, et al. Kineret^{TM} (anakinra) (recombinant interleukin-1 receptor antagonist): a large, placebo controlled efficacy trial of Kineret in patients with erosive rheumatoid arthritis disease. [Abstract] Ann Rheum Dis 2002;61(Suppl 1):173.

31. NICE. Anakinra for rheumatoid arthritis. Available at www.nice.org.uk/pdf/TA072 guidance.pdf. Accessed February 2, 2006.

32. Jiang Y, Genant HK, Watt I, et al. A multicenter, double-blind, dose ranging, randomised, placebo-controlled study of recombinant human interleukin-1 receptor antagonists in patients with rheumatoid arthritis: radiologic progression and correlation of Genant and Larsen scores. Arthritis Rheum 2000;43(5):1001–1009.

33. Shaw T, Quan J, Totoritis MC. B Cell therpay for rheumatoid arthritis: the rituximab (anti-CD20) experience. Ann Rheum Dis 2003;62(Suppl II):55–59.

34. Edwards J, Szczepanski L, Szechinski J, et al. Efficacy of B-cell targeted therapy with rituximab in patients with rheumatoid arthritis. N Engl J Med 2004;350:2572–2581.

35. Cohen SB, Greenwald M, Dougados MR, et al. Efficacy and safety of rituximab in active RA patients who experienced an inadequate response to one or more anti-TNFα therapies (REFLEX study). ACR/ARHP Annual Scientific Meeting, November 13-16, 2005, San Diego, CA. Abstract 1830.

36. Goldblatt, F, Isenberg D. New therapies for rheumatoid arthritis. Clin Exp Immunol 2005;140(2):195–204.

37. Mima T, Saeki Y, Oshima S, et al. Transfer of rheumatoid arthritis into severe combined immunodeficient mice. The pathogenic implications of T cell populations oligoclonally expanding in the rheumatoid joints. J Clin Invest 1995;96:1746–1758.

38. Genorese MC, Becker JC, Schiff M, et al. Abatacept for rheumatoid arthritis refactory to tumor necrosis factor-alpha inhibition. New Engl J Med 2005;353:1114–1123.

39. Kremer JM, Dougados M, Emery P, et al. Treatment of rheumatoid arthritis with the selective co-stimulation modulator abatacept: twelve month results of a phase IIb, double blind randomised, placebo-controlled trial. Arthritis Rheum 2005;52:2263–2271.

40. Weinblatt M, Combe B, White A, et al. Safety of abatacept in patients with active rheumatoid arthritis receiving background non-biologic and biologic DMARDs: one year results of ASSURE trial. EULAR 2005, June 8–11, 2005, Vienna, Austria. Abstract OP0012.

41. Maini RN Anti-IL-6 receptor therapy: rationale and early results in rheumatoid arthritis. EULAR 2004, June 9–12, 2004, Berlin, Germany. Abstract SP0074.

42. Woo P, Wilkinson N, Prieur A, et al. Proof of principle of the efficacy of IL-6 receptor blockade in severe systemic juvenile idiopathic arthritis. EULAR 2005, June 8–11, 2005, Vienna, Austria. Abstract OP0086.

43. Singh R, Robinson D, El-Gabalawy, Hani S. Emerging biological therapies in rheumatoid arthritis: cell targets and cytokines. Curr Opin Rheum 2005;17:274–279.

44. McKay J, Chwalinska SH, Boling E, et al. Belimumab, a fully human monoclonal antibody to B-lymphocyte stimulator, combined with standard care of therapy reduces the signs and symptoms of rheumatoid arthritis in a heterogeneous subject population. 2005 ACR/ARHP Annual Scientific Meeting, November 12–17, 2005, San Diego, CA. Abstract 1920.

45. Kaplan M. Eculizumab (Alexia). Current Opin Investig Drugs 2002;3(7):1017–1023.

46. Natalizumab in the treatment of rheumatoid arthritis in subjects receiving methotrexate. Available at www.clinicaltrial.gov/ct/show/NCT00083759. Accessed February 20, 2006.

47. Chaudhuri A. Lessons for clinical trials from natalizumab in multiple sclerosis. Br Med J 2006;332:416–419.

48. Chustecka Z. Progress with new drugs for RA. Available at www.jointandbone.org/printArticle.do?primary101696. Accessed February 20, 2006.

49. Suntharalingam G, Perry M, Ward S, et al. Cytokine storm in a phase 1 trial of the anti-CD28 monoclonal antibody TGN1412. N Engl J Med 2006;355:1018–1028.

Chapter 4
Study Design and End Points for Rheumatoid Arthritis Trials

Pieter Geusens and Colin G. Miller

Introduction

Rheumatoid arthritis (RA) is a chronic autoimmune inflammatory disease that primarily affects the synovium of the peripheral joints, resulting in pain, stiffness, swelling, loss of function, and destruction of bone and cartilage.

RA is a heterogeneous disease. The presentation, course, and prognosis in individual patients are variable, at the level of clinical expression as well as at the level of structural damage.

The aims of treatment of RA are therefore multiple: reduction in signs and symptoms, prevention of disability, prevention of structural damage, and induction of remission.

Drugs currently available in the treatment of RA can be classified as symptom-modifying (simple analgesics, nonsteroidal anti-inflammatory drugs [NSAIDs]) or as disease-modifying antirheumatic drugs (DMARDs). Selection of patients for a trial and for evaluation of symptomatic efficacy of therapeutic interventions is primarily based on a combination of clinical assessments. When treatments aiming to slow down or to prevent joint damage are evaluated, the resulting degree of joint damage, including bone and cartilage destruction, needs to be assessed.

Numerous measures have been developed to cover the wide range of aspects of disease activity in RA. These include clinical, laboratory, and imaging, mainly radiographic measures, but increasingly also using magnetic resonance imaging (MRI) and ultrasound.

Measures in RA can be classified as process and outcome measures. Outcome is defined as the end result of disease (death, disability, discomfort, iatrogenic events, and economic impact) [1]. Process measures are the clinical, symptomatic, and biomarker (both imaging and biochemical) changes that occur over time. Some of the process measures are related to outcome and can as such be helpful in selection of patients for trials and in predicting long-term outcome (Table 4.1) [1]. They are

P. Geusens

Department of Rheumatology, University Hospital, Maastricht, The Netherlands *and* Biomedical Research Institute, University Hasselt, Diepenbeek, Belgium

D.M. Reid, C.G. Miller (eds.), *Clinical Trials in Rheumatoid Arthritis and Osteoarthritis*,   51
© Springer-Verlag London Limited 2008

Table 4.1 Core domains and subdomains in longitudinal observational studies

Domain	Type*	Examples[†]
Core domains		
Health status		
Quality of life (QOL)/Health status instruments (HSI)	O	HUI, NHP, WHO-QOL RA-QOL/SF-36, AIMS, HLI, CLINHAQ, etc.
Symptoms	O, PC	VAS and multidimensional pain fatigue and sleep scales, etc.
Physical function	O, PC	HAQ, MHAQ, FSI, etc.
Psychosocial function	O, PC	Affect, socialization, social support, etc.
Disease process		
Joint tenderness/swelling	O, PC	Short and long swelling and tenderness scales, Ritchie and modified Ritchie index, self-report joint examination scales
Global	O, PC	VAS scales; patient's severity and/or activity; physician's activity, and/or severity
Acute phase reactants	O, PC	CRP, ESR
Damage		
Radiographic or imaging	O, PC	Sharp, Sharp–van der Heijde, Larsen, etc.
Deformity	O	Radiographic or by physical examination
Surgery	O	Total joint replacement, other arthropathies
Organ damage	O, PC	Extra-articular manifestations of RA: nodules, iritis, vasculitis, etc., pulmonary, renal damage, etc.
Toxicity/adverse reactions	O	Drug toxicity, adverse reactions to medical and surgical interventions
Mortality	O	Number and causes of death
Important but not core domains		
Work disability	O	Work disability, sick leave, days lost from work
Costs	O	Utilization, direct and indirect costs, charges

Source: From Reference 1.

HUI, Health Utilities Index; NHP, Nottingham Health Profile; WHOQOL, World Health Organization Quality of Life; HLI, Health and Lifestyle Index; VAS, visual analog scale; CLINHAQ, Clinical Health Assessment Questionnaire; SF-36, Medical Outcome Survey Short Form-36; FSI, Functional Status Index; CRP, C-reactive protein; AIMS, Arthritis Impact Measurement Scale; ESR, erythrocyte sedimentation rate.

*O, outcome; PC, predictor or covariate. Depending on the purpose of the study, these variables may be measured once or many times but are usually measured multiple times.

[†]These examples are provided for clarification only. OMERACT IV did not recommend any specific instruments in view of the limited data available on their use in longitudinal observational studies (LOS).

Table 4.2 OMERACT IV recommendations for reporting of longitudinal observational studies

Item	Information to be specified
Study rationale	State research question and importance.
Study design	Prospective, retrospective, or mixed.
Sources of and selection of cases	True population-based, catchment population or consecutive series. Describe calendar time, geographic, referral, and access factors.
	Case-control studies: method of case and control identification and selection.
Timing of recruitment	Describe timing of recruitment in relation to disease onset: cases followed from disease onset, cases followed from first presentation, or prevalent cases.
Inclusion criteria	Describe minimal criteria and when criteria were satisfied?
Assessment measures	Provide data on reliability and validity of instruments and study assessments.
Assessment methods	Describe principal and subsidiary outcome measures. Indicate means of follow-up data collection (clinical examination, clinic interview, questionnaire, mail, or telephone).
	Report number of observers, nature of training, observer variability and blindness.
Baseline clinical data collected	Specify data collected at baseline. Distinguish between items ascertained from routine medical records and those collected prospectively using a standard proforma.
Description of demographic and baseline	Describe demographic and baseline characteristics of participants.
Follow-up data collection	Specify frequency of follow-up, decision rules about timing of assessments. Full description of missing patients at each stage of follow-up. Indicate means of follow-up data collection (clinical interview, questionnaire, mail, or telephone).
Analyses	Describe missing data and missing subjects.
	Specify strategies used to limit missing data and to analyze missing data and loss to follow-up.
	Indicate the power to detect clinically meaningful change. If a statistical model is generated, indicate performance in a validation sample.
	Describe key model assumptions.
	Where appropriate, perform sensitivity analyses to account for loss to follow-up. Use appropriate time-dependent-variable–based analyses and survey methods.
	Describe rationale for statistical methodology.
	Biases and potential problems: identify and discuss possible sources of bias and misinterpretation.

Source: From Reference 1.

then used as surrogate markers of disease activity. Several attempts have been made to combine these measures in an index of disease activity.

Based on individual end points and combined measures, a core set has been proposed to follow the course of the disease and the response to treatment, including measures of remission. There is increasing consensus on several methodological aspects of clinical trials that are specific for RA, and many groups have contributed to its development such as the World Health Organization (WHO), the International League Against Rheumatism (ILAR), the European League Against Rheumatism (EULAR), the American College of Rheumatology (ACR), and the Outcome Measures in Rheumatoid Arthritis Clinical Trials (OMERACT) group. This has resulted in a core set application for governmental organizations, such as the Food and Drug Administration (FDA) in the United States and the European Agency for the Evaluation of Medicinal Products (EMEA) in Europe, which acknowledge such measures to be used in clinical trials for licensing purposes [2, 3].

We will review some specific, mainly clinical, end points used primarily when conducting and interpreting clinical trials in RA (Tables 4.2 and 4.3). Extensive and more detailed information is available at Web sites of scientific organizations [1, 4, 5] and governmental authorities [2, 3] around the world that are continuously updated with new methods of evaluating disease activity and treatments in RA.

Table 4.3 Core and potentially important variables: Demographics, covariate, and predictors

Variable	Requirement	Measurement time
Age	*	O
Sex	*	O
Education	*	O
Ethnicity	*	O
Disease duration	*	O
Comorbidity	*	O
Arthritis and nonarthritis treatment	*	O, M
Occupation	*	O, M
Referral setting	*	O
Social status	*	O
HLA/DNA		O
Rheumatoid factor		O, (M)
Smoking status		O
Marital status		O, (M)
Body mass index		O, M
Pregnancies		O, (M)
Oral contraceptive/hormonal status		O, M
Income		O, M
Access to and/or financing of health care		O
Family history		O, (M)

Source: From Reference 1.

O, measure once; M, measure many times; (M), can be measured many times but is usually measured just once.

*A core variable suggested for all studies. Items with no asterisk should be collected dependent on the disease under study and the study aim and possibilities.

Patient Selection

As the etiology of RA remains unknown, no specific test is available for the diagnosis. Classification criteria have been developed in order to include well-defined patients with RA. The most widely used classification is based on the ACR criteria (Table 4.4) [5]. The ACR criteria use a combination of clinical (swelling, stiffness), immunologic (rheumatoid factor), and radiographic measures (bone erosions) for the diagnosis of RA.

In most studies, patients are selected above a well-defined degree of disease activity. The parameters of disease activity will be discussed in more detail later in this chapter. They mostly include a minimum number of swollen and painful joints, an increased erythrocyte sedimentation rate (ESR) or C-reactive protein (CRP), positive rheumatoid factor, and/or the presence of joint erosions.

Table 4.4 ACR 1987 criteria for the classification of acute arthritis of RA

Criterion*	Definition
1. Morning stiffness	Morning stiffness in and around the joints, lasting at least 1 hour before maximal improvement
2. Arthritis of three or more joint areas	At least three joint areas simultaneously have had soft tissue swelling or fluid (not bony overgrowth alone) observed by a physician. The 14 possible areas are right or left PIP, MCP, wrist, elbow, knee, ankle, and MTP joints
3. Arthritis of hand joints	At least one area swollen (as defined above) in a wrist, MCP, or PIP joint
4. Symmetric arthritis	Simultaneous involvement of the same joint areas (as defined in no. 2) on both sides of the body (bilateral involvement of PIPs, MCPs, or MTPs is acceptable without absolute symmetry)
5. Rheumatoid nodules	Subcutaneous nodules, over bony prominences, or extensor surfaces, or in juxta-articular regions, observed by a physician
6. Serum rheumatoid factor	Demonstration of abnormal amounts of serum rheumatoid factor by any method for which the result has been positive in <5% of normal control subjects
7. Radiographic changes	Radiographic changes typical of rheumatoid arthritis on posteroanterior hand and wrist radiographs, which must include erosions or unequivocal bony decalcification localized in or most marked adjacent to the involved joints (osteoarthritis changes alone do not qualify)

Source: From Reference 1.

PIP, proximal interphalangeal; MCP, metacarpophalangeal; MTP, metatarsophalangeal.

* For classification purposes, a patient shall be said to have rheumatoid arthritis if he or she has satisfied at least 4 or these 7 criteria. Criteria 1 through 4 must have been present for at least 6 weeks. Patients with two clinical diagnoses are not excluded. Designation as classic, definite, or probable rheumatoid arthritis is *not* to be made.

Table 4.5 Typical inclusion and exclusion criteria for a study with NSAIDs in RA

Inclusion criteria

    Male and female patients aged $\geq$18 years

    Symptomatic RA as confirmed by the ACR criteria for the classification of RA

    Class I, II, or III according to the ACR revised criteria for functional status classification

    Symptoms for $\geq$3 months and requiring regular NSAID therapy

Exclusion criteria

    $\geq$3 DMARDs

    Systemic corticosteroids ($>$7.5 mg/day of prednisone or equivalent)

    Use of gastroprotective medication

    Low-dose aspirin ($\leq$325 mg/day) for cardiovascular prophylaxis

    A history of GI events such as ulceration or bleeding

    Known hypersensitivity to NSAIDs

    Significant medical problems

    Pregnancy

    Nursing women

    Women not using reliable contraceptive protection

Table 4.6 Typical inclusion and exclusion criteria for a study with new DMARD in RA

Inclusion criteria

    Age $>$18 years

    Disease duration 6 months to 20 years

    Adult-onset RA (ARA [American Rheumatism Association] class I–III)

    At least three swollen joints

    At least one of following:

        ESR $>$28 mm/h, CRP $>$20 mg/L, morning stiffness $>$45 minutes

    Less than satisfactory response to $>$1 DMARD other than methotrexate (MTX)

    Less than satisfactory response to MTX

Exclusion criteria

    Previous treatment with drug under investigation (or drugs of similar class)

    Previous use of investigational drugs

    Current use of oral glucocorticoids

    Relevant comorbidity, including infections and cancer

Depending on the drug and the aim of the study, some patients are excluded from participation. Typical inclusion and exclusion criteria in studies of NSAIDs and DMARDs are shown in Tables 4.5 and 4.6, respectively.

Types of Clinical Trials

Several study designs are available. They are based on timing (cross-sectional or longitudinal) and the presence and characteristics of the control population (cohort, case-controlled, randomized and controlled, crossover, or factorial). They all have their strengths and weaknesses, and their application depends on the aims of the study and the availability of patients and controls [1].

Cross-sectional trials are usually used to investigate prevalence (i.e., the number of patients with RA in the population at a given time) or incidence (i.e., the number of new cases of the disease within a population at a given time). They are open to bias because, in the first example above, the cases and controls may be different in other ways (e.g., if the control population is younger, the difference in prevalence of the disease may be due to age). Other factors such as body weight, smoking habits, or previous drug history may be confounding the results. The majority of clinical trials in RA trials are of a longitudinal nature because of the potential of confounding variables.

There are a number of different types of longitudinal study:

1. Randomized controlled trials (RCTs). The majority of trials in RA will fall into this category. Patients are randomized to treatment or control (placebo or active comparator) and monitored over a number of years. The length of follow-up will depend on regulatory requirements (1 to 6 months for NSAIDs, 1 to 2 years for DMARDs) and the end point chosen. Investigators and patients will normally be blinded to the treatment (double blinding), although in some trials with intravenous delivery, it may only be possible to blind investigators to the treatment (single blinding).
2. Factorial designs. These are RCTs where more than one treatment are tested alone and in combination against each other and against placebo. Although the majority of trials are the traditional RCT, in RA, this kind of trial design is becoming more prominent. It ensures that all patients receive at least monotherapy, which is now an ethical requirement.
3. Cohort studies. In such studies, a group of patients is selected because of risk or because of exposure to a factor being studied. Phase IV postmarketing trials in RA are a type of cohort study. Patients who are at risk of developing the disease or who have established RA are treated with a licensed, effective treatment and followed to measure long-term side effects and to see if any improvement is maintained over a long period.
4. Case-controlled studies. In case-controlled studies, a group of patients with RA, for example, are identified as cases. A control group is selected who do not have the disease but are similar to the control group in other factors. For example, the controls may be matched for age, body mass index (BMI), and critical blood assays. Such a study might follow the change in joint stiffness over a number of years in controls (who might be expected to develop joint stiffness as they start to exhibit symptoms of the disease) and cases (who might be expected to stabilize or demonstrate improvement in stiffness). Clearly, in evaluating new treatments, such studies may well introduce bias because of poor matching between cases and controls. In such studies, it is important that the investigator evaluating the end points is blinded to the patient group.
5. Crossover trials. A crossover trial is one where patients are randomized to treatment or control and then, after a fixed time followed by a period of washout for the active drug, patients are swapped from treatment to control or vice versa. Such trials are not often used in bone-related studies because of the length of

time treatments take to have a measurable outcome and the length of washout period that would be required.

There are four main types of intervention trials with drugs, from phase I to phase IV. Phase I studies to assess drug safety and initial dose finding in normal or disease subjects are beyond the scope of this chapter. Phase II and III studies are longitudinal RCTs. The controls consist of patients on placebo with or without specified other therapies, such as analgesics, NSAIDs or DMARDs. Phase IV studies are more and more being undertaken to determine safety and long-term efficacy. This chapter is most relevant to phase II and phase III trials in the setting of a RCT.

The primary and secondary end points of clinical trials in RA depend on the type of intervention. Symptomatic treatments with NSAIDs will be tested for their ability and speed to decrease pain, stiffness, and swelling, to increase function, and to maintain this amelioration with maximal safety. In studies with NSAIDs, the effects of new drugs are compared with placebo or other already approved NSAIDs. Rescue medication for pain consists of paracetamol at a prespecified maximum daily dose.

On top of this, treatment with DMARDs will be tested for their ability to slow down, prevent, or even restore structural joint damage, restore function, and induce remission in the medium- to long-term. In studies with DMARDs, the effects of new drugs are compared with other drugs or added to ongoing treatment. Placebo-controlled studies are performed in short-term studies in phase II. Phase III placebo-controlled studies can be difficult to perform as effective DMARDs are already available in daily clinical practice. This dilemma can be overcome by using a placebo arm during a limited time period of the total study duration (e.g., 4 to 6 months) and then switching to active medication.

End Points

The choice of end points in clinical trials for RA has a long history. Over the past few decades, many groups have studied the value of end points in terms of relevance to the disease and the population under investigation; acceptability to the scientific community and regulatory authorities; responsiveness to change; reproducibility; availability; and reliability and acceptability to patients [1].

The OMERACT has labeled measures on the basis of (1) validity (is the assessment measuring what it is intended to measure?) and (2) discrimination for reliability and responsiveness to change (is it unchanged when the phenomenon does not change, i.e., does it have a low measurement error, and does it change when true change occurs?) [1].

The main end points in trials in RA are clinical, serologic, and imaging, mainly radiographic, but increasingly also MRI and ultrasound. Several composite measures are available that combine different components of the disease. Furthermore, core sets have been developed for evaluation of RA, which are considered the minimum frame in which clinical trials should be performed.

Single End Points

Several end points have been extensively studied for application in clinical trials. They each reflect one aspect of the disease and have been extensively tested for applicability in trials.

Clinical End Points

Pain

Pain is the major problem for most patients with RA. Many scores have been developed, including numerical and verbal rating scales, the visual analog scale (VAS), questionnaires, and behavioral observation methods. VAS is most frequently used because of its sensitivity to change, but the technique is difficult to understand for elderly and illiterate patients. The arthritis impact measurement scales (AIMS) is also sensitive to change. The most frequent measure of pain includes a horizontal VAS on a continuous 10-cm line, a categorized scale (Likert scale), or a horizontal numerical scale (Fig. 4.1). It is important to specify the aspect of pain that is being assessed (pain at rest or on activity) and the time interval over which pain is evaluated (e.g., last 24 hours, last week, on movement, at rest, at night). Pain evaluation is also part of several multidimensional health status instruments (Health Assessment Questionnaire [HAQ], AIMS).

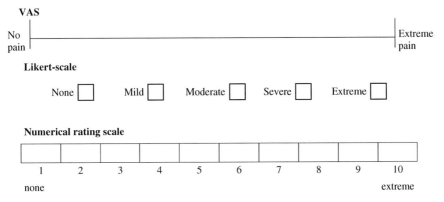

Fig. 4.1 Types of pain scales

Morning Stiffness

Long-lasting morning joint stiffness is a typical complaint of patients with RA. The duration of morning stiffness is often used as an inclusion criterion in clinical trials of RA, as it reflects the inflammatory component. It is also useful for follow-up.

Impairment Measures

Joint Counts

Many different joint counts of clinical signs of inflammation of the synovium (redness, heat, pain, swelling, and functional restriction) are available. They differ in the number of joints included, whether joints are measured separately or combined, and whether joints are graded for severity or size. The degree of joint tenderness and swelling gives information on different aspects of the disease. Most trials now include clinical evaluation of tenderness (tender joint count [TJC]) and swelling (swollen joint count [SJC]) in 28 joints (EULAR) or in 68 joints (ACR). The use of a homunculus (mannequin) is convenient to chart individual joint involvement (Fig. 4.2).

Joint counts are observer-dependent. Training for joint evaluation is therefore indicated in order to minimize intra- and interobserver and between-center differences in clinical trials. Blinding of evaluators from those who have access to source documents can be necessary (e.g., in dose-escalating studies).

Global Disease Activity

Global disease activity can be evaluated in the same way as VAS, on a continuous line of 10 cm, or in a Likert or numerical scale. This can be performed by the patient and by the physician. It is still debatable whether physician global assessment adds to the patient's global assessment, but the physician can consider additional aspects or may have insight into the patient's over- or under-perception of symptoms.

Function/Disability

Physical/Functional Disability

Disability can be measured by several methods, based on clinical judgment, observed patient performances, or self-administered assessments. The most frequently used self-reported questionnaires are the AIMS and HAQ. Others are the McMaster-Toronto arthritis scale (MACTAR), Functional Status Index (FSI), Patient Elicitation Form (PEF), Activity of Daily Living Scale (ADLS), Keitel Index, Lee Index, and so forth. No single instrument has consistently outperformed the others. It is recommended to choose one of these instruments in the core set in order to improve uniformity among trials.

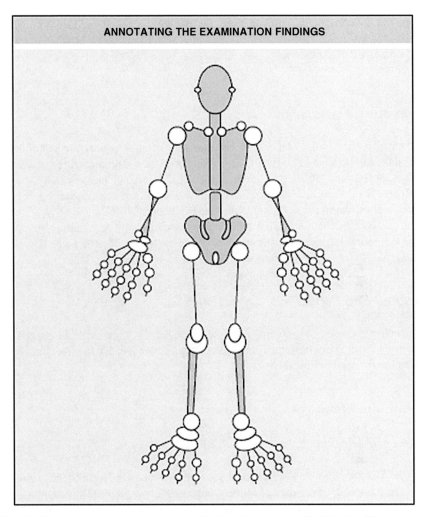

Fig. 4.2 Homunculus (mannequin) for recording joint involvement. (Published in Rheumatology (3rd Edition), MC Hochberg, AJ Silman, JS Smolen, ME Weinblatt and MH Weisman, Fig. 68.3, p. 126, Copyright Elsevier (2006).)

Grip strength can be measured by the use of a sphygmomanometer or a standard device. Because of the variability, the mean of repeated measurements (two to three repeats) of both hands are calculated.

Health Outcome Measures

Several health outcome measures are used in RA. Examples of global measures are the Global Outcome Survey Short Form-36 (SF-36), the Health Utilities Index (HUI), the Nottingham Health Profile (NHP), the World Health Organization Quality of Life (WHOQOL), the Health and Lifestyle Index (HLI), and the Clinical Health Assessment Questionnaire (CLINHAQ). Examples of more disease-specific measures, covering mainly one or more aspects, are the EQ-5D and Euroqol VAS. Additional available measurement tools focus on fatigue, work productivity survey, employment status, walk time, quality of sleep (MOS sleep), and analgesic consumption.

Laboratory Assessment

The most frequently used laboratory measures for disease activity are acute-phase reactants (APRs), such as ESR and CRP. They correlate with clinical disease activity indices, are sensitive to change, and may predict radiographic progression.

Recent data indicate a role for markers of bone and cartilage turnover, such as C-terminal cross linking telopeptide of type 1 collagen (CTX-1) and of type 2 collagen (CTX-2). Other laboratory assessments such as matrix metalloproteinases, cytokines, soluble receptors, the receptor activator of the nuclear factor kappa-B ligand (RANKL), and osteoprotegerin (OPG) are under investigation.

Imaging End Points

The radiographic end points are discussed in Chapter 7 and MRI in chapter 9. Ultrasound examination of the joints is an emerging noninvasive method that needs validation for use in clinical trials.

Composite Measures

Indices of Disease Activity

In order to reflect the many aspects of RA, composite measures have been developed based on combinations of the above-mentioned single end points. The advantages of combining the single components in one index are the unambiguous interpretation of disease activity, comparability between trials, and increased power. These composite measures can be used to measure current disease activity or change in disease activity and are continuous or ordinal.

Current Disease Activity

One of the most used disease activity measure is the disease activity score (DAS). The DAS index is a composite measure and is most commonly used as DAS28(ESR), which includes 28 joints, with the following calculation:

$$DAS28 = 0.56 \times \sqrt{(TJC)} + 0.28 \times \sqrt{(SJC)} + 0.70 \times \ln(ESR) + 0.014 \times \text{general health}$$

in which TJC is total joint count and SJC is swollen joint count. The DAS28 can also be calculated with the use of CRP in stead of ESR (DAS28CRP).

There are several other disease activity measures available, but they are less used in clinical trials. Examples are the Mallya/Mace index and the Stoke index, which need further validation. The RA disease activity index (RADAI) is a highly reliable and valid self-administered measure of disease activity for clinical, health services, and epidemiologic research. The simplified diseases activity index (SDAI) puts more weight on swollen joints.

Improvement Criteria

Based on preparative work of the ACR, EULAR, and OMERACT, the WHO/ILAR has proposed a core set of end points measures in RA clinical trials that includes pain, patient global assessment, physical disability, swollen and tender joints, physician global assessment, acute-phase reactants, and radiographic assessments (for studies with DMARDs) (Table 4.7).

For treatment evaluation, a time component should be included in the measure (i.e., change in disease activity during a certain period). Response can be measured for groups or for individual patients. Individual response criteria quantify the numbers of patients actually responding and the extent of amelioration. This is important additional information to mean group values as end points of clinical trials.

Individual response criteria, based on clinical variables, have been proposed by the ACR and the EULAR. In the ACR response criteria, an improvement is defined as 20% or more based on tender and swollen joint counts and 20% or more improvement in three of the five remaining ACR core-set measurements (patient and physician global assessments, pain, disability, and an APR) (ACR20), assessed by validated methods using standardized techniques. Other cutoffs at 50% (ACR50) or 70% (ACR70) have been developed from these same score measures (Table 4.8).

The EULAR response criteria are based on both the baseline status and changes in DAS and graded as good, moderate, or no improvement. There is a high level of agreement between ACR and EULAR improvement classification, and their validity is equivalent. The discriminating potential of the criteria between treatment groups is comparable [6]. For individual patients, agreement is good at the level of ACR20

Table 4.7 Core set of end points measures in RA clinical trials (WHO/ILAR)

1. Pain
2. Patient global assessment
3. Physical disability
4. Swollen joint count
5. Tender joint count
6. Physician global assessment
7. Acute phase reactants
8. Radiographic (for studies >1 year)

Source: From Reference 1.

Table 4.8 Individual response criteria, based on clinical variables proposed by the ACR and the EULAR

ACR	
≥ 20% improvement in	Tender joint count, and Swollen joint count, and At least three of the following:
	ESR or CRP
	Investigator assessment of global disease activity
	Patient assessment of global disease activity
	Patient assessment of pain
	Physical disability

Disease activity measure	Method of assessment
1. Tender joint count	ACR tender joint count, an assessment of 28 or more joints. The joint count should be done by scoring several different aspects of tenderness, as assessed by pressure and joint manipulation on physical examination. The information on various types of tenderness should then be collapsed into a single tender-versus-nontender dichotomy.
2. Swollen joint count?	ACR swollen joint count, an assessment of 28 or more joints. Joints are classified as either swollen or not swollen.
3. Patient's assessment of pain	A horizontal visual analog scale (usually 10 cm) or Likert scale assessment of the patient's current level of pain.
4. Patient's global assessment of disease activity	The patient's overall assessment of how the arthritis is doing. One acceptable method for determining this is the question from the AIMS instrument: "Considering all the ways your arthritis affects you, mark 'X' on the scale for how well you are doing." An anchored, horizontal, visual analog scale (usually 10 cm) should be provided. A Likert scale response is also acceptable.
5. Physician's global assessment of disease activity	A horizontal visual analog scale (usually 10 cm) or Likert scale measure of the physician's assessment of the patient's current disease activity.
6. Patient's assessment of physical function	Any patient self-assessment instrument which has been validated, has reliability, has been proven in RA trials to be sensitive to change, and which measures physical function in RA patients is acceptable. Instruments which have been demonstrated to be sensitive in RA trials include the AIMS, the HAQ, the Quality (or Index) of Well Being, the MHIQ, and the MACTAR.
7. Acute-phase reactant value	A Westergren erythrocyte sedimentation rate or a C-reactive protein level.

Source: From References 1, 5 and 6.
* ACR = American College of Rheumatology; ESR = erythrocyte sedimentation rate; CRP = C-reactive protein; AIMS = Arthritis Impact Measurement Scales; RA = rheumatoid arthritis; HAQ = Health Assessment Questionnaire; MHIQ = McMaster Health Index Questionnaire: MACTAR = McMaster Toronto Arthritis Patient Preference Disability Questionnaire.

Table 4.8 (continued)

EULAR

Current DAS	Decrease in ≤DAS			Current DAS28	Decrease in DAS28		
	>1.2	>0.6 and ≤1.2	≤0.6		>1.2		≤0.6
≤2.4	Good	Moderate	None	≤3.2	Good	Moderate	None
>2.4 and ≤3.7				<3.2 and ≤5.1			
>3.7				>5.1			

response, when EULAR overall, SDAI overall, or HAQ 0.22 criteria are applied. However, agreement between ACR50, EULAR good, SDAI major, and HAQ 0.5 response was found to be poor [7]. This should be considered when response criteria are used for clinical decisions.

Remission Criteria

Complete remission is not frequent in RA but is the ultimate goal of DMARDs. Remission criteria have been developed by the ACR, OMERACT, and the EULAR (Table 4.9).

Table 4.9 Remission criteria according to the ACR, OMERACT, and EULAR

ACR
Five or more for at least 2 consecutive months:
    No morning stiffness
    No fatigue
    No joint pain (by history)
    No joint tenderness or pain on motion
    No soft tissue swelling in joints or tendon sheets
    Normal ESR

OMERACT
Tender joint count of 0 and a swollen joint count of 0, and an ESR no greater than 10 mm.
If this condition is not met:
    DAS28 ≤ 2.85
    Or:
    5 of 7 criteria:
        1. Pain (0–10) < or = 2
        2. Swollen joint count (0–28) < or = 1
        3. Tender joint count (0–28) < or = 1
        4. Health Assessment Questionnaire (HAQ, 0–3) < or = 0.5
        5. Physician global assessment of disease activity (0–10) < or = 1.5
        6. Patient global assessment of disease activity (0–10) < or = 2
        7. ESR < or = 20

Core Set

A long history of meetings and reports of several groups has led to the development of a core set of measures that should be used in clinical trials (WHO/ILAR, FDA, ACR, OMERACT). It should be stressed that the core set is a minimum requirement. In addition, other outcomes should be considered (psychosocial function, patients' preferences, treatment dropouts, side effects, and costs). It is of interest to note that development and evaluation of core sets is a dynamic process. As an example, a pooled index of patient self-report questionnaire Core Data Set measures appeared to be as informative as ACR20 responses, DAS scores, and pooled indices of all and assessor-derived Core Data Set measures for distinguishing between active treatment and placebo treatment in one recent RA clinical trial [8].

Furthermore, some outcomes of importance to patients are not currently measured, and there are no measures available to capture them. Existing measures need to be calibrated to take account of the differing importance of outcomes at different stages of disease and variations in the magnitude of change within the same outcome that indicate treatment efficacy [9].

Adverse Events

Evaluation of adverse events is a hallmark of every RCT, as part of good clinical practice. However, the recent controversies about the effects of NSAIDs and selective cyclooxygenase (COX)-2 inhibitors on the incidence of cardiovascular events has underlined the need for large-scale and long-term NSAID safety studies and also continued observation in phase IV surveys [10]. Furthermore, the introduction of biological agents such as TNF blockers and B-cell inhibitors, which are closely linked with the defense against infections and cancer, has shown that infectious diseases and cancer should be monitored closely, including reporting such events when these products are marketed [11] (see Chapter 12). Several programs are under development to centralize such data during long-term follow-up.

Conclusion

On the background of good clinical practice and generally accepted principles of performance of clinical trials, specific measures have been developed for evaluation of patients with RA. These include single end points, composite measures, and core sets. These measures are considered of pivotal importance in clinical trials of RA and are endorsed by leading scientific and governmental organizations. Their development and refinement is, however, a dynamic process that continuously requires further follow-up.

References

1. Wolfe F, Lassere M, van der Heijde D, et al. Preliminary Core Set of Domains and Reporting Requirements for Longitudinal Observational Studies in Rheumatology. J Rheumatol 1999;26:484–489. Available at: http://www.jrheum.com/omeract/1-5toc.html. Accessed on December 21, 2007.
2. FDA. Guidance for industry clinical development programs for drugs, devices, and biological products for the treatment of rheumatoid arthritis (RA). Available at www.fda.gov/cder/guidance/index.htm. Accessed 16 November 2006.
3. Committee for the proprietary medicinal products (CPMP). Points to consider on clinical investigation of medicinal products other than NSAIDS for the treatment of rheumatoid arthritis. Available at: http://emea.europa.eu/pdfs/human/ewp/055695en.pdf. Accessed on December 21, 2007.
4. Dougados M, Betteridge N, Burmester GR, et al. EULAR standardised operating procedures for the elaboration, evaluation, dissemination and implementation of recommendations endorsed by the EULAR standing committee. Ann Rheum Dis 2004;63:1172–1176.
5. Felson DT, Anderson JJ, Boers M, et al. American College of Rheumatology. Preliminary definition of improvement in rheumatold arthritis. Arthritis Rheum. 1995;38(6):727–735. Available at: http://www.rheumatology.org/publications/guidelines/ra-improvement/Prelim_ definition_improve_%20RA.asp. Accessed on December 21, 2007.
6. van Gestel AM, Anderson JJ, van Riel PL, et al. ACR and EULAR improvement criteria have comparable validity in rheumatoid arthritis trials. American College of Rheumatology European League of Associations for Rheumatology. J Rheumatol 1999;26(3):705–711.
7. Gülfe A, Geborek P, Saxne T. Response criteria for rheumatoid arthritis in clinical practice: how useful are they? Ann Rheum Dis 2005;64(8):1186–1189.
8. Pincus T, Strand V, Koch G, Amara I, Crawford B, Wolfe F, Cohen S, Felson D. An index of the three core data set patient questionnaire measures distinguishes efficacy of active treatment from that of placebo as effectively as the American College of Rheumatology 20% response criteria (ACR20) or the Disease Activity Score (DAS) in a rheumatoid arthritis clinical trial. Arthritis Rheum 2003;48(3):625–630.
9. Carr A, Hewlett S, Hughes R, Mitchell H, Ryan S, Carr M, Kirwan J. Rheumatology outcomes: the patient's perspective. J Rheumatol 2003;30(4):880–883.
10. Drazen JM. Cox-2 inhibitors – a lesson in unexpected problems. N Engl J Med 2005;352:1131–1132.
11. Bongartz T, Sutton AJ, Sweeting MJ, Buchan I, Matteson EL, Montori V. Anti-TNF antibody therapy in rheumatoid arthritis and the risk of serious infections and malignancies: systematic review and meta-analysis of rare harmful effects in randomized controlled trials. JAMA 2006;295:2275–2285.

Chapter 5
Study Design and End Points in Ankylosing Spondylitis Clinical Trials

Désirée van der Heijde

Introduction

There have been an increasing number of research efforts and clinical trials for ankylosing spondylitis (AS) over the past several years. Multiple new agents are under development for use in AS, and many pharmaceutical companies conducting research and development of these new agents are interested in ultimate approval, especially as disease modification could become one of the new treatment goals in AS. Therefore, it is relevant to have some knowledge and insight in the design and end points of clinical trials in AS. The purpose of this chapter is to give an overview of (1) study design, (2) scope of patients, (3) type of end points to consider, (4) instruments for the various end points, and (5) assessment of response/improvement

This chapter incorporates the latest insight in trial design and outcome assessment. It is anticipated that the contents of this chapter will facilitate the selection of outcome variables and design of trials, including the analyses and presentation of the data. This will, in turn, lead to a more uniform approach to trial design and conduction, allowing a more appropriate comparison of results across trials that will ultimately lead to more informed health care providers and better evidence-based treatment options for patients.

Study Design

Trial Design

The majority of AS trials are randomized controlled trials (RCTs), and this is indeed the most appropriate trial design. Patients are randomized to treatment or

D. van der Heijde,
Professor of Rheumatology, Leiden University Medical Center, Department of Rheumatology, Leiden, The Netherlands

D.M. Reid, C.G. Miller (eds.), *Clinical Trials in Rheumatoid Arthritis and Osteoarthritis*,   69
© Springer-Verlag London Limited 2008

control (placebo or active comparator) and monitored over a certain period of time. Investigators and patients will normally be blinded to the treatment (double blindings).

Duration of Follow-up

The length of follow-up will depend on the end point(s) chosen. Until recently, only drugs that had symptom-modifying properties were available for treatment of AS, therefore the end points of trials investigating these drugs were signs and symptoms. The duration of these trials was short, usually around 6 weeks. This short-term duration does not permit a full documentation of the efficacy profile and the tolerability of the investigated drugs. Dougados et al. [1] suggest that a trial duration of 1 year might be of optimal value compared with a 6-week assessment in order to define better the efficacy and tolerability of nonsteroidal anti-inflammatory drugs (NSAIDs) in AS. Recently, the first trials with anti-TNF agents have been performed. End points of these trials were again sign and symptoms. However, the results were so impressive that it is considered that these agents may have disease-controlling properties. To determine whether anti-TNF agents are really disease-controlling antirheumatic therapy (DC-ART) in AS, it is necessary that these agents control the disease, which means in AS preventing structural damage and maintenance of physical function. Because axial involvement is central to the pathogenesis and course of disease, reference is made here only to structural changes with the axial skeleton. For the detection of chronic spinal changes, conventional radiography is the method of choice. With a 2-year follow-up, progression can be seen in a considerable number of patients and the observed progression may be of sufficient magnitude to be able to demonstrate a reduction on radiographic progression. Therefore, studies that claim prevention of radiographic progression in AS should be of at least 2 years duration.

Handling Missing Data

As the duration of a trial will be longer, there will be an increase in the number of patients that are lost to follow-up. Therefore, it is important that the protocol should prespecify the method of handling missing data. The optimal analysis of a trial is the intention-to-treat (ITT) analysis. An ITT analysis requires that missing data are substituted; for this the last observation carried forward (LOCF) technique is used for assessment of signs and symptoms. For the assessment of structural damage, another imputation method should be selected as the LOCF method would systematically underestimate radiographic progression.

Moreover, it is recommended that studies examine the robustness of obtained results from different plausible and prespecified methods of handling missing data; for example, by substituting the mean value of the specific arm, or right the opposite, substitution of the missing values in the treatment group by the mean value of the other arm, and so forth.

Sample Size Calculation

The sample size calculation depends on the primary outcome measure. This can be a proportion (e.g., x percent of patients show a y improvement of measurement z) or can be quantitative (e.g., a comparison of the mean value of a measurement between the treatment group and the placebo group).

For a sample size calculation, it is required to set values for the type I and II errors. The type I error is the risk that the trial will give a false-positive result. This is indicated with the symbol α and is usually set at 5%. The type II error is the risk that the trial will give a false-negative result. This is indicated with the symbol β and is often set at 20%. The value $1 - \beta$ is known as the power of the study and will therefore usually be 80%. The risk of false-positive and false-negative results can be reduced by reducing α and β, but this will lead to trials with larger number of patients. However, one must realize that the danger of small trials is the possibility that the trial will have insufficient patients to show a statistically significant effect; in other words, the trial is underpowered. To prevent dropout becoming a significant problem, one should adjust the number of included patients to ensure that the number completing the trial is adequate. This adjustment can be based on a review of the literature for the number of dropouts of other trials using similar study drugs.

In sample size calculations, more assumptions beside the setting of α and β must be made. For studies with a proportion as primary outcome, the magnitude of response in the treatment and placebo groups must be determined, and in studies with a quantitative measure, the difference in means between treatment and control groups expected at the end of trial with the standard deviation (SD) of both groups must be determined. To determine these values, it is sensible to use prior knowledge of other trials and the natural course of disease. If all values are determined, they can be put in formulas to calculate sample sizes; these formulas can be found in many textbooks but also on the Internet, for example at http://calculators.stat.ucla.edu/powercalc/.

Evaluation and Presentation of Results

In order to evaluate a treatment, there are at least three possibilities: (1) require a significantly greater difference in X of Y relevant measures for active treatment versus placebo groups, (2) perform multivariate analysis, or (3) use a patient-specific definition. As primary outcome, this third possibility (patient-specific definition) is preferred when available. The results expressed at an individual level might reflect either the concept of improvement ("to be better," "to be a responder") or the concept of low disease activity state after therapy ("to be in a good condition"). Both concepts are important to consider in the evaluation of the clinical relevance of the observed results in clinical trials. For both concepts, the presentation of the results can refer either to a composite index or to single variables (for this purpose, the continuous variable, e.g., change in pain has to be converted to a dichotomous variable, e.g., yes/no improvement in pain for the concept of improvement, yes/no for low level of pain for the concept of low disease activity state). Such definition of the cutoff should refer to the evaluation of the minimal clinically important difference (MCID) for the concept of improvement and the evaluation of low disease activity state (LDAS) for the concept of "to be in a good condition." All the protocols have to prespecify such cutoffs. For the presentation of the results of all the secondary analyses and in particular for all the collected variables, it is recommended to present the mean and SD at entry and at the final visit, the mean change and SD in each single variable, the percentage of patients with a clinically relevant change in each single variable, and the percentage of patients with a low disease activity state at the end of the trial.

Most of the studies should include not only the collection of the data at baseline and at the final visits but also that during intermediate visits. The data collected during such intermediate visits are of great importance in order to (1) facilitate the LOCF technique when using an ITT analysis; (2) permit the calculation of the mean change in a continuous variable during the trial for a single patient (which is more informative than the calculation of the change between final and baseline); and (3) permit the use of a life-table analysis for the dichotomous variables.

Scope of Patients

Patients participating in a clinical AS trial must have definitive AS. Fulfilling of the modified New York criteria [2] has been used for years as an inclusion criterion of AS trials. These criteria consist of three clinical and one radiographic criteria (Table 5.1).

Table 5.1 Modified New York criteria

Clinical criteria

- Low back pain of at least 3 months duration improved by exercise and not relieved by rest.
- Limitation of lumbar spine in sagittal and frontal planes.
- Chest expansion decreased relative to normal values for age and sex.

Radiographic criterion

- Unilateral grade 3 or 4 sacroiliitis or bilateral grade 2 sacroiliitis on radiographs of the SI joints.

A patient is classified as having definite AS if the radiographic criterion and at least one clinical criterion are present. A hallmark of the diagnosis is radiographic sacroiliitis. The disadvantage of this requirement of radiographic sacroiliitis is that radiographic sacroiliitis is frequently a late sign of disease in some cases and may not be present in early disease even in an otherwise typical patient. Currently, research is performed to establish other imaging techniques, especially magnetic resonance imaging (MRI), for earlier diagnosis of sacroiliitis. But more studies are needed to determine if patients with abnormalities of the sacroiliac joints on MRI should be regarded as having sacroiliitis and therefore having met the radiographic criterion. Including a subset of patients with these features in clinical trials would improve the understanding of the disease and is therefore recommended.

To investigate whether a certain intervention can lead to improvement, a patient should have a certain level of disease activity, functionality, and so forth, that can improve, or in case of structural damage, radiographic progression that can be inhibited. Depending on the hypothesis under investigation, inclusion and exclusion criteria must be made.

There is no general agreement about such inclusion criteria, but there is some agreement about exclusion criteria. Features associated with AS such as psoriasis, inflammatory bowel disease, and other comorbidities should not be exclusion criteria in trials. Both patients under the age of 18 years and those whose symptoms started prior to this should be not excluded if they fulfill the entry criteria otherwise. Also, the absence of HLA-B27 should not be an exclusion criterion for clinical trials.

Type of End Points to Consider

In 1995, the international Assessment in Ankylosing Spondylitis (ASAS) Working Group was formed [3]. ASAS defined core sets for the following three settings: DC-ART, symptom-modifying antirheumatic drugs (SMARDs)/physical therapy, and clinical record-keeping. The domains for all three core sets are physical function, pain, spinal mobility, spinal stiffness, fatigue, and patient global assessment. The core sets for clinical record-keeping and DC-ART were extended with the domains acute-phase reactants, peripheral joints, and entheses. The DC-ART core set includes also radiographic assessment (Fig. 5.1). For each domain within the core sets, one or several instruments are available for assessing the patient. The core sets ensure that a minimum of required information is collected. Other data are likely to be needed, depending on the underlying research question or the particular clinical situation. The ASAS Working Group selected specific instruments for each core set [4]. This selection procedure was undertaken to diminish the large number of assessments to create uniformity and comparability in AS clinical trials. The end points discussed in this chapter are in agreement with the work of ASAS.

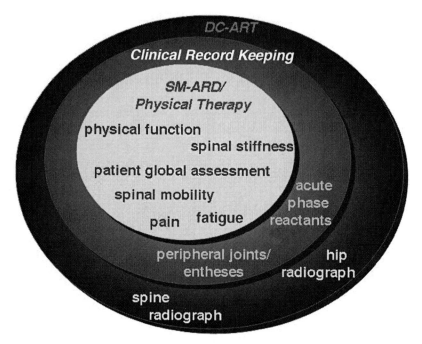

Fig. 5.1 ASAS core sets

Instruments for Various End Points

In this section, the different instruments selected by the ASAS Working Group for each core set are discussed. Many instruments use a visual analog scale (VAS): a horizontal 10-cm line with two anchors. The left anchor represents the best situation (a score of 0) and the right anchor represents the worst situation (a score of 10). Patients are asked to put a vertical mark at the position on the line that best represents their symptoms. The distance between the left anchor and the vertical mark is measured and recorded to one decimal point. An alternative to a VAS is a numerical rating scale (NRS), which consists of a row of numbers from 0 to 10. Patients are asked to put a cross through the number that best represents their symptoms. The anchors (0 and 10) have the same meaning as on the VAS. A NRS has several advantages over a VAS:

- It is better understood and accepted by patients.
- The results are immediately obvious without measuring.
- There are no extra sources of measurement error.
- It can be assessed by telephone.

Domains and Instruments for All Core Sets

Patient global assessment: The patient is asked to place a mark on a VAS or an NRS to represent their response to the question: "How active was your spondylitis on average last week?"

Pain: Patients are asked two questions about the pain experienced on average over the previous week. The first question is "How much spine pain did you experience due to ankylosing spondylitis?" and the second is "How much spine pain did you experience *at night* due to ankylosing spondylitis?" Patients indicate their response on a VAS or NRS.

Spinal stiffness: The patient is asked: "On average last week, for how long after you woke up did you experience stiffness in your spine?" This is recorded in minutes or on a VAS that has a maximum score of 2 hours. Often also the intensity of spinal stiffness is assessed by the following question: "How would you describe the overall level of morning stiffness you have had from the time you wake up?" The final result for spinal stiffness is the average of duration and intensity of morning stiffness.

Fatigue: One general question is asked about the average level of fatigue in the previous week: "How would you describe the overall level of fatigue/tiredness you have experienced?" This, too, is answered on a VAS or NRS.

A frequently used instrument to assess disease activity and that contains a number of the above-mentioned items is the Bath Ankylosing Spondylitis Disease Activity Index [5]. This is an index combining information on back pain, pain of the peripheral joints, pain of the enthesis, fatigue, and morning stiffness.

Physical function: Two indexes are available to assess functional capacity: the Bath Ankylosing Spondylitis Functional Index (BASFI) [6] and the Dougados Functional Index [7]. The BASFI consists of 10 questions answered on a VAS or NRS. The final score is the average of the scores on the 10 questions, ranging from 0 (no limitation in function) to 10 (maximal limitation). The Dougados Functional Index has 20 questions, which are answered on a 3-point or 5-point verbal rating scale and summed to give a total score. The answers are scored 0, 1, and 2 or 0, 0.5, 1, 1.5, and 2, respectively, to ensure that the final score always falls in the range 0 to 40. Both functional indexes have been shown to be valid and sensitive in differentiating between groups of patients with a different level and/or improvement in physical function. There seems to be little difference between the two instruments in their sensitivity to change.

Spinal mobility: Assessment of the spinal mobility domain involves the use of the following five instruments:

- Chest expansion. The patient is asked to rest his or her hands on or behind his or her head. The difference between maximal inspiration and expiration is then measured anteriorly at the fourth intercostal level (e.g., 5.1 cm). The better of two such measurements should be recorded.
- Modified Schober test. The physician makes a mark on the patient's skin on the imaginary line between the superior and posterior iliac spine. A second mark is then made 10 cm higher than the first mark. The patient is asked to bend forward

as far as they can, and the distance between the two marks on the skin is measured. The increase in the distance is noted (e.g., if 14.3 cm is the distance measured between the lines when the patient is bent forward maximally, the recorded result would be 4.3 cm). The better of two tries is recorded.

- Occiput-to-wall test. The patient stands with the heels and back against a wall and with hips and knees as straight as possible. The chin should be held at the usual carrying level. The patient is asked to try as hard as they can to touch their head against the wall. The distance between the wall and the occiput is then measured in centimeters (e.g., 9.6 cm). The better of two tries is recorded.
- Lateral spinal flexion. The patient stands as close to a wall as possible, with the shoulders level. The distance between the patient's middle fingertip and the floor is measured with a tape measure. The patient is asked to bend sideways as far as they can without bending the knees or lifting the heels while keeping the shoulders against the wall. The new distance from middle fingertip to floor is measured and the difference between the two is noted. The better of two tries is recorded for full left and right lateral flexion. The mean of the left and right values gives the final result for lateral spinal flexion (expressed in centimeters to the nearest 0.1 cm).
- The patient sits with shoulders to the wall. A goniometer is placed at the wall above the patient's head. The patient rotates his or her head as far as possible, keeping shoulders still and ensuring no neck flexion or side flexion occurs. The examiner aligns the goniometer branch parallel to the sagittal plane of the head. The average of left and right rotation gives the result for cervical rotation in degrees.

Added Domains and Instruments for the Core Sets Clinical Record-Keeping and DC-ART

Acute-phase reactants: The erythrocyte sedimentation rate (ESR) after 1 hour using the Westergren method and C-reactive protein (CRP) were selected. Keep in mind that normal results do not exclude inflammation as a significant proportion of patients with AS do not have elevated ESR or CRP.

Peripheral involvement: The 44-swollen-joint count should be assessed. Joints included are acromioclavicular joints, humeroscapular joints, sternoclavicular joints, elbows, wrists, metacarpophalangeal joints, proximal interphalangeal joints, knees, ankles and metatarsophalangeal joints.

Enthesitis: A few validated enthesitis scores are available for clinical studies but none of these has yet been selected as the instrument of preference.

Added Domain and Instruments for the Core Set DC-ART

For the radiographic assessment of AS, three methods are available. Lateral views of the cervical and the lumbar and anteroposterior (AP) views of the lumbar spine are recommended by ASAS to be able to perform all available scoring methods. There seems to be no reason for imaging of the thoracic spine by x-rays due to technical problems related to the anatomy of the chest with superimposed lung tissue. Available scoring methods for spinal changes in AS detected by conventional spinal radiography are the Bath Ankylosing Spondylitis Radiography Index (BASRI), the Stoke Ankylosing Spondylitis Spine Score (SASSS), and the modified SASSS [8–10]. The BASRI is a global grading system from 0 to 4 for the Sacroiliac joints, the AP and lateral lumbar (combined) and lateral cervical spine separately. This gives a total score range between 0 and 12. The SASSS scores all four corners of the lumbar vertebrae (0 to 3) on the lateral lumbar spine giving a total range between 0 and 72. The modified SASSS scores only the anterior sites of the lumbar and cervical vertebrae (lateral views) resulting in a score range between 0 and 72. A recent study showed that the modified SASSS is the preferred method to use [11]. With a 2-year follow-up, progression can be seen in a considerable number of patients, and the observed progression may be of sufficient magnitude to be able to demonstrate a reduction in radiographic progression.

Assessment of Response/Improvement

The preferred evaluation of treatment effect is to present a patient-specific definition, as already mentioned in the paragraph about study design. This means that for each patient, it has to be determined whether the patient has improved and can be considered as a responder. Therefore, criteria have been developed to assess the response of an individual with AS [12]. These ASAS response criteria are based on the domains physical function, morning stiffness, patient global assessment, and pain. In summary, three of the four domains should each improve by at least 20% and a minimum of 1 unit on a 10-point scale, and the remaining domain should show less than 20% worsening and less than a 1-unit deterioration. The ASAS response criteria were developed based on studies with NSAIDs and should be used in the evaluation of signs and symptoms. To assess clinical response for agents that possess disease-modifying capabilities, no final selection could be made. Based on limited trial data combined with expert opinion, the following two definitions of clinical response performed equally well [13]:

1. ASAS 40 response criteria: At least 40% improvement and an absolute change of 2 units in three of four domains (using the same domains as the ASAS response criteria) without any worsening in the fourth domain.
2. ASAS 5/6 response criteria: 20% improvement in five of six domains (same four domains as the ASAS response criteria plus two extra domains: spinal mobility and acute-phase reactants).

The advantage of the ASAS 40 response criteria is its simplicity. The disadvantage is that it implies a greater quantitative but not a conceptually qualitative difference in terms of response. The advantage of the ASAS 5/6 response criteria is that there is an impact on the domains of acute-phase reactants and spinal mobility that otherwise do not need to change for symptom modification. The disadvantage is that it is not well established what the clinical meaning of a 20% change in the additional two domains implies. Most preferred are the ASAS 5/6 response criteria, but for the time being it is recommended that both criteria sets should be used to further the knowledge of this concept. It should be noted that in addition to this clinical response, also an effect on function and structural damage needs to be present before the disease-controlling property of a drug can be fully demonstrated.

In addition to the response criteria, partial remission criteria have been proposed to indicate the presence of very low levels of disease activity [12]. Partial remission is defined as a value below 2 (on a 10-point scale) in all four domains (function, morning stiffness, patient global assessment, and pain). An advantage of the partial remission criteria is that the factor time can be incorporated; for example, partial remission remaining for at least 1 year. By applying both the response and partial remission criteria to clinical trials, more information is available on the percentage of patients benefiting from therapy.

Conclusion

A RCT in AS should use the ITT analysis with a prespecification of the missing data analysis. The results should be presented at an individual level at which the concept of improvement (responder) can be used as the primary criterion. For the presentation of the results of all the secondary analyses and in particular for all the collected variables, it is recommended to present the mean and SD at entry and at the final visit, the mean change and SD in each single variable, the percentage of patients with a clinically relevant change in each single variable, the percentage of patients with a low disease activity state at the end of the trial, and the percentage of patients fulfilling the ASAS partial remission criteria at the end of the trial. The domains and instruments that are recommended to be included in each trial are presented.

References

1. Dougados M, Gueguen A, Nakache JP, Velicitat P, Veys EM, Zeidler H, Calin A. Ankylosing spondylitis: what is the optimum duration of a clinical study? A one year versus a 6 weeks non-steroidal anti-inflammatory drug trial. Rheumatology 1999;38(3):235–244.
2. van der Linden S, Valkenburg HA, Cats A. Evaluation of diagnostic criteria for ankylosing spondylitis. A proposal for modification of the New York criteria. Arthritis Rheum 1984;27(4):361–368.
3. van der Heijde D, Bellamy N, Calin A, Dougados M, Khan MA, van der Linden S. Preliminary core sets for endpoints in ankylosing spondylitis. Assessment in Ankylosing Spondylitis Working Group. J Rheumatol 1997;24(11):2225–2229.
4. van der Heijde D, Calin A, Dougados M, Khan MA, van der Linden S, Bellamy N. Selection of instruments in the core set for DC-ART, SMARD, physical therapy, and clinical record

keeping in ankylosing spondylitis. Progress report of the ASAS Working Group Assessment in Ankylosing Spondylitis. J Rheumatol 1999;26(4): 951–954.

5. Garrett S, Jenkinson T, Kennedy LG, Whitelock H, Gaisford P, Calin A. A new approach to defining disease status in ankylosing spondylitis: the Bath Ankylosing Spondylitis Disease Activity Index. J Rheumatol 1994;21(12):2286–2291.

6. Calin A, Garrett S, Whitelock H, Kennedy LG, O'Hea J, Mallorie P, Jenkinson T. A new approach to defining functional ability in ankylosing spondylitis: the development of the Bath Ankylosing Spondylitis Functional Index. J Rheumatol 1994;21(12):2281–2285.

7. Dougados M, Gueguen A, Nakache JP, Nguyen M, Amor B. Evaluation of a functional index for patients with ankylosing spondylitis. J Rheumatol 1990;17(9):1254–1255.

8. Averns HL, Oxtoby J, Taylor HG, Jones PW, Dziedzic K, Dawes PT. Radiological outcome in ankylosing spondylitis: use of the Stoke Ankylosing Spondylitis Spine Score (SASSS). Br J Rheumatol 1996;35(4):373–376.

9. Creemers MCW, van't Hof MA, Gribnau FWJ, van de Putte LBA, van Riel PLCM. A radiographic scoring system and identification of variables measuring structural damage in ankylosing spondylitis. Thesis, University of Nijmegen, The Netherlands; 1993.

10. Kennedy LG, Jenkinson TR, Mallorie PA, Whitelock HC, Garrett SL, Calin A. Ankylosing spondylitis: the correlation between a new metrology score and radiology. Br J Rheumatol 1995;34(8):767–770.

11. Wanders A, Landewé R, Spoorenberg A, et al. What is the most appropriate radiologic scoring method for Ankylosing Spondylitis? A comparison of the available methods based on the outcome measures in rheumatology clinical trials filter. Arthritis Rheum 2004;50(8):2622–2632.

12. Anderson JJ, Baron G, van der Heijde D, Felson DT, Dougados M. Ankylosing spondylitis assessment group preliminary definition of short-term improvement in ankylosing spondylitis. Arthritis Rheum 2001;44(8):1876–1886.

13. Brandt J, Listing J, Sieper J, Rudwaleit M, van der Heijde D, Braun J. Development and preselection of criteria for short-term improvement after anti-TNFα therapy in ankylosing spondylitis. Ann Rheum Dis 2004;63(11):1438–1444.

Chapter 6
Trial Design and Outcomes in Osteoarthritis

Nigel Arden

Introduction

As we continue to learn more about the pathophysiology of osteoarthritis, the number of potential new treatments will continue to increase, as will the need for research into its management. Over the past couple of decades, many excellent clinical trials in osteoarthritis have been performed; however, the study design and presentation of many trials has been inconsistent and often suboptimal. This leads to considerable difficulties when trying to assess the benefits of an individual treatment by assimilating a number of studies or when trying to make a comparison across different treatments. Some of these limitations reflect the design of the study (too small, patient selection, outcome measures), and others simply represent the presentation of the results in publications (details of study design, effect sizes).

In terms of the practicing clinician, the greatest limitation of clinical research into osteoarthritis is that the majority of studies are designed to assess whether a treatment works in a relatively homogenous group of patients with osteoarthritis. Clinicians want to know whether the treatment will work in a specific patient and therefore need to know the predictors of response to answer the more clinically important question of "in who does it work?" In this chapter, I will discuss the important steps that have been made by international cooperations to address these important issues.

Study Design

The traditional design for assessing the efficacy of a new treatment is a randomized, double-blind, placebo-controlled clinical trial. This design minimizes the chance of bias and will assess whether the new treatment is better than placebo. Once this has been established, a randomized, double-blind comparator trial should be performed to compare the efficacy of the new treatment with other existing therapies.

N. Arden
Senior Lecturer in Rheumatology, MRC Unit, Southampton General Hospital, Southampton, UK

D.M. Reid, C.G. Miller (eds.), *Clinical Trials in Rheumatoid Arthritis and Osteoarthritis*, 81
© Springer-Verlag London Limited 2008

There are several forms of randomized controlled trials (RCTs). The favored design is a parallel group trial whereby participants are allocated to a treatment group for the whole study period. An alternative is the crossover design whereby each participant receives both treatments in a random order. This has the advantage of requiring a smaller number of patients to detect an effect. There are, however, several problems with this design, the most important is that if drugs have a prolonged or permanent effect, the subjects have to have a "washout period" between treatment arms to avoid a carryover effect; this design is therefore not suitable for trials of slow-acting symptom-modifying drugs or structure-modifying drugs. The N of 1 trial where patients receive the study drugs in a random order on more than one occasion has been proposed but suffers from the same limitations as the crossover design.

Osteoarthritis is rarely treated by a single treatment modality, and therefore there is increasing interest in the factorial parallel group RCT. This design is often used to assess a combination of two different treatments $(A + B)$; there are four groups receiving treatments as shown in Fig. 6.1. This will answer several questions: Are treatments A and/or B better than placebo? Is either treatment superior to the other? Are both treatments together better than either alone?

There are several treatments for osteoarthritis where it is either impossible or unethical to blind patients or to use placebos; these include treatments such as surgery, education, or some forms of exercise therapy. In these situations, other designs can be used including randomized but not blinded parallel-group trial studies or occasionally in the case of total joint replacement observational studies such as cohort studies may need to be used.

Scientific versus Pragmatic Trials

An important early decision when designing a clinical trial is whether it should be a scientific or a pragmatic study. A scientific study design is used early on in the development of a treatment to assess its efficacy, whereas pragmatic designs are used later in development to asses the effectiveness, cost-effectiveness, and clinical

The factorial Design	
Group 1	Pl A + Pl B
Group 2	A + Pl B
Group 3	Pl A + B
Group 4	A + B

A = Drug A
Pl A = placebo to drug A
B = Drug B
Pl B = placebo to drug B

Fig. 6.1 The factorial design. A, drug A; Pl A, placebo to drug A; B, drug B; Pl B, placebo to drug B

Table 6.1 Scientific and pragmatic trials

	Scientific	Pragmatic
Measures	Efficacy	Effectiveness
Scientific validity	Good	Limited
Generalizability	Limited	Good
Patient selection	Well defined and homogenous	Representative of clinical population
Control group	Often placebo	Often usual clinical care + placebo
Exclusion criteria	Many	Few
Identify predictors of response	Limited	Good
Concomitant analgesics	Usually restricted	Usually unlimited
Intra-articular injections	Not allowed	Often allowed
Cost-effectiveness analyses	Limited use	Useful

predictors of response. Table 6.1 highlights the important differences between the two designs.

Study Duration

The duration of follow-up will depend on the therapy being assessed and the primary outcome measures. For an analgesic or nonsteroidal anti-inflammatory (NSAID) trial, 6 weeks would be the minimum duration to demonstrate its efficacy and adherence. For slower-acting symptom-modifying drugs and intra-articular therapies, 3 to 6 months would be required to demonstrate efficacy although longer may be required if assessing cost-effectiveness. A duration of 3 years is optimum for studies of structure-modifying drugs; although shorter periods can be used, it will require a greater number of patients to achieve the same statistical power.

Patient Selection

Scientific trials, early in a treatment development stage, tend to recruit well-defined patients and exclude patients with comorbidities in an effort to reduce the size and therefore costs of the study. A further technique often used in NSAID trials is the flare design: to enter the study, participants have to be on a NSAID, which is discontinued at the screening visit. Only those whose pain flares by a predetermined level are entered into the study, therefore including only patients who are responsive to NSAIDs. Whereas this is undoubtedly a scientifically valid and cost-effective approach to trial design, it induces several limitations. The results are not generalizable to the whole population of patients with osteoarthritis and more importantly neither is any estimation of effect size, NNTs, or cost effectiveness.

For trials of structure-modifying agents, symptomatic patients are usually selected on their radiographic grade. Traditionally, the Kellgren and Lawrence

Table 6.2 Kellgren and Lawrence grading of osteoarthritis

(a) Radiologic features on which grades were based

1. Formation of osteophytes on the joint margins or, in the case of the knee joint, on the tibial spines.
2. Periarticular ossicles; these are found chiefly in relation to the distal and proximal interphalangeal joints.
3. Narrowing of joint cartilage associated with sclerosis of subchondral bone.
4. Small pseudocystic areas with sclerotic walls situated usually in the subchondral bone.
5. Altered shape of the bone ends, particularly in the head of the femur.

(b) Radiographic criteria for assessment of osteoarthritis

Grade 0	None	No features of osteoarthritis
Grade 1	Doubtful	Minute osteophyte, doubtful significance
Grade 2	Minimal	Definite osteophyte, unimpaired joint space
Grade 3	Moderate	Moderate diminution of joint space
Grade 4	Severe	Joint space greatly impaired with sclerosis of subchondral bone

grading scale (Table 6.2) [1] has been used for knee osteoarthritis studies with grades II and III commonly being included. As most trials used JSN as the main outcome measure, a minimum joint space width is usually added into the inclusion criteria.

There is increasing interest in performing clinical trials in patients with knee pain or knee osteoarthritis defined by clinical criteria (Table 6.3) [2] without performing knee radiographs. Up to 50% of patients diagnosed with knee osteoarthritis in clinical practice will not fulfil the above radiographic criteria and are usually excluded from clinical trials. This therefore limits the generalizability of current clinical trials to a large proportion of patients in practice. These inclusion criteria are not suitable for structure-modifying drugs or early phase II or III studies of symptom-modifying drugs but are particularly suited to interventions such as home exercise regimens or phase IV trials of symptom-modifying drugs.

Control Arm

The choice of control groups will vary according to the trial question. In an early phase II or III study, it will invariably be a placebo group. However, it is becoming increasingly difficult to justify a placebo arm ethically when proven treatments are available. Trials of symptom-modifying drugs are therefore often performed against a comparator drug, but if against a placebo, participants are allowed free access to analgesics such as paracetamol. The use of free access to analgesia may introduce a conservative bias, as increased usage in the placebo group will minimize any treatment effect. To minimize this bias, participants are often asked to exclude escape analgesia for 48 hours before each assessment; however, this is becoming increasingly difficult to justify to an ethics committee. The alternative is to measure

Table 6.3 American College of Rheumatology (ACR) criteria for osteoarthritis of the hand, hip, and knee

	Clinical		Osteoarthritis is present if the items present are:
Hand	1.	Hand pain, aching, or stiffness for most days or prior month.	1, 2, 3, 4 *or* 1, 2, 3, 5
	2.	Hard tissue enlargement of ≥2 of 10 selected hand joints.*	
	3.	MCP swelling in ≤2 joints.	
	4.	Hard tissue enlargement of ≥ 2 DIP joints.	
	5.	Deformity of ≥1 of 10 selected hand joints.	
	Clinical and radiographic		
Hip	1.	Hip pain for most days of the prior month.	1, 2, 3 *or* 1, 2, 4 *or* 1, 3, 4
	2.	ESR ≤ 20 mm/h (laboratory).	
	3.	Radiograph femoral and/or acetabular osteophytes.	
	4.	Radiograph hip joint-space narrowing.	
	Clinical		
Knee	1.	Knee pain for most days of prior month.	1, 2, 3, 4 *or* 1, 2, 5 *or* 1, 4, 5
	2.	Crepitus on active joint motion.	
	3.	Morning stiffness ≤30 minutes in duration.	
	4.	Age ≥38 years.	
	5.	Bony enlargement of the knee on examination.	
	Clinical and radiographic		
	1.	Knee pain for most days of prior month.	1, 2 *or* 1, 3, 5, 6 *or* 1, 4, 5, 6
	2.	Osteophytes at joint margins (radiograph).	
	3.	Synovial fluid typical of osteoarthritis (laboratory).	
	4.	Age ≥40 years.	
	5.	Morning stiffness ≤30 minutes.	
	6.	Crepitus on active joint motion.	

MCP, metacarpophalangeal; DIP, distal interphalangeal; ESR, erythrocyte sedimentation rate.
*Ten selected hand joints include bilateral second and third DIP joints, second and third proximal interphalangeal (PIP) joints, and first carpometacarpal (CMC) joint.

use with an analgesia diary with this data then used as a secondary outcome measure and also as a covariate in multivariate statistical analyses of the primary outcome measure.

For structure-modifying drugs, where there is little evidence for structure modification with currently available agents, it is still acceptable to use a placebo. A bigger issue for these studies is whether participants taking glucosamine sulfate or chondroitin sulfate should be excluded from these studies, because of their proposed structure-modifying effects. As the prevalence of usage increases, this will become an ever-increasing problem because of problems of recruitment and also of the generalizability of any study that does not include them. One option is to include participants on a long-term stable dose but to stratify recruitment according to usage.

Sample Size

The determination of the sample size is a crucial step in the design of a clinical trial. It is essential that the study recruits enough patients to definitively determine the efficacy of the intervention, but ideally it should be large enough to also detect predictors of response to treatment. It is important to allow for dropouts from the study, which can be as high as 25% in studies of more than 12 months duration. To perform a sample size calculation, it is important to set the type I (α) and type II (β) error rates; the standard type I error is 0.05 and the type II error should ideally be 0.10, which means that the study has 90% power to detect the specified effect. There is still little agreement on how to define the difference between the studied treatments that the study should aim to detect. The Outcome Measures in Rheumatoid Arthritis Clinical Trials (OMERACT) group has considered this issue in some detail and come up with several options [3]. There are a number of options that use the minimum statistically detectable difference of the outcome tool used. More clinically useful are definitions based on clinical improvement, including the minimum perceptible clinical improvement (MPCI) and the minimum clinically important difference (MCID) [4]. OARSI has recently published responder criteria [5], which may in the future be used to perform dichotomous sample size calculations.

Outcome Assessment

Outcome measures used in clinical trials need to be valid, reliable, and responsive to change. OMERACT has defined a core set of outcome measures that should be measured in all osteoarthritis trials, with a list of additional optional measures [3] (Fig. 6.2). Measures of pain, physical function, and patient global assessment should be measured as outcome measures for all clinical trials. A list of commonly used instruments for the assessment of each of these measures is shown in Table 6.4. Imaging of the index joints should be performed in all studies of 12 months or greater; as an outcome measure for studies of structure-modifying drugs; and as a safety measure for other studies.

OMERACT Core Concept
Figure 1 from[3]

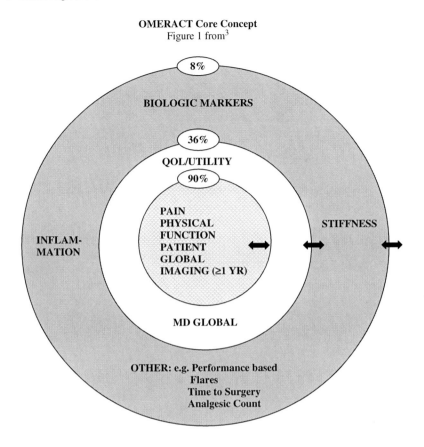

%voting for inclusion in core set	Placement	Consequence
≥90%	INNER CORE ⟶	"CORE SET"
≥36% - <90%	MIDDLE CORE ⟶	Q OL/UTILITY (Strongly Recommended)
8% - <36%	OUTER CORE ⟶	OPTIONAL

Fig. 6.2 OMERACT core concept (From Bellamy N, Kirwan J, Boers M, Brooks P, Strand V, Tugwell P, et al. Recommendations for a core set of outcome measures for future phase III clinical trials in knee, hip, and hand osteoarthritis. Consensus development at OMERACT III. J Rheumatol 1997;24:799–802.)

The use of additional analgesics should be recorded and used as a secondary outcome measure for all studies in which they are allowed. Studies assessing cost-effectiveness should also record usage of all other medications and therapists in order to obtain a total costing to the health service. In studies of structure-modifying

Table 6.4 Commonly used instruments for the assessment of measures

	Pain	Stiffness	Function	Health status
Knee and hip	WOMAC [7]	WOMAC	WOMAC	SF-36
	Lequesne	Lequesne	Lequesne [8]	EuroQol [9]
Hand	AUSCAN [10]	AUSCAN	AUSCAN	SF-36
			Cochin [11]	EuroQol

drugs, joint surgery should be recorded during the study, and preferably with long-term follow-up after the study has finished.

Radiographs of the index joint are currently the primary outcome measure of choice for studies of structure-modifying drugs. Change in joint space width is the preferred measure of disease progression for hips and knee osteoarthritis, and much work has been performed to define the most reproducible technique of assessing width (see Chapter 14). Although there is not yet agreement on a single technique, there is general consensus that for the knee, the patient should be weight bearing with the knee in a semiflexed position. Much work is being performed to assess the role of MRI as an outcome measure, however currently it cannot be recommended as the sole primary outcome measure. There is currently much interest in the role of biochemical markers of cartilage and synovial turnover as outcome measures, however although the results look interesting, they are not yet suitable as a primary outcome measure.

Compliance

It is essential to know if the participants are compliant with the study protocol. What used to be termed *compliance* is now split into two separate entities: *continuance* is whether the patient remains on the treatment regimen, and *adherence* is the degree to which the patient adheres to the regimen (i.e., how many of the prescribed tablets do they take). Adherence is usually regarded as acceptable if the participant takes at least 80% of the prescribed medication. There are several methods of measuring adherence: drug diary, tablet counting, direct observation of ingestion, and plasma monitoring. The last two techniques are not suitable for large-scale clinical trials, and most studies will use one of or both diaries or tablet counting.

Statistics

The intention to treat (ITT) analysis, where all patients analyzed are included in the final analysis irrespective of whether they were adherent or completed the trial, is the traditional method of analyzing clinical trials as it is the least susceptible to bias. There are several methods for dealing with noncompleters; there is, however, no consensus on which is the best. The most commonly used is the last observation carried forward technique, where the last observation recorded is used as the study end point. Another techniques is to use the best, worst, and last observation carried forward to give a spread of possible end points within which the true value should lie. More recently utilized are imputation techniques, whereby the last observation measured is used to predict the final result based on other participants in the trial. A completers analysis can be performed in participants fully adherent to the protocol to give an estimate of the best effect of the intervention. Although this can provide useful information, it should always be accompanied by an ITT analysis.

Many studies measure outcomes at several time points providing the opportunity for more complex and informative statistical approaches. It is possible to use techniques such as repeated measure analysis of variance (ANOVA) to measure all time points to give an idea of the cumulative effect of the intervention over the whole study period. For dichotomous outcome, it also allows the use of survival analyses, which allow for the time to event rather than just the presence of the event.

Presentation and Dissemination

For a clinical trial to change clinical practice, it must be well presented to provide all of the information that the reader or health care provider requires. The Consort guidelines detail the basic requirements for publication and have been adopted by the majority of medical journals [6]. It is important that all clinical trials are published, including negative trials, to avoid publication bias.

Study Organization

It is important when designing the study protocol to include all of the professions that will be involved at the very beginning. As well as rheumatologists and orthopedic surgeons, this should include physiotherapists, general practitioners, statisticians, and health economists. It is very important to perform a pilot study before finalizing the protocol of the study. This should test all of the proposed outcome instruments used in the study and the logistics of the day-to-day operation. Most importantly, it should address the issue of recruitment rates, which is the most common downfall of large studies. With increasing legal requirements relating to the conduct of clinical trials, it is important to appoint an independent data monitoring and ethics committee in the early stages of the trial in addition to the trial steering committee.

Conclusion

The past two decades have seen a major advance in the design of clinical trials in osteoarthritis. This is largely due to the standardizing of outcome measures and trial reporting. This will allow for greater evaluation of existing and novel therapies for osteoarthritis in the future.

References

1. Kellgren JH, Lawrence JS. Radiological assessment of osteo-arthrosis. Ann Rheum Dis 1957;16:494–502.
2. Cooper C. Osteoarthritis and related disorders: epidemiology. In Klippel JH, Dieppe PA, eds. Rheumatology. London: Harcourt Publishers Ltd; 2000:8.2.1–8.2.8.
3. Bellamy N, Kirwan J, Boers M, Brooks P, Strand V, Tugwell P, et al. Recommendations for a core set of outcome measures for future phase III clinical trials in knee, hip, and hand osteoarthritis. Consensus development at OMERACT III. J Rheumatol 1997;24:799–802.
4. Bellamy N, Carr A, Dougados M, Shea B, Wells G. Towards a definition of "difference" in osteoarthritis. J Rheumatol 2001;28:427–430.
5. Dougados M, Leclaire P, van der HD, Bloch DA, Bellamy N, Altman RD. Response criteria for clinical trials on osteoarthritis of the knee and hip: a report of the Osteoarthritis Research Society International Standing Committee for Clinical Trials response criteria initiative. Osteoarthritis Cartilage 2000;8:395–403.
6. The CONSORT Statement. 2004.
7. Bellamy N, Buchanan WW, Goldsmith CH, Campbell J, Stitt LW. Validation study of WOMAC: a health status instrument for measuring clinically important patient relevant outcomes to antirheumatic drug therapy in patients with osteoarthritis of the hip or knee. J Rheumatol 1988;15:1833–1840.
8. Lequesne MG, Mery C, Samson M, Gerard P. Indexes of severity for osteoarthritis of the hip and knee. Validation–value in comparison with other assessment tests. Scand.J Rheumatol Suppl 1987;65:85–89.
9. Hurst NP, Jobanputra P, Hunter M, Lambert M, Lochhead A, Brown H. Validity of Euroqol—a generic health status instrument—in patients with rheumatoid arthritis. Economic and Health Outcomes Research Group. Br J Rheumatol 1994;33:655–662.
10. Bellamy N, Campbell J, Haraoui B, Gerecz-Simon E, Buchbinder R, Hobby K, et al. Clinimetric properties of the AUSCAN Osteoarthritis Hand Index: an evaluation of reliability, validity and responsiveness. Osteoarthritis Cartilage 2002;10:863–869.
11. Poiraudeau S, Chevalier X, Conrozier T, Flippo RM, Liote F, Noel E, et al. Reliability, validity, and sensitivity to change of the Cochin hand functional disability scale in hand osteoarthritis. Osteoarthritis Cartilage 2001;9:570–577.

Chapter 7
Ethical Considerations

Derek Pearson and Colin G. Miller

Introduction

Whenever a clinical trial is being designed, the ethical implications have to be considered. All trials have to fulfill the general guidance issued in the Declaration of Helsinki, Edinburgh Amendment 2000 [1]. This has been enshrined in good clinical practice (GCP) guidelines that have been produced by the International Committee for Harmonization (ICH), although at the time of writing have still not been fully adopted by the Food and Drug Administration (FDA) for the United States [2] or the Committee for Proprietary Medicinal Products (CPMP) within Europe [3]. It has now been taken into law in Europe in the form of the European Clinical Trials Directive [4]. The GCP guidelines cover issues that researchers must consider such as:

1. The anticipated benefit of the trial to the individual subject and society must outweigh the foreseeable risks and inconveniences.
2. The protection of the trial subject, which should be the most important consideration.
3. The responsibilities of the local institutional review board/independent ethics committee (IRB/IEC).
4. The responsibilities of the investigator and sponsor.
5. The informed consent of the trial subjects.
6. The study protocol and investigator's brochure and the essential documentation required to undertake a clinical trial.

In the treatment of rheumatoid arthritis (RA) and osteoarthritis (OA), there are a few further nuances that have to be considered and carefully evaluated above and beyond the usual considerations.

D. Pearson
Clinical Director, Medical Physics, City Hospital, Nottingham, UK

D.M. Reid, C.G. Miller (eds.), *Clinical Trials in Rheumatoid Arthritis and Osteoarthritis*,
© Springer-Verlag London Limited 2008

Who Does What?

The proper conduct of research requires those involved to be fully aware of their responsibilities. These should be clearly understood, and for large, complex studies, such as those in RA and OA, clear, well-documented agreements should be in place that outline these responsibilities.

- *The sponsor*: Usually a pharmaceutical company (see later), responsible for ensuring:

  1. The scientific quality of the research;
  2. Any and all necessary regulatory approval is obtained;
  3. IRB/IEC approval is obtained by each site, or through a central IRB;
  4. Arrangements are in place to manage and monitor the research.

  The sponsor may delegate aspects of this to a site management organization (SMO) or contract research organization (CRO). Problems arise in identifying a single sponsor (particularly in Europe, given the requirements of the Clinical Trial Directive) for trials organized, for example, by university-employed staff working within hospitals on hospital patients. Local agreements should clearly document who is acting as sponsor in these circumstances.

- *The principal investigator*: Most multicenter trials will have a lead center, where the principal investigator has developed the proposal for research into a new molecular entity (NME) in conjunction with the sponsor. They are responsible for ensuring that the research proposal is ethical and scientifically sound, seeking IRB/IEC approval, conducting the research according to the agreed protocol, ensuring the health, safety, and welfare of the trial subjects, and feeding the results of the research back to the trial subjects.
- *The local investigator* at each center in a multicenter trial is responsible, at that center, for conducting the research according to the agreed protocol, ensuring the health, safety, and welfare of the trial subjects, and feeding the results of the research back to the trial subjects.
- Institutions where local and principal investigators are based must ensure that research is managed and monitored properly.

Sponsorship: Who's Paying the Bill?

Essentially, the local investigator must ensure that his primary concern is for the individual patient. However, they or their employer generally get reimbursed by the sponsor on a per patient recruited basis. This obviously provides an immediate dichotomy of interests particularly for the SMOs. There is a potential for SMOs in particular to see individuals as income rather than as patients. This could lead down the avenue toward competitive recruitment or differential payment for different levels of recruitment in order to improve accrual to the trial [5]. This, in turn, may lead to investigators recruiting subjects who would not be appropriate for the trial in order to gain greater financial reward from the trial. On the other hand, many trial subjects will gain access to a far more thorough clinical workup and evaluation than they would in the average clinic or health care system. There is evidence of improved outcome for patients participating in oncology trials [6], whether in the treatment or placebo group.

The same issue is true of testing drugs in the lesser developed countries (e.g., Eastern Europe, Latin America). Here there is quite often a lack of health care, and patients are motivated to participate because of the extra doctor visits and access to medication that would not otherwise be available.

The cost of developing new therapies for RA is increasing as the ability to find new patients is becoming more challenging because of the many new medications now becoming available. In the field of OA, the costs are still being evaluated as companies wrestle with which end points to use. If it is purely a clinical end point, then studies will be extensive in time and number of patients required. However, the option of using an imaging surrogate will make the costs more palatable. At the time of writing, a Phase III program for the treatment and/or prevention of RA or OA will be in the region of US$500 million to US$800 million. However, both markets are continuing to grow rapidly, so there is a potentially huge payback.

Placebo or Not Placebo?

With any new therapeutic field, the initial studies can be, ethically, placebo controlled. Although a placebo may not be in the best interest of the individual subject, without a thorough investigative program the potential benefit of a NME is also unknown, and therefore in this situation, patients can be considered to be ethically treated both on placebo and active treatment. However, once a good accepted treatment becomes available for the routine patient, then it becomes ethically questionable as to whether new placebo-controlled studies should be performed. The current version of the Declaration of Helsinki [1] states:

> The benefits, risks, burdens and effectiveness of a new method should be tested against those of the best current prophylactic, diagnostic, and therapeutic methods. This does not exclude the use of placebo, or no treatment, in studies where no proven prophylactic, diagnostic or therapeutic method exists.

For the patient with RA, this stage has now been reached [7, 8], certainly in the so-called Western world. All future NMEs will have to be active comparator studies, and in fact studies have been carried out against methotrexate for a number of years. For OA, there are not any recognized disease-modifying treatments so that placebo-controlled studies can be contemplated.

For the evaluation of the new biologics for the treatment of RA (e.g., etanercept, infliximab, and adalimumab) that have recently become available, the numbers of subjects required for the primary studies was of the order 500 to 800 patients. This is because these new drugs were considerably more efficacious than the standard treatment of methotrexate. In the future, as these drugs become the standard medication of choice, all new NMEs will have to use these compounds as comparators. It is difficult to imagine that anything new will have a dramatically improved efficacy, certainly from a clinical end point. With the advent of new biomarkers, it may be possible to distinguish NMEs from these new standards, but the numbers of subjects required for these studies will be large if development is in countries where the these compounds are approved. This scenario is also untenable from a cost situation. It is also ethically questionable to have such large numbers of subjects taking a nonproven therapy when scientifically there may be other ways of providing information on drug safety and efficacy. It may be acceptable to demonstrate that a NME is as good as, rather than better than, existing therapies using a surrogate end point, such as radiographic erosion score in RA, because there may be other aspects of the treatment that give one product advantages over another product (e.g., cost, fewer side effects, greater acceptability to the patient).

Therefore, the optimal route, from a subject recruitment perspective, for the pharmaceutical industry is to run the clinical trials in the so-called developing countries. It could be argued that in less developed countries the individual patient is still in a better position to be enrolled in a placebo-controlled clinical trial because there may not be the infrastructure or health care capital to treat patients with RA or OA. However, this position raises the questions of ethics regarding the acceptability of treating patients in one county rather than another when it comes to clinical trials. We do not have a uniform world of health policy, and each country has its own view of health and its treatment thereof. Therefore, it may be possible to perform trials ethically in one country but not in another, although any sponsor has an ethical and moral responsibility in the planning of a trial regardless of the country in which it is conducted. They are also driven by the need to obtain FDA approval for any NME under development and will therefore carry out trials in countries covered by ICH GCP.

For the treatment of OA with disease-modifying osteoarthritis drugs (DMOARDs), there is still not an accepted standard available, and the challenge is that there are no proven surrogate markers, although the FDA accepts radiographic evidence of joint space narrowing, at the time of writing this is still not proven in a clinical submitted to this agency. However, pain medication is now standard of care, and it therefore would be ethically challenging not to allow analgesics in these trials.

Randomization

The randomized controlled trial (RCT) currently appears to be the "holy grail" when designing a clinical trial. It is said to eliminate bias on entry to the trial. Nonrandomized trials are thought to demonstrate a greater treatment effect than RCTs. There is a growing debate that patient preference and motivation should be taken into account when designing clinical trials [9–11]. This is much more like real life as patients get more and more involved in decisions about their care. With the use of imaging as a surrogate end point, blinding can now be performed at a higher level, with the radiologist being blinded to treatment and temporal sequence. This may provide a new paradigm for evaluating efficacy, as with most studies having to be comparator studies, it may be better to take into account patient preference. "A well designed non-randomised study is preferable to a small, poorly designed and exclusive RCT" [9]. Results of literature surveys comparing nonrandomized and randomized studies have shown that the treatment effect is not necessarily larger in the nonrandomized studies and is not significantly different from the differences between RCTs. Future ethical review may well consider patient preference as there are increasing moves to include patient and lay representatives on IRB/IECs.

Who Can Take Part?

In designing a Phase III RCT, researchers must ensure that the study population is representative of the disease population. This requires careful consideration of the inclusion and exclusion criteria. If these are too strict, the result of the trial may not be generalizable. Recruitment methods often rely on a high level of literacy among patients, which results in study participants being well-educated, middle-class patients who have easy access to health information through the press and other media. This raises the ethical issue of the availability of new, effective treatments for RA and OA to those excluded from clinical trials. New treatments are often costly and are not provided by local health services.

Patients are also excluded because of administrative reasons, often on the grounds of ethnicity. Trial sponsors are often unwilling to fund the translation of patient information into other languages and, even when translators are available locally, use the argument that they are unsure that patients have fully understood the information so cannot ensure properly informed consent has been given. Translation of the patient consent form has to be carefully undertaken to ensure language differences do not effect the character of the patients being recruited and hence meet the original inclusion/exclusion criteria. Therefore, it is recommended that for all translation work, each document is also back-translated into the original language to ensure the same meaning and nuances remain.

Are the inclusion and exclusion criteria for a trial biased so that only those patients who show greater potential to benefit are included? The pharmaceutical companies need to use those individuals with advanced disease to prove efficacy, at least in the first instance. If the data gets watered down too much with patients who are at the early stages of the disease, then more patients have to be recruited and the study has to be longer. However, more of these "prevention" programs are being undertaken after the initial treatment trials have proved efficacy. This therefore overcomes cost significantly more, but the ethics of treating a larger number of subjects with significant disease with a nonproven NME has to be considered. This is one of the reasons for phase IV clinical trials. The sponsors obtain the initial data for regulatory approval through phase III trials and then use phase IV studies to see if the treatment effect of a NME is maintained in a wider population. Furthermore, the cost of phase IV studies is considerably less because fewer measurements and end points have to be recorded.

Researchers should take care to review inclusion and exclusion criteria when attempting to generalize research to a wider population. Multicenter trials, particularly those based in primary care, should ensure that the choice of centers is representative of the population.

Trial Procedures

When conducting clinical trials in any therapeutic field, there are usually a battery of clinical examinations, tests, or assessments that have to be performed. These extend from extra physical examinations or drawing more blood than is routinely performed to having more images taken, be they ultrasound, x-ray, magnetic resonance imaging (MRI), and other minimal-risk measurements (e.g., height measurements). This may involve the subject in extra visits to the hospital or clinic resulting in additional expense and inconvenience. The IRB/IEC will expect the sponsor to cover traveling expenses, and some trials offer a small inconvenience allowance payable at the end of the study or paid on a *pro rata* basis if the patient drops out before the end. This is not normally considered coercive if the amount paid is reasonable for completing a major trial over a number of years, for example. Most IRB/IECs will support the use of newsletters and small "thank you" gifts at the anniversary of recruitment, say, to encourage patients to stay in the trial.

Trial subjects should be made aware of the tests and investigations that are additional to normal treatment within the informed consent process. A flowchart outlining the trial procedures can be helpful, for example (Table 7.1). This should include a clear, lay explanation of any procedures and risks involved. The IRB/IEC will make an assessment of the additional investigations from an ethical standpoint. This might include, for example, weighing the drawing of 20 ml of blood every 3 months for biochemical markers (generally acceptable) against the large number of blood samples that may be required in Phase I pharmacokinetics studies where there may be concern at the volume of blood taken.

One area of concern is the radiation dose given to patients. For a trial evaluating RA, it is common to have bilateral hand and foot radiographs taken every 6 months. In OA, radiographs of the hip or knees would be taken at similar intervals, although in both disease states MRI might become the image assessment of choice for future studies. Table 7.2 outlines the potential radiation dose that a patient could receive. At baseline, the complete radiologic assessment is not dissimilar to a routine clinical workup a physician may request for a patient. The radiation dose should also be specified in the informed consent, but one has to be careful to ensure a certain overage is written in for allowance of repeat films for quality issues.

Table 7.1 A typical study flowchart for assessments in RA studies

Procedure	Screening	Baseline	3 month	6 months	12 months	18 months	24 months*	36 years	4 years	5 years
Clinical assessment	X	X	X	X	X	X	X	X	X	X
Health questionnaire	X	X	X	X	X	X	X	X	X	X
Lumbar spine x-ray	X									
Hand x-ray	X		(X)†	X	X		X		X	
Foot x-ray	X		(X)†	X	X	X	X		X	
MRI (if being evaluated)		X	X	X	X	X	X			
Blood tests including FBC, ESR	X	X	X	X	X	X	X	X	X	X
Study medication		Throughout								
Adverse event monitoring		Throughout								

ESR, erythrocyte sedimentation rate; FBC, full blood count.

* A 24-month time point is typically the last time point required for initial submission to the FDA and other agencies. Follow-up time points are currently required by FDA for the new biologics.

† Radiographs would only be taken to compare with MRI. If MRI scans are not being taken, radiographs are not needed.

The additional radiation dose and the associated risks have to be explained to the patients in simple terms. It is best to use the effective dose (ED; mSv) rather than entrance skin dose (ESD; mGy) or organ dose (mGy) as it can be related to the additional risk that the subject is exposed to. The main radiation risk from x-ray or computed tomography (CT) investigations is cancer induction. Table 7.2 also gives the lifetime risk of fatal cancer for patients aged 16 to 69, based on a risk coefficient of 5% Sv^{-1} [12–14]. To apply this to pediatric patients, double the risk; for geriatric patients, divide by 5. To put these risks in context, approximately 1 in 3 of the population will develop cancer in their lifetime and 1 in 4 will die from cancer.

Three categories of radiation risk have been proposed [15], with levels corresponding levels of benefit to society:

> Category I: Trivial risk (below 0.1 mSv) requiring minor benefit to society from the research.
> Category II: Minor to intermediate risk (0.1 to 10 mSv) requiring intermediate to moderate benefit to society from the research. This has been subdivided into:
>
> - Category IIa: 0.1 to 1 mSv minor risk;
> - Category IIb: 1 to 10 mSv intermediate risk.
>
> Category III: Moderate risk (above 10 mSv) requiring substantial benefit to society.

If subjects receive x-rays of the hands and feet, most RA trials fall into category I (trivial risk). The IRB/IEC must consider the benefit to society from the research in the light of additional radiation dose. This is not likely to be a problem if the trial limits the use of x-rays to the hands and feet. If the study design is poor,

Table 7.2 The typical effective dose and estimated lifetime risk of fatal cancer from common radiographic and DXA examinations

	Typical effective dose	Estimated lifetime risk of fatal cancer
Thoracic AP spine radiograph	0.4 mSv	1 in 50,000
Lumbar AP spine radiograph	0.7 mSv	1 in 29,000
Thoracic lateral spine radiograph	0.3 mSv	1 in 67,000
Lumbar lateral spine radiograph	0.3 mSv	1 in 67,000
Hand x-ray		
Foot x-ray		
MRI	0	
X-ray of knee		
X-ray of femur		
Forearm DXA		
QCT spine		

AP, anteroposterior; DXA, dual X-ray absorptiometry; QCT, quantitative computerized tomography.

however, with insufficient patient numbers or a poor research hypothesis, the study should be rejected. With the move to develop drugs for those conditions that are less prevalent, like ankylosing spondylitis, the radiation dose is significantly increased with the number of spine films that are required. This moves these kinds of studies into category II or category III, depending on the number of x-rays taken. However, because there have not been the drugs available until recently to treat these kinds of rheumatic diseases, this is arguably an acceptable risk.

A further aspect of this is how to explain the radiation risk to trial subjects as part of informed consent. Many use the chest x-ray as a unit of radiation risk (ED 10 to 20 µSv), but this is unhelpful as it is not an expression of the additional risk. Perhaps it is better to explain the risk in terms of the equivalent number of days or months of natural background radiation. This is, on average, 2.4 mSv per annum or 7 µSv per day in the United Kingdom. Thus, hand x-ray might be equivalent to a few hours of natural background, whereas a lumbar spine x-ray is approximately 3 months of natural background. This, at least, associates the risk with something that patients can grasp.

Genetic testing of blood samples is becoming increasingly common, particularly because of the genetic factors associated with RA and the development of genetic markers of response to treatment [16–18]. The IRB/IEC will review the study to ensure that safeguards are in place to protect the interests of the patient in this sensitive area. Where genetic testing is part of a study, there should be a clear hypothesis for the test. It is not acceptable to take a blood sample and retain it indefinitely to test the sample for a whole range of genes as new tests become available. The patient should be made aware of the genetic test in the patient information sheet. They should be told if the blood sample is going to be stored for future use, and further informed consent should be obtained is a new genetic test becomes available. Will the patient be told the result of the genetic test? Generally, results of such tests should not be fed back to the patient as genetic testing in RA and OA is speculative and nonspecific at present, although this is rapidly changing. If there is feedback, it is unlikely that there will be any genetic counseling required, but investigators may want to consider how to approach other family members if the study is to be widened. Now that specific cell lines are the object of patents, this is clearly a sensitive area. Trial subjects may need to be made aware of the transfer of samples to external organizations for genetic testing, particularly those that may develop patents commercially. Trial subjects should be made aware that they will not gain from the commercial development of cell lines or patents that result from genetic testing of their samples. A clear statement as to the implications of genetic testing should be included on the consent form. The UK Medical Research Council (MRC) guidelines "Human Tissue and Biological Samples for use in Research - Operational and Ethical guidelines 2001" are helpful here [19].

In many countries, including the United Kingdom, the use and storage of blood and tissue samples has become a major issue following a number of scandals involving the retention of organs and tissue samples without appropriate consent. The MRC guidelines above [19] provide an example of good practice. They consider issues such as:

- Ownership of the tissue sample. The research subject will not have the right to benefit from any profits arising from use of the sample.
- Confidentiality.
- How results from tests on blood and tissue samples will be fed back to the research subjects.
- Consent to access medical records.
- Controls that are required if the sample is to be stored for use in future research trials.
- Who is responsible for acting as custodian of the sample.
- Consent for genetic testing.

In many situations, institutions are establishing research tissue banks with proper consent arrangements in place to alleviate the burden of consenting the patient into a number of studies.

One other aspect that is in its infancy is the ability to profile patients to their susceptibility to treatment. Obviously, this has far-reaching consequences if we can tailor the NMEs to fit a particular profile of individual. The challenge is that patients with more unusual profiles may never receive therapy that is of minimal benefit or might not show the significant response to the therapy that the pharmaceutical company is wanting to show.

There are also early results in animal models and Phase I trials that suggest that gene therapy will be feasible in RA [20, 21]. This raises a whole raft of ethical issues including the use stem cells in the development of new treatments [22], although treatments proposed in RA have concentrated on the use of adult stem cells to date. In some countries, IRB/IEC approval for gene therapy studies will come from a specific committee that ensures that trial subjects involved in gene therapy are followed up for many years to ensure that there are no unforeseen adverse events associated with the gene therapy, whether a somatic or genetic effect.

Ethical Review

The role of the IRB/IEC is to protect the patient and ensure the scientific integrity of the study. When reviewing a study, they will consider the following issues:

1. Has the trial a clear research question?
2. Is the trial designed so that it is capable of answering that research question?
3. What are the arrangements for recruitment?
4. Are arrangements in place to deal with the interference in the management of patient care?
5. Are there adequate arrangements in place for identifying and monitoring adverse events?
6. Is the patient information adequate and written in clear, nontechnical language? Is it coercive in any way?

7. Are the consent arrangements adequate? Do patients have a "cooling off" period between receiving the patient information and being asked to consent?
8. Do the benefits of the research outweigh the risk to the patients?
9. Are the financial arrangements ethical? Are the indemnity and compensation arrangements adequate if a serious adverse event is linked to the study? Are the amounts and arrangements for rewarding investigators and trial subjects appropriate?

In RA and OA clinical trials, one of the key questions the IRB/IEC will consider when reviewing the scientific validity of the trial is the choice of end point and study size (see Chapters 13 to 16).

In the United States, the National Commission for the Protection of Human Subjects of Biomedical and Behavioral Research in 1974 was charged with the task of identifying the basic ethical principles involving the conduct of human subjects involved in clinical research [23]. The three basic principles that the commission published in the Belmont report are

1. Respect for persons. Individuals are capable of making informed choices about taking part in research. Researchers must acknowledge this and seek to protect individuals who may not be able to take informed decisions because of illness or other incapacity. The application of this is in ensuring trial subjects receive adequate information about the trial that allows them to make an informed choice as to whether to take part.
2. Beneficence ("do no harm"). Not only should investigators respect the decisions of the individual, but there is an obligation to protect them from harm and secure their well-being, that is, maximize the benefit while minimizing the harm
3. Justice. The selection of trial subjects should be fair and be representative of the population who is likely to benefit from the research. The burden of research should not fall on any one patient group more than others. Investigators should ensure that subjects are not recruited to multiple trials at the same time.

The FDA guidelines pertaining to ethical standards for research on human subjects is primarily based on this report. However, an IRB/IEC not only has to weigh these ethical considerations but also the competing principle of the social benefits derived from scientific research.

In a multicenter trial, the committee will also consider the suitability of the local investigator, the institution in which the trial is to be carried out, and the suitability of the local research subjects. They will ensure that patients are not recruited into multiple studies in centers where many clinical trials are operating at the same time.

The IRB/IEC will usually have lay members as members. A clear, nontechnical lay summary of the project is vital. The lay members see their role as protecting the patients' interests and will undertake review from the patients' viewpoint.

The European Clinical Trials Directive [4] sets a statutory time period for dealing with applications to the IRB/IEC. An ethical opinion has to be given within

60 days of an application. For multicenter trials, only one ethical opinion has to be obtained for each member state of the European Union. Clinical trials involving NMEs have to be registered in the European Clinical Trials system, which can be accessed online at http://eudract.emea.eu.int/. Each member country must also establish a list of approved IRB/IECs, much like the IRB Registration and Assurance process run by the Office of Human Research Protections in the United States (http://www.hhs.gov/ohrp/).

Informed Consent

Clear patient information is a priority. Many studies are rejected by IRB/IECs simply because of poor patient information. It is wise to spend time producing a good patient information sheet. Take advice from those who are involved in the production of patient leaflets and do not assume that something that is obvious to you will be obvious to the patient. Guidance is available from the FDA (Table 7.3) [24]. A sample patient information sheet for an example trial is shown in Appendix 1 of this chapter. It is based on the current guidelines issued by the Central Office of Research Ethics Committees (COREC; http://www.corec.org.uk) in the United Kingdom. It is broken into sections, rather than being a large block of text. Patients should be invited to take part in the trial in the opening paragraph. The language should be nontechnical and the risks and benefits of participating in the trial clearly stated. Explain what will happen to the patient if he or she takes part and give details of any investigations that may be involved in the trial. A picture of the equipment to be used can be helpful as many patients have no idea of what MRI equipment, for example, is like. The information should explain any financial arrangements, explaining that the local investigator may be receiving funds from the sponsor to carry out the trial. Patients should be made aware of their rights, any compensation available to them if something goes wrong, and the fact that participation in the trial may affect insurance policies, including health insurance. There is a requirement for IRB/IEC approval of a study to be included in the patient information. A study has shown, however, that patients understand that the role of the IRB/IEC is to ensure that patients come to no harm [25]. Informing them of IRB/IEC involvement in the review process may imply to patients that the trial is safe and likely to be of benefit.

As well as providing a patient information sheet specific to the trial, it may be useful to include some general information on RA or OA, with contact information on local and national self-help groups.

Patients may be recruited to a study via advertisements in primary- or secondary-care clinics and through local radio, television, and newspapers. Advertisements should be reviewed by the IRB/IEC. To ensure informed consent is achieved, an invitation to an initial information session at the local hospital may be extended, where a general talk on the disease could be given as well as a talk on the trial. Only then should subjects be given the formal patient information, to be contacted at a

Table 7.3 Basic elements of informed consent

1. A statement that the study involves research, an explanation of the purposes of the research and the expected duration of the subject's participation, a description of the procedures to be followed, and identification of any procedures that are experimental.

2. A description of any reasonably foreseeable risks or discomforts to the subject, including the risks associated with the NME, the risk of not being on active treatment, the risks of additional investigations, DXA, and multiple x-rays.

3. A description of any benefits to the subject or to others that may reasonably be expected from the research. Therapeutic research may be of no direct benefit and may not reduce the subject's risk of fracture, but there may be societal benefit if the study adds to knowledge of the disease or to treatment of the disease.

4. A disclosure of appropriate alternative procedures or courses of treatment, if any, that might be advantageous to the subject.

5. A statement describing the extent, if any, to which confidentiality of records identifying the subject will be maintained and that notes the possibility that the Food and Drug Administration, other regulatory authorities, or the trial sponsors may inspect the records.

6. For research involving more than minimal risk, an explanation as to whether any compensation and an explanation as to whether any medical treatments are available if injury occurs and, if so, what they consist of, or where further information may be obtained.

7. An explanation of who to contact for answers to pertinent questions about the research and research subjects' rights, and who to contact in the event of a research-related injury to the subject.

8. A statement that participation is voluntary, that refusal to participate will involve no penalty or loss of benefits to which the subject is otherwise entitled, and that the subject may discontinue participation at any time without penalty or loss of benefits to which the subject is otherwise entitled.

Additional Elements of Informed Consent

9. A statement that the particular treatment or procedure may involve risks to the subject (or to the embryo or fetus, if the subject is or may become pregnant) that are currently unforeseeable.

10. Anticipated circumstances under which the subject's participation may be terminated by the investigator without regard to the subject's consent.

11. Any additional costs to the subject that may result from participation in the research.

12. The consequences of a subject's decision to withdraw from the research and procedures for orderly termination of participation by the subject.

13. The approximate number of subjects involved in the study.

later date once they have been given time to consider their involvement in the trial. Such a complex recruiting process can be expensive and time consuming and result in only limited [26] recruitment, but it ensures that patients are well informed and raises the awareness of the problem of the disease in the local community.

It is important that subjects demonstrate that they fully understand the information they have received. The consent form is, therefore, important. An example of good practice is given in Appendix 2 of this chapter. Investigators should ensure subjects complete the form for themselves. It is unlikely in RA and OA trials that patients will be unable to consent, so this issue of relative or caregiver assent need not be considered.

Dissemination

The dissemination of trial findings is key to the ethical conduct of research and is fraught with the danger of bias. The IRB/IEC will want to know how the findings are to be disseminated as part of the review process. Researchers have a responsibility to ensure that the findings are available for publication in peer-reviewed journals, even if the findings are negative. This is one area of bias as fewer negative studies are published or take longer to reach publication [27, 28]. The use of overoptimistic language in the report, the ease of publication of reports from high-profile clinicians and high-profile centers, and the abuse of the peer-review process all add to the bias at publication. A well-structured report in a peer-reviewed publication is the only way to reduce the risks of such bias (see Chapter 9).

Conclusion

The ethics of performing clinical trials are complex and variable. Some of the further considerations in the field of RA and OA have been provided and need to be evaluated for each protocol. It is important for the trialist to consider this aspect of the trial prior to submission to the ethics review committee or institutional review board.

References

1. Recommendations guiding medical doctors in biomedical research involving human subjects. Adopted by the 18th World Medical Assembly, Helsinki, Finland, 1964, and revised by the 52nd World Medical Assembly, Edinburgh, 2000. Available at http://www.wma.net/e/policy/b3.htm.
2. International Conference on Harmonization. Guidelines for good clinical practice. Federal Register 1997;62:25691–25709. Available at http://www.fda.gov/cder/guidance/959fnl.pdf.
3. The Committee for Proprietary Medicinal Products. Step 5 note for guidance on good clinical practice (CPMP adopted July 96): CPMP/ICH/135/95. available at http://www.emea.eu.int/pdfs/human/ich/013595en.pdf.
4. European Parliament. Directive 2001/20/EC of the European Parliament and of the Council of 4 April 2001. Approximation of the laws, regulations and administrative provisions of the Member States relating to the implementation of good clinical practice in the conduct of clinical trials on medicinal products for human use. Available at http://eudract.emea.eu.int/docs/Dir2001-20_en.pdf.
5. DuVal G. Institutional ethics review of clinical study agreements. J Med Ethics 2004;30(1): 30–34.
6. Weijer C, Freedman B, Fuks A, Robbins J, Shapiro S, Skrutkowska M. What difference does it make to be treated in a clinical trial? A pilot study. Clin Invest Med 1996;19(3):179–183.
7. Garcia-Porrua C, Gonzalez-Gay MA. Ethical aspects of new medicines targeted at treatment of RA. Ann Rheum Dis 2001;60(3):304.
8. Kreutz G. European regulatory aspects on new medicines targeted at treatment of rheumatoid arthritis. Ann Rheum Dis 1999;58(Suppl 1):I92–95.
9. Britton A, McKee M, Black N, et al. Choosing between randomised and non-randomised studies: a systematic review. Health Techol Assessment 1998;2(13).

10. Brevin CR, Bradley C. Patient preferences and randomised clinical trials. BMJ 1989;299: 313–315.
11. Cooper RG, Grant AM, Garratt AM. The impact of using a partially randomised patient preference design when evaluating alternative managements for heavy menstrual bleeding. Br J Obstetr Gynaecol 1997;104:1367–1373.
12. International Commission on Radiation Protection. Recommendations of the International Commission on Radiation Protection. ICRP Publication 60. Ann ICRP 1991;21:1–77.
13. Watson SJ, Jones AL, Oatway WB, Hughes JS. Ionizing radiation exposure of the UK population UK Review.HPA-RPD-001. Available at: www.hpa.org.uk/radiation/publications/hpa/ hpa_hpa_reports/2005/hpa_rpd_001.htm.
14. Huda W, Gkanatsios NA. Radiation dosimetry for extremity radiographs. Health Phys 1998;75(5):492–499.
15. European Commission. Radiation Protection 99. Guidance on medical exposures in medical and biomedical research. Luxembourg: Office for Official Publication of the European Communities; 1998.
16. Aho K, Heliovaara M. Risk factors for rheumatoid arthritis. Ann Med 2004;36(4):242–251.
17. Klareskog L, Alfredsson L, Rantapaa-Dahlqvist S, Berglin E, Stolt P, Padyukov L. What precedes development of rheumatoid arthritis? Ann Rheum Dis 2004;63(Suppl 2):ii28–ii31.
18. Barton A, John S. Approaches to identifying genetic predictors of clinical outcome in rheumatoid arthritis. Am J Pharmacogenomics 2003;3(3):181–191.
19. Human tissue and biological samples for use in research - operational and ethical guidelines 2001. Available at http://www.mrc.ac.uk/pdf-tissue_guide_fin.pdf.
20. Evans CH, Gouze JN, Gouze E, Robbins PD, Ghivizzani SC. Osteoarthritis gene therapy. Gene Ther. 2004;11(4):379–389.
21. Trippel SB, Ghivizzani SC, Nixon AJ. Gene-based approaches for the repair of articular cartilage. Gene Ther 2004;11(4):351–359.
22. Jorgensen C, Gordeladze J, Noel D. Tissue engineering through autologous mesenchymal stem cells. Curr Opin Biotechnol 2004;15(5):406–410.
23. U.S. Department of Health and Human Services. Protection of human subjects. Belmont Report: notice of report for public comment. Federal Register 1979;44:23191–23197. Available at http://www.hhs.gov/ohrp/humansubjects/guidance/belmont.htm.
24. 21 Code of Federal Regulations 50.20. General requirements for informed consent. Available at http://www.fda.gov/oc/ohrt/irbs/.
25. Kent G. The views of members of local research ethics committees, researchers and members of the public towards the roles and functions of LRECs. J Med Ethics 1997;23:186–190.
26. Grainge MJ, Coupland CA, Cliffe SJ, Chilvers CE, Hosking DJ. Cigarette smoking, alcohol and caffeine consumption, and bone mineral density in postmenopausal women. The Nottingham EPIC Study Group. Osteoporos Int 1998;8:355–363.
27. Jadad A. Randomised controlled trials. London: BMJ Books; 1998.
28. Fries JF, Krishnan E. Equipoise, design bias, and randomized controlled trials: the elusive ethics of new drug development. Arthritis Res Ther 2004;6(3):R250–255.

Appendix 1

Rheumatology Department, St. Elsewhere's Hospital
A Randomized, Double-Blind, Placebo-Controlled
Trial of Etanercept in Rheumatoid Arthritis
Investigators: Dr. Smith, Dr. Jones

You are being invited to take park in a research study. Before you decide, it is important for you to understand why the research is being done and what it will involve. Please take time to read the following information carefully and discuss it with friends, relatives, and your primary care physician if you wish. Ask us if there is anything that is not clear or if you would like more information. Take time to decide whether or not you wish to take part.

Thank you for reading this.

What Is the Purpose of the Study?

The purpose of the study is to test the effectiveness of etanercept in controlling your rheumatoid arthritis (RA) when compared with the current standard treatment (methotrexate). The study will take 12 months to complete. During that time, you will either be taking etanercept by injection twice a week and a dummy drug (placebo) as a tablet by mouth once a week or you will be taking methotrexate as a tablet by mouth once a week and a placebo injection twice a week. Six hundred patients are being recruited to the study worldwide.

Why Have I Been Chosen?

You have been diagnosed with RA in the past 3 years

Do I Have to Take Part?

It is up to you to decide whether or not to take part. If you do decide to take part, you will be given this information sheet to keep and be asked to sign a consent form. If you decide to take part, you are still free to withdraw at any time and without giving a reason. This will not affect the standard of care you receive.

What Will Happen to Me if I Take Part?

This study will last for 12 months. At the start of the study, you will need to come to the Rheumatology Department at St. Elsewhere's Hospital for a screening visit. At this visit, we will ask you a number of questions about your medical history, diet, smoking, and exercise and give you some more general information about RA, diet, and exercise. We will take 10 mL (2 teaspoons) of blood to measure chemicals that are markers of disease activity in RA and look for genetic factors that may affect RA. You will also have an x-ray of your hands and feet. unless you have had x-rays of these joints within the past 3 months. The screening visit will take approximately 2 hours. At the end of the screening visit, it may be decided that you are not suitable to continue in the study because of your medical history. You will be paid traveling expenses at the end of the visit.

If you are suitable to continue in the study, you will be asked to attend for a second visit within 1 month of the screening visit. The format of the visit will be similar to the screening visit, but no more x-rays will be taken. At that visit, you will be randomly assigned to the etanercept group or the methotrexate group. Neither you nor your doctor will not know which group you are in, but you have a 2 in 3 chance of receiving etanercept. Your doctor will be able to find out which group you are in if necessary.

If you are in the etanercept group, you will receive etanercept by injection twice a week. You will be shown how to give this injection yourself. You will also be asked to take a dummy tablet (placebo) by mouth once a week. If you are in the methotrexate group, you will also be shown how to inject yourself with a dummy injection. This is so you do not know which treatment you are getting. You will take methotrexate tablets by mouth once a week.

The study lasts for 12 months, and you will need to come to clinic every 2 months for approximately 1 hour. During the study, we will take further x-rays of the affected joints.

The blood samples taken throughout the study will be stored by Dr. Jones for use in future research studies in the Department of Rheumatology. Your samples will be treated as a gift and you will not have any right to share in the profits that might arise from the research use of the samples. Some of the projects may be carried out by researchers outside the Department of Rheumatology. If that is the case, you will not be able to be identified from the sample. Some of these projects may include further genetic testing if new genes are identified that are associated with RA. We will not tell you the results of these tests.

You will be given reasonable traveling expenses for attending the clinic and an inconvenience allowance of $100 after completing the study. If you do not complete the study, the inconvenience allowance will be paid on a *pro rata* basis (e.g., $50 after 6 months).

What Do I Have to Do?

It is important that you take the trial medication as directed by the doctor in clinic. You will be given instructions as to how to take the medicine and give the injection. There are no other precautions that you have to take, and you can take any other medication you normally use. You will be given general information about living with RA, including advice on diet and exercise, but it is up to you to decide whether or not to follow this advice.

What Is the Drug That Is Being Tested?

The drug being tested is called etanercept and has been used for a number of years in patients with chronic RA without significant side effects. This is the first time the drug has been tested in patients with early RA. You will given a card (similar to a credit card) with details of the trial on it, and you should carry the card at all times.

What Are the Alternatives for Treatment?

Other forms of treatment are available that are known to help in early RA. You can discuss these with your general practitioner or the clinic doctor if you wish.

What Are the Side Effects of Taking Part?

Etanercept has been used successfully to reduce disease activity in patients with long-standing RA. The reported side effects of taking etanercept are as follows. A third of patients reported injection-site reactions. Other side effects include abdominal pain, respiratory infection, nausea, and headache. In very rare cases, where patients were taking other immunosuppressive drugs, serious infections were reported that required patients to stop taking etanercept. If you experience any of these, please report it to the doctor organizing the study

What Are the Possible Disadvantages and Risks of Taking Part?

The disadvantages of taking part are that you have a 1 in 3 chance of not receiving the study drug and having to give yourself unnecessary placebo injections. The x-rays involve exposing you to additional radiation. The additional radiation dose is very small, equivalent to less than a few days of natural background radiation.

If you have private medical insurance, you should check with the company before agreeing to take part in the trial. You will need to do this to ensure that taking part will not affect your medical insurance.

What Are the Possible Benefits of Taking Part?

Taking part in this trial may be of no direct benefit to you. The information we get from this study may help us to treat RA in the future.

What if the New Information Becomes Available?

Sometimes during the course of a research project, new information becomes available about the drug that is being studied. If this happens, your research doctor will tell you about it and discuss with you whether you want to continue in the study. If you decide to withdraw, your research doctor will make arrangements for your care to continue. If you decide to continue in the study, you will be asked to sign an updated consent form.

Also, on receiving new information, your research doctor might consider it to be in your best interests to withdraw you from the study. He or she will explain the reasons and arrange for your care to continue.

What Happens When the Research Study Stops?

At the end of the study, you will not be able to continue on the study drug. You will be able to discuss treatment options with your general practitioner or the research doctor. Occasionally, the company sponsoring the research may stop it. If this is the case, the reasons the study has been stopped will be explained to you.

What if Something Goes Wrong?

Compensation for any injury caused by taking part in this study will be in accordance with the guidelines of the Association of the British Pharmaceutical Industry (ABPI). [The sponsor], without legal commitment, will compensate you without you having to prove that it is at fault where it is likely that such injury results from giving [trade name] or any other procedure carried out in accordance with the protocol for the study. [The sponsor] will not compensate you where such injury results from any procedure carried out that is not in accordance with the protocol for the study. Your right at law to claim compensation for injury where you can prove negligence is not affected. You can also use the standard complaints mechanism and contact the St. Elsewhere's Complaints Officer at [telephone number].

Will My Taking Part in This Study Be Kept Confidential?

If you consent to take part in the research, you will be identified by study number alone. Any of your medical records may be inspected by the [sponsor] for purposes of analyzing the results. They may also be looked at by people from the [sponsor] and from regulatory authorities to check that the study is being carried out correctly. Your name, however, will not be disclosed outside the hospital. Your general practitioner will be told that you are taking part in the study.

What Will Happen to the Results of the Research Study?

The results of this study will be published in a journal, and a copy of the results will be available on request after the study has closed.

Who Is Organizing and Funding the Research?

[Sponsor] are funding this study, which is being organized through the Rheumatology Department at St. Elsewhere's Hospital.

Contact for Further Information

If you want to discuss this further, please contact Dr. Smith at [contact details].
    Thank you for taking the time to read this information.

Appendix 2

CONSENT FORM
Rheumatology Department, St. Elsewhere's Hospital
A Randomized, Double-Blind, Placebo-Controlled Trial
of Oral Estrogen/Progestin in the Prevention of Bone Loss in
Postmenopausal Women
Investigators: Dr. Smith, Dr. Jones

The patient should complete the whole of this sheet herself.

	Please cross out as necessary
• Have you read and understood the patient information sheet?	YES/NO
• Have you had opportunity to ask questions and discuss the study?	YES/NO
• Have all the questions been answered satisfactorily?	YES/NO
• Have you received enough information about the study?	YES/NO

Who have you spoken to?   Dr./Mrs./Ms. ....

- • Do you understand that you are free to withdraw from the study

• At any time?	YES/NO
• Without having to give a reason?	YES/NO
• Without affecting your future medical care?	YES/NO
• Do you agree to take part in the study?	YES/NO

- • Do you agree that the blood samples taken in this project can be stored by Dr. Jones on behalf of the Rheumatology Department for possible use in future research projects that may be carried out by other researchers?   YES/NO
- • Do you agree that the blood samples taken in this project can be used in genetic research aimed at understanding the genetic influences on rheumatoid arthritis, which will be unlikely to affect you personally.   YES/NO

Signature (Patient)   Date

Name (In block capitals)

I have explained the study to the above patient and she has indicated her willingness to take part.

Signature (Doctor)   Date

Name (In block capitals)

Chapter 8
Organization of the Clinical Trial by the Sponsor

Colin G. Miller

Introduction

There is a standard set of start-up, ongoing monitoring, and close-out requirements or procedures for all clinical trials. These generic requirements are discussed in other texts and are not the remit of this book. However, because of the nature of this therapeutic area, it is important to consider the particular extras and details that have to be evaluated. The aim of this chapter is to briefly discuss these items and to ensure the sponsor is aware of these items in a timely manner. All too often, the novice will overlook an important detail until it becomes a critical issue. Hopefully, this will ensure these kinds of errors are avoided.

As a definition, sponsor is the company developing the product, which is usually either a pharmaceutical or Biotechnology company. However, these companies may also commission a thrird party such as a contract research organization (CRO) to conduct the trial or the clinical trial program.

Regulatory Guidance

Regulatory approval of a new product is the ultimate goal within the pharmaceutical industry. Therefore, knowledge of the rules and guidelines are critical prior to embarking on any clinical program. Furthermore the global market has to be considered, so the high cost of developing any new molecular entity (NME) needs to address most of the world's markets in one program. No longer can companies afford to run studies to attain approval in a single country. This chapter will not address the generic good clinical practice (GCP) issues per se but only the ones related to the field of rheumatoid arthritis and osteoarthritis.

C.G. Miller
Senior Vice President, Medical Affairs, Bio-Imaging Technologies Inc., Newtown, Pennsylvania USA

D.M. Reid, C.G. Miller (eds.), *Clinical Trials in Rheumatoid Arthritis and Osteoarthritis*,   113
© Springer-Verlag London Limited 2008

At the time of writing, the regulatory field is changing significantly within the United States and hence globally in the area of rheumatoid arthritis (RA) and osteoarthritis (OA), and it is suggested the reader refers to the RA guidelines as the end points are similar in approach [1] (It should be noted that the RA guidelines are equally old but are final and not still in the draft stage.) However, there is a significant discussion in the guidelines about the various end points, be it a rating score like the WOMAC or OMERACT scores (see Chapters 4, 5, and 6) imaging (see Chapters 13, 14, and 15), or biomarkers (see Chapters 11 and 16).

In the guidelines for RA, there are several specific end points that are discussed and the acceptance for surrogate end points [2]. Radiographs are described as potentially acceptable with an example given that "a significant effect on radiographic progression might be the demonstration, in a randomized controlled trial, of maintenance of an erosions-free state in a large majority of patients when control patients develop multiple erosions." However, in the previous paragraph, it also states that "sponsors are urged to consult with the relevant U.S. Food and Drug Administration (FDA) staff before embarking on a clinical program based on these regulations." This is reiterated in several places throughout the document, particularly with respect to potential labeling indications and the phase III studies. Therefore, based on this information, for both OA and RA studies, the sponsor should have planned to meet with the FDA in advance of phase III to ensure the study design will meet the FDA's current requirements for the labeling indication that is being sought. Therefore, rather than discuss the draft guidelines in any further detail here, the author has provided the reference to them at the FDA Web site [2], and any sponsor should anticipate a face-to-face meeting with the FDA and in the same vein the corresponding European agencies early in the clinical development program.

Surrogate Markers

As part of the planning stages of the clinical trial, the sponsor needs to consider the organization of the radiographs, the magnetic resonance imaging (MRI) and computed tomography (CT) scans, and, if they are being collected, the samples for the biochemical markers.

If the study is part of a submission to a regulatory agency, then a central blood lab and imaging core laboratory (ICL) will have to be selected, as all the recent submissions to the FDA have comprised central collection, evaluation, and submission to the agency. Even if the study is not for regulatory submission, an ICL is highly cost-effective, not only in saving the direct cost of data entry but also by ensuring a higher quality of data. By personal experience, if an ICL is not involved, between 3 % and 25 % of the data could be invalid or analyzed incorrectly. Cost is one component of this issue; the other is the ethical implications of having lost patient data that could have been salvaged.

Medical Imaging

As imaging end points have now become the accepted standard surrogate for both RA and OA trials the ICL will be able to provide input into study design and logistics management. Time points need to be carefully considered, as they will vary depending upon whether MRI or plain radiographs and the expected pharmacological effects on the cartilage and bone. Furthermore for the x-ray film, consistency is the key, and it has now become standard practice to ensure the same standard at each investigator site by supplying the film and x-ray cassettes, where digital x-rays are not available. Furthermore this helps to provide inter-site blinding for the reader, which is discussed below and in Chapter 8. Choosing an ICL should be carefully considered. Historically, the images used to be handled by academic centers. Now there are professional, dedicated ICLs set up to provide this kind of service. Sponsors should visit the ICL center before initiating any contract with them, although all too often this step is, disappointingly, missed in the interests of time. Sponsors would not expect to conduct a study at a trial site that they have not visited, so likewise, the same level of detail should be applied to the ICL. Although you may not be familiar with all the types of imaging methodologies that are required, a good ICL should be able to show you around their facilities and to demonstrate the software for all the imaging requirements you anticipate using in your study. Furthermore, the staff at the ICL should be able to answer any technical questions and give you a basic understanding of the measurement techniques. Because image submissions are now a *de facto* standard for RA studies of "biological compounds" for submission to the FDA, it is important for the ICL to explain how this is accomplished, perhaps showing an example of an anonymized submission that had previously been submitted. If the software cannot be demonstrated or questions are left unanswered, it would suggest that your study might be the launch of a new service for the ICL—probably not what you want for your study! Many places advertise their experience generically and either may not have experience in the relevant therapeutic area or it was acquired by personnel in a previous company. Another question to ask is how many technologists do they employ and what is their experience in performing work with RA or OA studies. If they only have one technologist, what happens if he or she leaves midway through the trial? The choice of reader, be they radiologist or rheumatologist, is also important, and the use of those experienced reading these types of studies with the scoring system you wish to employ is critical. In a large phase III study in RA, it may require more than 200 days of reading by expert rheumatologists to complete the study. This requires careful evaluation and the selection of a team of readers. Behind the scenes, the logistics required to successfully implement this type of study with the complex reading scheme involving multiple radiologists or rheumatologists needs to be evaluated. It will require a dedicated team with the necessary tracking and logistics support. If this team is not set up well, then it will not matter if you have the best readers in the world, the results from the imaging portion of the study will be a mess.

Finally, and probably the most critical, is that in recent years, the FDA has required all films to be read by two independent radiologists. This means they have to be from two different institutions and not from a site that is also one of the investigational centers. Hence only one in-house radiologist could be used in this scenario, and a second separate reader would also have to be selected. Reader training and selection is further discussed in Chapter 8.

Biochemical Markers

Laboratories for the assay of bone biochemical markers may need to be selected. There are several in the world that can perform these specialized assays and the choice is growing. Again, the sponsor should evaluate the laboratory by personal visitation and by going through their SOPs. As with the ICL, a systems audit should be possible to conduct without an in-depth knowledge of the technology being employed. Further details of the handling and management of laboratory samples is provided in Chapter 11.

Couriers

With all the data that has to be handled and sent to various laboratories, it is important to ensure a good courier system is in place for the study. Most of the laboratories or service providers described above will suggest a vendor based on their experience. Although you may have a preference for a particular courier company that may appear less expensive, it may well not be able to handle the requirements for the study. Generally, the laboratories handling this specialized kind of data have tried most courier companies, and experience will have taught which ones are better to use and which to avoid. It is strongly recommended that you stick with the courier companies recommended.

Investigator Meetings

These are now a standard part of the start-up procedure for any clinical trial. It is certainly advantageous and cost-effective (in the longer term) to have a representative of the laboratories (both imaging and biochemistry) give a presentation at the meeting, not only to provide an overview of their services but also to provide a data flow and answer any technical and specific questions. For some of the samples, there may be special storage and shipping requirements that need to be explained. Another facet of the training meeting to consider is whether to include training for the imaging technologists. Most ICLs recommend this for several reasons, which are detailed in Chapter 10. An alternative methodology that has been employed is to provide the technologists at the investigator site with a training compact disc (CD) with all the study requirements. These can be produced in a cost-effective manner and then distributed to all the site technologists. To ensure completion, a small exam can be built into the program that has to be submitted to the ICL prior to patient enrollment. Further incentives could be provided e.g. continuing education units (at least in the United States). This can alternatively be accomplished by a phone-in conference call. The latter can also be used as a stand-alone training opportunity.

The Internet is often used for training, particularly with the use of the interactive systems. However, it has to be remembered that the technologists at the site rarely have Internet access or their own e-mail. Their regular day is spent working the imaging equipment and therefore any Web-conferencing may be a logistics night-mare rather than a solution to provide training for the study.

Cross-Calibration of Scanners

For Phase II type studies using CT or MRI for complex algorithms, there may be the need for the calibration of the scanners to ensure the uniformity of the images being evaluated. (This is not required for imaging end points using planar radiographs). This can be performed either by a site visit by a representative of the ICL or by sending the phantom(s) around by courier. The cheapest methodology is obviously sending the phantom around by courier. The disadvantage is that this then takes some considerable time. As a rule of thumb, you should allow a week for each instrument per phantom that is on rotation. The reason for this length of time is purely logistical. Let's assume that the phantom is sent out by courier on Monday, it gets to the site Tuesday or Wednesday, and the site scans the phantom on Wednesday or Thursday. At best, it will be sent out again on the Wednesday or Thursday for arrival at the next site by Friday or the following Monday. This assumes that the site is primed and has allotted sufficient time for this to be accomplished. Obviously, this can be achieved, but there is very tight timing. It works more efficiently within the United States, where there are no borders to cross between countries, but becomes more problematic in Europe and further afield.

Site visits with a cross-calibration phantom, though quite costly, can provide some additional benefits:

1. A site audit from an imaging perspective, or prequalifying visit, can be performed.
2. Training can be given to the technologists there. This can help supplement the training from the investigator meeting, if the technologist attended, or be an alternative to the training that would have been performed at the meeting. This also allows the technologist to ask questions one-on-one rather than in the group setting, which some find intimidating. Furthermore, if more than one technologist is at the site, they can also be involved with the training, which they would otherwise miss out on at an investigator meeting.
3. Time is obviously a major gain. It should be possible, on average, to complete a site visit a day for one representative. It should therefore be possible for all but

the largest studies to have all the site visits completed either before or within a short time frame of patient recruitment at each site.

The choice of phantoms for cross-calibration is fairly limited. It should be remembered that phantoms are at best patient mimics that are designed to provide an assessment of how a machine is operating. However, there may be differences in requirements depending upon the end point and the ICL selected.

Inclusion and Exclusion Criteria

For many trials, there is often at least one inclusion and/or exclusion criterion based on imaging. Historically, this has always been left up to the investigator sites to determine, and for smaller studies, this is still the optimal methodology. However, for the larger phase III studies where there is pressure on the investigator site to recruit and a financial incentive to enroll patients, it has become more commonplace for the ICL to play a "policing" role and have the images evaluated for correct enrollment. Medical images are interpreted and therefore there is often no absolute right or wrong, but an independent opinion as to the disease state of the subjects being enrolled, particularly when the imaging involves a subtle interpretation. This step will ensure that when the study is complete, there is not an excessive number of subjects that were incorrectly enrolled according to the strict criteria being evaluated by the central readers.

Data Flow

Some serious consideration needs to be given to the data flow with respect to the biochemical and medical image data. The priorities will differ depending on the phase and complexity of the study. The central blood laboratory results will need to be sent back to the site in a timely manner, except for assays that are esoteric and have no effect on patient management. In general, there is no reason for the investigational sites to ever receive the results of the imaging data, at least during the course of the study, particularly if the study is double blind. From a patient safety viewpoint, the ICL may need to be monitoring and flagging any images that show a significant change from baseline that could be considered a patient management issue. These limits should be determined a priori at study start for these data and likewise for vertebral deformities. A data safety monitoring board (see below) should also be involved with setting out these guidelines and reviewing the data. However, this will depend greatly on the images being collected and the use of these at the investigational site for patient management.

There is often a discussion as to whether the sites should receive a copy of all the data at the end of the study. If the central laboratories and ICLs are considered the repository of all the data, then this should be sufficient to ensure data integrity and satisfy external audit. Some sponsors believe copies should be returned to the site, for complete data sets. This is a lot of extra work for both the center and the sites and does not guarantee everything will get back to the sites' central documentation. There is a different argument for patient management, when there is need for the treating physicians to know the full patient records for the study, depending on the trial and the treatment. There may also be ethical and safety factors to consider. For example, if an imaging radiograph has been acquired but is *not* available to the investigational site, it might be required to be repeated, putting the subject at risk due to excess radiation exposure.

The Data Monitoring Committee

The sponsor may appoint a data monitoring committee for the trial. Their role is to:

1. Receive the monitoring reports from the sponsors monitors.
2. Receive adverse event (AE) reports.
3. Monitor accrual rates into the trial.
4. Decide on changes to the inclusion and exclusion criteria.
5. Agree to changes in sample size.
6. Oversee interim analyses of the trial data.
7. Agree to early stopping of the trial if necessary.
8. Review individual patient data from a safety perspective (optional).

Ideally, the inclusion and exclusion criteria and sample size should not change as the trial progresses [3] (unless it has been designed *a priori* as part of a novel adaptive trial design). Such changes may be necessary in the light of the monitoring reports, AE reports, and accrual rates. Sample sizes can be changed, particularly in long-term trials, as new information about the magnitude of a possible treatment effect becomes available. Alternatively, the outcome of an interim analysis may allow the sample size to be changed.

Interim analysis should be handled with care! They should be planned in the protocol prior to the trial starting, rather than succumbing to the temptation to see how the results are coming along. The statistical methods should be defined in advance, and all the staff involved in the day-to-day running of the trial should remain blinded to the results of such analyses. Investigators should only be made aware of the changes to the protocol that arise because of the results of the interim analysis.

Stopping a trial early should only be considered on ethical grounds either on the basis of the safety data or if it becomes apparent that the power of the trial is not acceptable on the basis of an interim analysis. If it is intended to stop the trial because an adequate treatment effect has been demonstrated, then the interim analysis should be planned and included in the protocol.

Trial Audit

All trials sponsored by the pharmaceutical industry will be audited, and there is good documentation in the regulations as to how in general these should be conducted. However, the question arises as to how these audits might differ in a study in the arthritis areas compared with other therapeutic areas, and what, if anything, has been carried out differently by the FDA.

From a sponsor's perspective, audits should be carried out much earlier on in the study than for other therapeutic areas because of the very long nature of these studies. If there were issues at a site or a laboratory or ICL, it could go undetected for a significant period of time if these are not performed in a timely fashion. It has now become a recognized practice that the centralized facilities can become the holders of source data as well as the investigator sites themselves. This therefore negates the issue of having all the results returned to the sites for audits. However, the sequelae to this is the central facilities also need to be audited, and this is where the challenge comes in from the sponsor's point of view. Investigator site audits should pose no unusual problems to a seasoned auditor, the only difference may be the need to see the radiology department and review the documentation that is stored by the technologist there. These include the instructions or manuals detailing the imaging requirements present. For most studies, the technologists are involved in the transmission of the data to the ICL. Therefore, there should be some documentation present to show the transmission of all images. Furthermore, there is likely to have been some correspondence between the ICL and radiographers/radiologists during the course of the trial, which again should be documented. Finally, if instruction manuals for scan and image acquisition have been issued, are they in the department where the staff who are involved in obtaining the medical images have access to them and can be seen by the auditors?

How to handle the central ICL's and blood labs? A full systems audit should be performed and a review of the documentation for a sample of patients at both the biochemistry/blood laboratory and the ICL. The blood laboratories have to be accredited, and this at least ensures there is some standardization and compliance built into the system. The question then arises as to who is performing an audit on the ICL's data as it is an unusual auditor who can review medical images. A good ICL will have a second review process built into their data flow to ensure that two pairs of eyes look at each piece of data. Full systems audits can be completed and are now routine for ICLs as well as the blood laboratories.

It can be anticipated that the FDA will audit the blood laboratory or ICL, as these have been conducted fairly routinely in recent years. For RA, the FDA, as previously discussed, has often requested a complete set of digital images in a format in which they can review them. In many respects, this review of the images in the submission, along with the data logs from the ICL, has provided the necessary information for the FDA, and a further audit has not been required. It is unknown how the FDA will review OA data as no disease modifying ostearthritis drugs (DMOARDs) have been submitted at the time of writing.

Trial Closure

At the end of the trial, the trial monitors will ensure that each center has submitted all the required documentation on all trial subjects. The sponsor or CRO will then review all the data. The CRA should produce a final monitoring report for each participating center. It is then the responsibility of the sponsor to carry out the statistical analysis of the data and produce a final clinical study report and any peer-reviewed publications. Guidance on the format and content of clinical study reports is available [4] from the FDA. Chapter 12 deals with the analysis and presentation of results for peer-reviewed publication.

Conclusion

Whereas there is a standard set of tasks that have to be conducted in clinical trials, those in bone- or cartilage-related diseases require some unique extra details that have to be addressed. Arguably, the most critical of these is the assignment of an ICL and a biochemistry laboratory, as they will need to be ready to provide kits to the trial sites before patient enrollment. Furthermore, having these teams identified early in the trial process will provide some technical and consulting support for protocol development, if that is required.

All trials should have good documentation and audit trails, and this is critical in trials where medical imaging is an end point and an image review charter is required (see Chapter 10). Because of their nature, the trials will normally be running for several years, and even with a normal turnover of staff, this will mean that very few people involved in the trial at the start will still be working on it at the end. Therefore, without good documentation, it will be difficult for staff writing up the final reports to follow some of the decisions that were made and the rationale for them.

Because trials evaluating measurements of bone and cartilage are some of the longest in duration in the pharmaceutical world, it is therefore critical to ensure that there is good planning at the front end. Not only is it costly to repeat a trial, but also in this arena it could be a year or more before the errors in planning are finally noticed. From a sponsor's perspective, as with all trials, good up-front planning is critical to the good execution of the trial. With the handling of so many surrogate end points or biomarkers, it is critical that this is given the up-front planning that is needed to ensure the logistics are in place before the first patient is enrolled.

References

1. FDA. Guidance for industry: clinical development programs for drugs, devices, and biological products intended for the treatment of osteoarthritis (OA). Available at http://www.fda.gov/cber/gdlns/osteo.htm.

2. FDA. Guidance for industry: clinical development programs for drugs, devices, and biological products for the treatment of rheumatoid arthritis (RA). Available at http://www.fda.gov/cder/guidance/index.htm.
3. International Conference on Harmonization. Guidance on statistical principles for clinical trials. Available at http://www.fda.gov/cder/guidance/91698.pdf.
4. International Conference on Harmonization. Structure and content of clinical study reports. Available at http://www.fda.gov/cder/guidance/iche3.pdf.

Chapter 9
Organization of the Trial at the Investigator Site

Julie Shotton, David M. Reid, and Colin G. Miller

Introduction

Every day thousands of people volunteer to take part in clinical research trials. It is because of this willingness to participate in these studies that modern medicine is able to meet the challenge of continually identifying new improved treatments and cures. The investigational site is the critical point in the trial organization, as this is where the patient meets the study personnel. It is where all the planning and organization come together and practical execution takes place. Without good organization by site personnel, a great study can be turned into a disaster very quickly.

Subjects choose to participate in clinical research trials for a variety of reasons. Some enjoy the opportunity to further science; others desire early access to new, still experimental medications; some use clinical research to gain access to highly sought-after physicians or specialists.

New drugs, medical devices, surgical procedures, and physical and psychological therapies all need to be assessed as objectively as possible and compared with the possible alternative treatments. The aim is to discover which treatment is best in which circumstances and for which patients. Thus, the management of individual patients and the health of the population as a whole are improved. However, the challenge is to ensure the clinical management of the patient is optimized without the loss of study integrity.

Historically, medical doctors are the principle investigators (PIs) engaged in all the routine aspects of clinical research. Today, with the increasing demands on medical time, physicians are less involved in day-to-day implementation of clinical trials, and trial coordinators or study site coordinators (SSCs) are typically employed in the specialized research team. This has resulted in a novel role for nurses, that of trial coordinator or SSC. The SSC will recruit and schedule participants, implement protocols monitor positive or negative effects of the trial medication, evaluate outcomes, perform laboratory tests, advocate on behalf of participants, and interpret

J. Shotton
Previously Senior Research Nurse, Osteoporosis Research Unit, Department of Medicine & Therapeutics, University of Aberdeen, Aberdeen, UK

clinical data. Trial coordination is established through multidisciplinary teamwork with professionals such as nurses, radiographers, pharmacists, and medics. These key members will require appropriate input and authority from the lead physician and sponsor personnel for conduct of any medical issues.

Site Resources

The PI is responsible for all clinical research activities at the research center. One of the most important aspects of clinical studies is that the investigators commit to personal involvement and interest in the studies. They will have a clinical leadership role and will be one of the key factors in successful trial execution.

When the sponsor has selected the research center, it is up to the PI and the SSC to get the study up and running as soon as possible. To achieve this successfully, it is necessary to assess the availability of staff before each study, ensuring that there is high quality core staffing to coordinate the research activity. There is little point in agreeing to take on a study, only to discover there is not an adequate availability of resources. In OA and RA trials, the core staff would include medical, nursing, radiographers, pharmacists, secretarial, administrative, and laboratory staff.

All staff must be suitably trained and understand the principles of good clinical trial management. All clinical studies require procedures to be performed in specific ways, and the sponsoring company will usually provide manuals explaining these and should also provide specific training for staff.

The practical resource planning required for a successful study include examination rooms for conducting confidential patient interviews and physical assessments. Office equipment such as computing and communication equipment is essential. The processing of samples will require phlebotomy and laboratory shipping materials and an area to process those samples should be provided. The site will also require adequate storage areas for study materials. A locked calibrated refrigerator and freezer for laboratory samples is often required for storage of these samples. Secure storage for study medication is also required and may require refrigeration. In many centers, this is now handled directly by the pharmacy, so the communication and coordination with the pharmacy department has to be scheduled well in advance of the trial. With medical imaging being a critical end point in these studies, a further series of discussions needs to be conducted with the radiology department. Finally, it is important to also consider adequate working space for on-site visits from the pharmaceutical company representatives Clinical Research Associate (CRAs).

One of the most important tasks for the SSCs is to ensure the case report forms (CRFs) are accurately completed. The CRFs are the primary documents and the official records that pharmaceutical companies use to house the data collection from the investigator. More recently, there has been an increasing use of electronic data capture (EDC). EDC, though designed to improve the data flow, may in fact increase the workload for the SSC at the site, in particular if using slow Internet connections, and thus may further increase the cost to the sponsor. Therefore, it is essential that this is discussed thoroughly by the sponsor with the site staff prior to implementation. Clearly, accurate record keeping is of paramount importance for a clinical trial to be executed successfully. Therefore, the presence of a well-organized and experienced clinical study coordinator to assist the investigator and his or her staff in maintaining study-related documentation cannot be overestimated.

Study Budget and Clinical Trial Agreement

The study budget and clinical trial agreement is an important part of the study start-up at any center. Generally, a sponsoring pharmaceutical company will offer a budget taking into account all the local costs which include the following:

- Staff costs to complete study screening and all study visits. These costs should include payments for the time spent by all study site personnel including the PI, any subinvestigators, the study site coordinator, and other research staff including nurse, radiographer, and secretarial time. It is worth considering during the negotiations that study site personnel may also be required to attend pre–study investigator meetings and also to spend time with study monitors. Furthermore, trials in osteoarthritis (OA) and rheumatoid arthritis (RA) can often last up to 5 years, therefore it is important to allow for increases in cost of services and that a budget for this to be agreed upon with the sponsor.
- All study site investigations (i.e., those investigations not taken at central laboratories). Typically for an RA or OA study, these might include electrocardiograms (ECGs), erythrocyte sedimentation rate (ESR) or C-reactive protein (CRP) testing, and radiology investigations including x-rays or magnetic resonance imaging (MRI). This need to include the costs of copying images if the original needs to be sent to an imaging core laboratory (ICL).
- All pharmacy costs. Larger and more experienced research centers will have a standard start-up fee and individual charge for each prescription issued.
- All administrative and overhead costs. Individual institutions frequently seek to levy either an initial set-up charge for each trial initiated and/or a percentage overhead charge to cover the costs of carrying out the trial at the center, including the use of space and facilitates that are not otherwise covered.
- Any new equipment required for careful completion of the trial. On occasions, this may be supplied on a loan or even "donated" basis from the sponsoring company, but do remember to include any service or consumable costs for the equipment in the budget.
- Travel and other costs for subjects consenting to participate in the trial. Many studies ask for patients to come to their appointment in a fasting state, therefore there will be a requirement for the sponsor to support costs for the coordinator to provide drinks and snacks.
- Finally, any advertising, if required for patient recruitment, or ethics submission costs should be included.

Once agreement has been reached on the budget, including any start-up allowance, based on the percentage of the study fee the costs will generally be embedded in the clinical trial agreement, which requires to be signed off by the PI, his or her administrative authority, and, of course, the sponsoring pharmaceutical company.

Included with the study start-up documentation will be a letter of indemnification assuring the study site personnel and administrative authority that they will be covered for any liability from the study drugs during the trial period.

Ethics IRB and Informed Consent

All research involving human subjects must be reviewed and approved by an institutional review board (IRB) or ethics committee (for a full discussion on ethics, see Chapter 5). The IRB reviews the research protocol, the informed consent form, known information about the drug (including reports of unexpected adverse events), and any potential advertising planned for recruitment of subjects. The job of the IRB is to ensure that the protocol and recruitment techniques are ethical, the potential subjects are fully informed about the procedures, risk, benefits, and alternative treatments available before they agree to participate in the study, and that the subjects are not placed at unacceptable risk. Therefore, planning for the IRB approval needs to be taken into consideration well ahead of the trial start. The PI and SSC need to understand exactly the requirements of their local IRB to ensure a successful submission. No supplies or study drug can be shipped until this approval has been obtained.

As a study progresses, investigators must continue to provide updated information to their IRB, usually on an annual basis. In particular, the focus is upon additional safety information either in the form of updated letters or revisions to the original investigators' brochure supplied to the ethics committee at the time of application.

The prestudy documentation that the PI should collect and maintain includes a list of appropriately qualified persons who have been delegated significant trial-related duties including a copy of each individual's résumé or curriculum vitae (CV). A signed and dated résumé for the PI and each of the study site personnel will need to be submitted to the sponsoring company for their documentation and will need to be updated as it changes over time. The PI will also need to sign a copy of the protocol to acknowledge that he or she has read it and agreed to conduct the study as laid out in the document. If the study is being conducted under U.S. Food and Drug Administration (FDA) requirements, the Form 1572 [1] also has to be completed and signed. The sponsoring company should provide this form, which is signed and initialed by the PI and all the study site personnel and lists the responsibilities of all the study center research staff.

Finally, in Section 4.1 of the ICP good clinical practice (GCP) guidelines [2], there is a requirement that the investigator should permit monitoring and auditing by the sponsor and regular inspection by appropriate regulatory authorities. An investigator who is not prepared to accept these requirements should not be selected to conduct clinical research. This requirement will also require access to the base subject documentation, that is, their hospital or primary care records or case notes. Access to such records will also be needed by the sponsoring company's study monitors to enable verification of CRF data.

It is imperative that all source documentation pertaining to the study is retained, either by the site or by the pharmaceutical company, pending any federal licensing authority audit. Any amendments ought to be discussed with the site personnel. It is also essential that the correct version of the protocol is the one being adhered to. This can become difficult if the sponsor adds new visit schedules on a regular basis. Unless there is a clear indication of which protocol is being used mistakes can be made. The protocol will include a visit schedule for the subject study visits and will list the procedures required at these intervals. It must be followed accurately to allow correct information to be gathered that will ensure a scientifically robust study.

Study Initiation and Conduct

Immediately after submission of the final documentation, which can take some time, the supplies, such as patient kits, CRFs, and study files, will arrive. These study files will include the protocols which must be read and understood thoroughly by all participating staff. Most important for the trial coordinator is the patient evaluation and visit schedule. These give information on the types of investigations/assessments that are to be carried out at each visit. Taking time to familiarize oneself with these schedules is vitally important. There may be changes in the visit schedules and also there may be extensions to the trial. The coordinator must be kept informed of any of these changes or this may impact the planning of patient visits. Whereas some visits may be straightforward other visits may require input from the PI, radiographers, pharmacy, and secretarial staff.

It is also advisable prior to the documents and kits arriving to discuss storage space. The documents can often be bulky and lack of space may become an issue.

Good clear lines of communication at this stage are paramount to a well-run trial. This is an excellent time to make any staff aware of any changes in the protocol. A well-run trial relies on excellent teamwork and if this does not take place at the beginning of the trial problems are certain to arise. Each participating member of the staff must be completely aware of his or her role. In most cases, there will be an investigators' meeting prior to the start of the study. These meetings will involve key personnel and although these can often be held in glamorous locations, they are very intensive with little time for sightseeing!

Handling of Blood Samples: Central versus Local Laboratories

For each study there may be involvement of both local and central laboratories. If local laboratories are used, then certification must be included in the study file these include:

1. A copy of current laboratory certification.
2. A list of the laboratory normal ranges.
3. A copy of the CV from the laboratory manager.

Before the trial begins, each center will receive laboratory kits (for both blood/urine samples and imaging, see Chapters 11 and 10, respectively, for more information on the role of each of these organizations). These kits will contain all supplies required for the collection of blood and urine (or other) samples. Each kit will also include a requisition form that must be completed consistently and accurately for each patient. If a requisition form has not been completed the central laboratory will usually contact the SSC and this can cause delay in analysis of results and in some cases may involve collection of further samples. This will not only be inconvenient to the patient but also will add to the costs of the study. The kits will also include a protocol, within the central laboratory manual. This specifies exactly the way in which the samples ought to be collected, for example after an overnight fast. This will also specify the types of samples and how to process, pack and store these samples.

The sponsor normally chooses the courier company for the collection and delivery of samples, and it is of utmost importance to have a reliable courier who will guarantee collection of samples at the agreed time. However this is not foolproof and problems can occur. If problems do occur the CRA must be informed immediately and the necessary interventions made; the sponsors pay the courier companies well and it is important to have this reflected in a quality service. All transport documentation must be completed as per the protocol.

There are many studies that require frozen samples to be sent to central laboratories. The trial coordinator will need to arrange an appropriate time for collection. Once again the sponsor ought to have organized the company who is providing the dry ice but it is important not to underestimate the logistical issues that can be encountered. The handling of dry ice must be by a fully trained person and the sponsor ought to provide training for this.

Once the central laboratories have received the samples the results will be faxed back to the sending investigator site. The PI will need to evaluate these results all of which must be within the range specified by the sponsor.

Many protocols have automatic exclusion criteria instructing the PI to withdraw a subject from the study if these results are outside these parameters. In some cases, these samples may be repeated particularly if there has been a problem with courier collection. Protocols may also instruct the investigator to withdraw a subject from the study if the disease under examination worsens significantly.

Pharmacy

Investigational clinical supplies must be received by a designated person at the study site and handled and stored safely and appropriately. These supplies must be kept in a secure location to which only the investigator and designated staff have access. Clinical supplies are to be dispensed only in accordance with the protocol. The trial coordinator is responsible for keeping accurate records of the clinical supplies received from the sponsor, the amount dispensed to and returned by the patients and the amount remaining at the conclusion of the study. It is also vital that the CRA is made aware of the "geography" of the recruiting center in comparison with the pharmacy. There are research centers that are not within the vicinity of the main hospital and appropriate transport must be set in place for delivery of the drug at the correct time and to the correct place.

Recruitment Methods

Patient databases are a productive way of finding suitable and willing patients who may consider taking part in a clinical trial. Through large epidemiologic studies and patient surveys particular groups of subjects can be found. Contacting such individuals within the United Kingdom must be within the provision of the 1998 data protection act. Subjects cannot be contacted unless they have previously given permission for this to occur. Recently in U.K. general practice, databases have been a useful source of such details, or in the United States the primary care physician (PCP) is a good source of information. The general practice can approach a patient to ascertain if they might consider taking part in a research study. If the patient agrees, the practice will forward the patient contact details to the PI. A further successful way of recruitment can be through identification of patients who regularly attend the appropriate outpatient clinic. Assessing a patient's interest in clinical trials is important as these patients could be contacted if a suitable clinical trial was imminent.

Potential subjects may often respond to advertisements as clinical trial participation has many benefits for the patients. The opportunity to receive new potentially more effective treatments does interest many volunteers. Equally important is the detailed monitoring and the close medical and nursing supervision that comes with participation in a trial. In countries where the local health care provision is limited or expensive, there are clear advantages to volunteers who will obtain free health care during the study period.

Newspaper advertisements are also a worthwhile way of recruiting volunteers. Where recruiting volunteers it is essential to include precise wording and age group requirement for the study. For example, leaving out the age range can result in many telephone calls and an influx of phone calls that produce no benefit to the recruitment efforts. Therefore, correct wording is absolutely essential and will ultimately help the selection process of suitable volunteers.

This form of recruitment will lead to a much larger workload and will increase the requirement for staffing. Secretarial time will be increased because of additional telephone calls. Medical and nursing time will also be increased during this busy screening period. Too often, these issues are not taken into account when planning the trial or the budget for the trial at the local center, resulting in unnecessary stress. The answer is to address this increased workload prior to advertising, allowing time for discussion and agreement, and any potential difficulties can then be addressed before the trial commences.

An additional problem with advertising is that it may create bias as the respondents to the advertisements are not necessarily representative of the population as whole. Newspaper advertising may encourage inappropriate responses by the public, and other responders may feel rejected if they are found to be unsuitable for the study. Posters and leaflets may also be a useful way of advertising. It should also be remembered that because that all advertising is part of the study documentation, it must be approved by the IRB or local ethics committee prior to its use.

Once a volunteer has responded to an advertisement and has received an explanation of the study, he or she may request to receive further information. It is very important at this stage to have experienced coordinators answering any queries and to begin the screening process; this will prevent enrolling a volunteer into the study only to fail at the later screening stage. It also ensures that potential subjects who are unsure can be reassured given the correct information, and they can then make a more informed decision as to whether to participate.

It can become demoralizing if recruitment for studies is slow, and it is important to have time to discuss difficulties in the early stages of recruitment. Often pressure mounts if the study is competitive. Competitive recruitment can develop via a couple of different scenarios: (a) Each site has a target and a timeline and unless a particular site meets its target, other more productive sites will have their allocated target number increased. (b) There are no set numbers of subjects required at each site but the more subjects sites can enroll the greater the income, with bonuses paid in some instances for faster recruitment. Once the enrollment figure is reached patient recruitment is stopped immediately. In both these scenarios there will be financial implications should the recruitment targets not be met.

Monitoring Adverse Events

Clearly, it is vital to have a commitment to ensure adequate medical care for any adverse events, including the identification of clinically significant laboratory values related to the trial. The investigator should also inform a subject when medical care is needed for any intercurrent illness of which the investigator becomes aware (ICG GCP 4.3.2) [2]. One of the important implications of this GCP requirement is that clinical laboratory reports generated during the course of the study must be reviewed promptly in order to ensure that clinically significant values are handled appropriately. Lack of evidence of such prompt review by a medically qualified individual is a frequent finding of audits and inspections of clinical trials.

Monitoring serious adverse events is by the very definition critical. The responsibility for reviewing and reporting serious adverse events rests with those who have the expertise, that is, the PI and subinvestigators who take medical responsibility for the patients.

There may also be a data safety monitoring committee (DSMC). The role of the DSMC is to evaluate trial data as well as relevant information from other studies, consider the safety of the patients in the trial, and recommend to the trial steering committee any changes that they think they should be made.

Informed Consent

The Declaration of Helsinki [3] requires that clinical research be conducted by scientifically qualified people and also requires the supervision of a clinically competent medical person. In terms of activities such as obtaining informed consent, the declaration states that a medically qualified person should perform this process. Volunteers interested in becoming part of a research study should first read the informed consent document carefully. These volunteers must have the opportunity to ask the study personnel any additional questions before agreeing to participate.

Participation in research means that the patients' care and safety must be a priority. Patients must be respected and fully involved in decisions about their care. In any research project all participants must be fully informed of the risks and benefits of taking part. Volunteers must have all required procedures explained to them in a language they can understand. Just as with obtaining agreement from patients in any clinical context, consent must be truly informed. Researchers must be sure that participants are given enough information to make a decision and that they are competent in understanding that information. Participants must never be coerced and they must be able to make an informed decision without feeling any obligation. Therefore, for informed consent patients must:

- Be able to give consent.
- Be given enough information to enable a decision.
- Act under their own free will and not under the strong influence of another person.
- Be able to ask exactly what the treatment will involve.
- Understand what are the benefits.
- Understand if there are any alternative therapies.
- Be able to ask what the risks are, if any.
- Understand what will be the next steps if they decide to decline study participation? (Nothing as far as their medical care is concerned and any other treatments if available should be offered).

It is also important that informed consent be taken before any treatment or care is given, including any screening investigations. Most studies require that the volunteer has 24 to 48 hours to read the information sheet. Having considered this information, the patient's decision to participate or not must be respected and not debated by the study staff. Further, it must also be made clear to the patient that they have the right to withdraw their consent at any time during the trial and that this withdrawal will not affect the usual standard of medical care.

Subject Retention and Compliance

Once a patient has consented to the study, it is of equal importance to retain that patient and ensure their compliance to the study drug. It is impossible to accurately say how compliant a patient has been unless there is an honest open line of communication from the initial screening period. Many patients will be anxious and if the study schedule and dosing instructions are not accurately explained, the result is misunderstanding or noncompliance. Therefore, a good relationship between the study staff and patient is paramount. Undoubtedly compliance is vital if there is to be accurate data collected; however, a site coordinator who is open and friendly and easily accessible is more likely to have patients willing to comply. It is also important to attempt to have the same person in attendance at each visit as consistency is very important. Obviously, if noncompliance becomes an issue and will affect the end results, a patient may have to be withdrawn from the study.

Retention is crucial as pharmaceutical studies can last for 3 years or more. There may an additional problem in retaining volunteers, in that participants may be in full-time employment. Consequently, site staff must be willing to work around these commitments to make it possible for these patients to attend all follow-up visits. It is therefore vital that volunteers have had the visit schedule explained in detail. Most employers are willing to allow time off for their employees who are taking part in research studies.

Pharmaceutical companies often supply the volunteer with a regular newsletter and small tokens, such as calendars, pens, or diaries. It is also important to send Christmas and birthday cards as a small "thank you" to volunteers who are continuing in the trial. The SSC needs to be very organized to ensure these important details are not missed.

Advocacy

The study coordinator should become the volunteers' advocate during the course of the trial and at the same time will gain commitment to the trial from the patients. In health care, the concept of advocacy has become increasingly important over recent years, as consumers demand better quality, better responsiveness, and easier access to services. The UKCC code of Professional Conduct (UKCC 1992) [4] states that advocacy will "promote the interests of individual patients or clients and serve the interests of society." The advocate will be the "communicator" and transmit and exchange information with the client, family, physician, and other health care professionals. The coordinator will also keep the volunteer informed by disclosing pertinent information voluntarily and on request. They must also provide information advise and check the understanding of the volunteer and repeat information, invite questions, describe options and reinforce the idea that the patient has a choice.

In addition, the trial coordinator must empower the patient volunteers by supporting them and providing advice on health care. They must be able to provide contacts to access other agencies, such as local support groups. Study coordinators need excellent communication and relationship skills good listening skills and assertiveness skills. Finally, the coordinator must be responsible for safeguarding the volunteer from what they might consider poor practice.

Study Closeout

There is normally a "buzz" during study start-up and anticipation in getting the study under way. At the end of the clinical trial fatigue may set in and the final closeout procedures can be overlooked or not completed adequately. However, this is an important step in ensuring a well-conducted study is drawn to a good conclusion and can prevent a good deal of rework if the study center is selected for audit, particularly an FDA audit.

After conclusion of all patient visits, the trial paperwork and documentation needs to be carefully reviewed and then archived. Duplicate documentation can be destroyed, but all originals and CRFs need to be collated, chronologically filed, or filed in patient number sequence and stored for up to 15 years according to EU GCP guidelines. This needs to be completed with the guidance of the sponsor to ensure everything required is stored and maintained appropriately. If there are difficulties in providing archiving space for final study documentation at the study center many pharmaceutical sponsors will arrange and pay for independent off-site archiving, although such an arrangement is best negotiated at the study planning stage rather than at the end of the study.

All remaining drug supplies need to be accounted for and either sent back to the sponsor or destroyed after all the appropriate disposition records have been completed. Equipment that has been provided on a loan basis will need to be returned (e.g., centrifuges, imaging phantoms or positioning aids, or even fax machines).

The study is not complete until the final documentation or letter of close-down has been received by the sponsor. It is at this time that the study can be fully closed down.

Conclusion

The successful running of a clinical research trial requires the presence of a dedicated team of health care professionals with varied expertise. It requires working together in a cooperative manner coordinated by the clinical trial coordinator.

An involved and enthusiastic principal investigator is essential. It is paramount to develop good working relationships with the pharmaceutical company representatives, particularly the clinical research associates. The research staff has responsibilities to the sponsoring company and even greater responsibilities to their patients. In a well-organized research study, these two sets of responsibilities should not conflict. Good organization and attention to detail is vital for the successful management of a clinical trial. The amount of paperwork is enormous and can seem unending. Getting it right at every stage will help. It is particularly important that good relations are established between the study subjects and the staff at the local centers and the CRA who will monitor them. This will ensure that there is adequate recruitment, good compliance with treatment, and good communication between the sponsor and the investigators.

References

1. Information for Sponsor-Investigators Submitting Investigational New Drug Applications (INDs). US Food and Drug Administration. Available at http://www.fda.gov/cder/forms/1571–1572-help.html.
2. ICH Harmonised Tripartite Guideline for Good Clinical Practice E6(R1). International Conference on Harmonisation of Technical Requirements for Registration of Pharmaceuticals for Human Use. Available at www.ich.org/cache/compo/276-254-1.html
3. World Medical Association Declaration of Helsinki. Ethical Principles for Medical Research Involving Human Subjects. Available at http://www.wma.net/e/policy/b3.htm.
4. United Kingdom Central Council for Nursing, Midwifery and Health Visiting. Code of professional conduct for the nurse, midwife and health visitor. London: UKCC; 1992.

Chapter 10
Role of the Imaging Core Laboratory in Rheumatoid Arthritis and Osteoarthritis Clinical Trials

Mark D. Endres and Anna M. Baratelle

Introduction

Radiographic imaging end points in rheumatoid arthritis (RA) and osteoarthritis (OA) efficacy clinical trials have become commonplace over the past several years. Independent review of the radiographic images rather than on-site readings is used to determine efficacy. Ultimately, the independent review scores along with the images will be submitted to the regulatory agencies. In addition to submitting the imaging results to the regulatory agencies, the images will be submitted as well. As such, many sponsors are outsourcing the management of the imaging component of the trial to imaging core laboratories (ICLs).

The draft FDA guidance for RA clinical trials [1] (Fig. 10.1.) states that radiographic claims should be based on comparison films taken at 1 year (and subsequently yearly points) with those taken at baseline. The films should be evaluated using a validated radiographic index. Modified Sharp scoring has been used in recent studies, including those submitted and approved by the FDA [2–6].

In the draft FDA guidance for OA clinical trials [7] (Fig. 10.2), both a delay in structural progression and a prevention of OA claim are described. There are, currently, outstanding issues within the guidance document that need to be better defined. Most studies currently focus on knee OA, and there is a growing body of literature suggesting both a semiquantitative approach to the evaluation and a fully quantitative approach using quantitative magnetic resonance imaging (qMRI) or radiographs.

The Imaging Core Laboratory

Prior to initiation of a clinical trial in RA or OA, the sponsor will need to select an ICL to assist them in the collection and independent review of the medical images. The use of an ICL will not only provide input into the design of the imaging protocol

M.D. Endres
Vice President, Global Business Development, Bio-Imaging Technologies, Inc., Newtown, Pennsylvania, USA

F. Prevention of Structural Damage

Prevention of structural damage is an important goal of RA therapy. Trials evaluating this outcome should be at least one year in duration.

The following are examples of outcome measures that could be used to support prevention of structural damage claims.

1. Slowing X-ray progression, using either the Larsen, the modified Sharp, or another validated radiographic index.

Radiographic claims should be based on comparisons of films taken at one year (and subsequent yearly points) with those taken at baseline. All randomized patients should have films at both time points, regardless of whether they are continuing treatment. Patients dropping out of the trial should have films taken at that time. Prespecification of the handling of dropouts is especially important in these trials.

2. Prevention of new X-ray erosions — maintaining an erosion-free state or preventing new erosions.

Trials evaluating this claim would ordinarily use a categorical endpoint to assign a status of progression or nonprogression to each patient, comparing the final state to the baseline state.

3. Other measurement tools (e.g., MRI)

Other measures, such as MRI (magnetic resonance imaging) or ultrasonography, could be employed. However, because of the technique's potential for identifying small, albeit statistically significant changes, the magnitude of the difference that would reflect actual patient benefit is unclear and needs to be established.

Fig. 10.1 An excerpt from the FDA guidance document (Section 2F) for RA studies

but will also improve the independent review results or statistical outcome of the medical image data as the data will be standardized and reader bias and reader variability reduced.

The role of the ICL is to:

- Assist the sponsor in protocol development with regard to imaging.
- Codevelop the imaging review charter.
- Standardize the image acquisition.
- Minimize the loss of image data.
- Collect and perform quality control (QC) of the images.
- Perform an independent analysis and review of the images.
- Provide the independent review results and images to the sponsor or regulatory authority.

Each of the above-mentioned roles will be discussed, in detail, throughout this chapter.

As a sponsor of a clinical trial, it is important to visit and evaluate the potential ICLs before deciding which one to partner with for the study. Having a thorough understanding of the ICL's capabilities and experience is vital for the success of the trial. A sponsor should be confident that the ICL they are using has experience in RA or OA studies and that the ICL employs registered technologists that will

B. Delay in Structural Progression

The structural measurement currently proposed is demonstrating a slowing in the loss of knee or hip JSN using x-ray; other validated structural measurements may be developed in the future. Whether parallel symptom evidence should be included in the claim depends on what JSN outcome is achieved (see below), but symptom endpoints (using measurement of pain, a patient global assessment, a self-administered questionnaire) should be collected regardless of the outcome anticipated. Trials to demonstrate structure improvement should last at least one year. The reason for this is that the concept *structural improvement* connotes an element of durability, even if future technology allows the demonstration of slowing of the loss of JSN in shorter time periods. At present, the imprecision of the JSN measurement often results in trials lasting even longer than one year.

At present, few data speak to the validity or likelihood of a product showing benefits in delaying structural progression, but not showing benefits in improving patient symptoms. Although most products affecting inflammation would not be expected to slow JSN without affecting symptoms, it is possible that certain classes of products developed in the future may do so. A claim of slowing JSN (i.e., showing structural improvement) might plausibly be dissociated from other claims when the mechanism of action of the product, and/or the size of the effect on slowing of JSN, are suggestive of future clinical benefits. In general, products will not be considered for approval or for separate claims if (1) they are not anticipated to have different effects on these parameters, or (2) they show only small improvements in JSN without demonstrated effects in symptoms. Trials of agents expected to show isolated benefits should be carefully designed to preserve type 1 error. In addition, measurements of symptoms should be collected in all trials regardless of expectations of effects on JSN, because their assessment is critical for the analysis of the overall risks and benefits of the product.

A hierarchy of claims for structural outcomes is shown here.

1. *Normalize* the x-ray. An x-ray that shows a normalization of JSN is possible, at least in principle, and it would be the most convincing outcome of an improvement in structural integrity. But given our current understanding of OA, this outcome does not seem attainable for any currently studied class of products.

2. *Improve the x-ray.* An x-ray that shows a reversal in the JSN (i.e., a widening of the joint space) at endpoint compared to baseline would reflect new or regrown cartilage (and not the cartilage hypertrophy sometimes seen early in OA). This outcome would be convincing and require no formal parallel evidence of improvement in clinical outcomes.

3. *Slow JSN by at least a prespecified amount.* The amount of slowing of JSN to demonstrate improvement of patient symptoms or function (i.e., the amount *clinically relevant*) remains unknown. Given that there exist important questions in this area, sponsors wishing to claim that their product slows JSN, but does not reduce symptoms should contact the Agency to discuss such a proposal, including the biological rationale, the relative amount of slowing of JSN they anticipate, and plans for studying long-term clinical outcomes. In general, sponsors seeking this claim should anticipate relatively large changes (<50 percent) in slowing JSN relative to the control arm.

Fig. 10.2 (continued)

C. Prevention of OA

Because the claim *prevention of the occurrence of OA*, using symptomatic and radiographic criteria, in new joints in patients with OA or in individuals at risk to develop OA in the future could be possible in principle, it is mentioned here. However, the practicality of this outcome would be challenging because OA can at times present radiographically first, and at times clinically first. Any trial used to demonstrate this outcome should first define the term *new OA*. Because one cannot repeatedly survey radiographically all possible OA sites, there are important unresolved assessment issues for designs capable of properly validating this claim. Furthermore, because this claim would be a chronic disease claim different in kind from all past approvals, it should have a more extensively and more formally documented safety database than previous submissions.

Fig. 10.2 An excerpt from the FDA guidance document (Sections 5B and 5C) for OA studies

be performing the quality control of the images taken at the sites, and that those technologists are well versed on the criteria they need to use when applying quality controls to the images. It is helpful for the ICL to have proven relationships with the independent expert reviewers. The independent expert reviewers are typically recognized opinion leaders in their respective therapeutic areas.

Assist the Sponsor in Protocol Development

During the development of the study protocol, it is important for the sponsor to review the imaging protocol with the ICL, along with the independent expert reviewers. There needs to be congruency with the imaging end points (both safety and efficacy) and the imaging acquisition requirements. If, for example, a study is being developed for RA, the anatomy and radiographic view may vary. A study protocol using the change in modified Sharp–van der Heijde score as a primary end point but only collecting hand radiographs, not feet, is an obvious incongruency between end point and image acquisition. An experienced ICL should have the capacity to recommend imaging protocols that have been used for previous RA/OA studies and acceptable to the regulatory authorities.

Codevelop the Imaging Review Charter

The U.S. Food and Drug Administration (FDA) has recently started to request that an independent review charter (IRC) be developed for studies where imaging will be a primary or secondary end point in a submission. The IRC provides a prospective definition of the imaging program and a complete description of the image management for the study. It is an unusual document in that it has to be signed off by both the sponsor and the ICL. Therefore, the development of the IRC should have a similar effort and emphasis as the development of the clinical trial protocol.

If the studies are being performed under a FDA special protocol assessment (SPA), the FDA will want to review the IRC prior to the initiation of the study and may provide input. For pivotal efficacy trials not under a SPA, the FDA will still require an IRC. However, timing of the submission of the IRC to the FDA is not as clearly defined as for the SPA process. In these cases, it is recommended that the IRC be submitted to the FDA prior to the independent review of the images.

A comprehensive IRC should contain the following information [8]:

- Executive summary
- Summary of image data to be collected
- How image data will be processed
- Scoring or measurement methodology
- Design process of the independent review database
- Independent review methodology
- Selection, compensation, and training of radiologists
- Special issues
- Process for exporting review results to sponsor
- Submission of images to FDA

Standardize the Image Acquisition

Standardization of the image acquisition and collection is essential to ensure high-quality image data with minimal variation. This decrease in variation has a profound effect on the statistical scatter of the results and therefore has a major impact on the statistical power of the study. The following site preparation activities can take place parallel to the study start-up activities the sponsor or contract research organization (CRO) are performing.

Investigator Meetings

For most large trials, sponsors hold investigator meetings. It is important that a representative from the ICL be invited to attend and present at this meeting to enable the clinical site study staff to understand the role of the ICL and establish communication lines. The ICL should be provided sufficient time at the meeting to review the imaging procedures, image data collection, archival, transfer, and administration procedures relevant to the imaging section of the study. It may also be beneficial for the sponsor to invite the study site radiology technologist (or radiologist) to the investigator meeting. The ICL staff can also provide specific training by holding a "breakout" session for the radiology technologists at the meeting. These sessions can be critical if the study site technologists are responsible for obtaining the images that will be evaluated to determine the primary efficacy or safety end point for the study. The breakout session will also provide the opportunity for the site technologists and ICL staff to interface and allow the site technologist to ask questions to personnel experienced with imaging in these types of trials. This also facilitates communication and cooperation at the site as they become an integral part of the study team [9].

Site Survey

In order to obtain important information on the site's imaging capabilities and its radiology staff, a study-specific site survey should be developed by the ICL. This can be sent via fax or e-mail to the study site coordinator to complete or delegate to radiology staff. The site survey should be designed to capture information on the radiology staff responsible for implementing the imaging protocol, the site's imaging equipment hardware, software, and image data archival and transfer capabilities. The sponsor will have the principal investigator and study coordinator information available, but the ICL needs to have the radiology contact information for each site. This information provides the ICL with the appropriate contact information in the event that technical or image quality issues arise with the site. The survey also provides information on the type of digital archival media required by the sites.

Site Training

Most ICLs will employ registered radiology technologists in the various imaging modalities (e.g., magnetic resonance imaging [MRI], x-ray, computed tomography [CT]) that can perform site visits. Specific training can be provided to the technologist(s) at each clinical site. This training can be an alternative to inviting the technologist to the investigator meeting. The site visit will allow training for all the technologists at the clinical site that may be involved with the study, as many times it is difficult for the site to dedicate one technologist to perform all the imaging for the study. Additional benefits of the site visits are the ability to further evaluate the imaging equipment at the site, to meet one-on-one with the site staff, and communicate the GCP requirements. Site visits can be costly because of the ICL staff's time and related travel expenses. Thus, the additional benefits or added value obtained from the site visits should be evaluated over the associated expense.

Other options for site training are compact discs (CDs), Web-based presentations, and/or telephone conference calls. The training CD study modules or Web-based presentations can be customized to the specific protocol and tailored to the specific study criteria. This CD will assist in training the technologists to the study protocol as well as the submission requirements of the ICL.

Imaging Study Kit

Standard x-ray radiography is the gold standard for RA and OA studies. However, more complex imaging such as MRI may also be used for exploratory end points. A knowledgeable ICL can assist the sponsor in developing an imaging protocol relevant to the study. Depending on the end points of the study, a specialized or advanced imaging protocol may need to be developed. To ensure the standardization of the image acquisition and to facilitate compliance with the sites, an imaging study kit should be provided to each clinical site prior to patient enrollment.

The imaging study kit should contain the following:

- Imaging guideline/manual
- Instructions on image archival
- Image data transmittal forms
- Instructions on transmitting the image data to the ICL
- X-ray film and cassettes (if relevant for RA studies)
- Archival media for image data (optical disk, CD-ROM, etc.)
- Labels for x-ray films and digital archival media
- Mailers and courier waybills

Sample Image Data

A simple way to ensure that the clinical sites understand the imaging protocol is for the ICL to request sample images from the sites using the required imaging protocol. This can also improve the imaging protocol compliance by requiring the sites to receive approval prior to enrolling patients. If the sample image data does not meet the protocol requirements, then repeat scans may be necessary until the site performs the acquisition correctly. This can help to prevent problems before the site actually begins to enroll patients and perform the medical imaging. It should be noted that the collection of sample image data can sometimes be challenged by the institutional review board (IRB) due to the radiation exposure to the patients. In these situations, sample image data obtained on phantoms may be acceptable.

Radiographic Acquisition

Hand and foot radiographs are the accepted standard in RA trials, rather than radiographs of all affected joints, because there is correlation between the damage seen on hand/foot radiographs and the damage in other joints [10].

For OA studies, knee radiographs are the accepted standard practice, however, hip radiographs have also been used in clinical trials [11].

Standardization of Image Acquisition

Clinical trial images must be of optimal radiographic quality and reproducible across time points to reduce variability of the results. If the image does not meet these two criteria, then scoring methods cannot accurately assess change over time for a subject, therefore decreasing the value of the data.

To standardize the image acquisition and reduce variability in RA studies, the use of the same x-ray film and cassette screen combination is required at all clinical sites. The film/screen combination recommended is a combination of single-emulsion fine-grain film with cassettes containing a single high-resolution screen [12].

All clinical sites should receive an imaging manual for their radiology department's use, which contains clear, concise instructions on how to obtain the images in a standardized method. This will ensure that patient positioning is consistent across patients and across time points. Detailed patient positioning instructions can be found in Chapters 13 and 14.

Image Collection

Once a patient's scans have been acquired at the clinical site, the medical images should be sent to the ICL for QC review. The specific time frame for the submission of image data for the study can vary on the protocol requirements. The timely submission of the images is important in order for the ICL to perform a QC assessment of the images and to provide feedback to the clinical sites to ensure quality is maintained. In some trials, repeat films may be required when the x-ray is of poor quality.

Each site may have varying methods of archiving the image data. Some sites will have the ability to archive the image data in a digital format to electronic media (CD-ROM, digital archival tape, optical disk, etc.) or print to sheets of film. For x-ray, the gold standard is still primarily film. It is important that the ICL have the ability to handle different image file formats and digitize film data. The digital data and film data need to be converted to the same image file format. For digital data, this is handled by making use of specific hardware and validated software. For film data, specialized high-resolution film scanners need to be used.

Image Quality Control

Images from all sites should be forwarded to an independent ICL and QC performed by a qualified person(s) within a few days of acquisition. This rapid QC ensures consistency in the acquisition across all sites and allows for ample opportunity for repeat films if required.

When the image data is received at the ICL, it is important that the image data be logged and tracked through the ICL processes. Upon receipt of the image data, the ICL should confirm they have received all the relevant imaging data for the patient, in addition to confirming the basic demographic information (site number, patient number, time point, date of scan, etc.). This can be achieved by making use of an image data transmittal form (DTF). The DTF is also used to provide an audit trail.

The ICL technologist will review the images for protocol compliance and technical adequacy (Tables 10.1 and 10.2). If image sets are missing data or are of poor quality, a query process should be established whereby a data clarification form (DCF) is returned to the site for explanation and resolution—sometimes repeating the radiograph or MRI scan. The tracking of the DCF is important in order to complete the audit trail. Upon submission of the new drug application (NDA),

Table 10.1 Quality control criteria for evaluating RA films

Was the standardized film used (when applicable)?
Were the x-rays performed as single exposures for each hand/foot?
Is the positioning optimal?

- Index finger aligned with radius
- No radial or ulnar deviation
- Hand/fingers flat on the cassette to prevent superimposition or rotation of the joints
- Foot placed flat to prevent medial or lateral rotation

Is all required anatomy on the image?
Is the radiographic technique optimal?
Does the follow-up time-point image match the baseline image:

- Is it the same patient?
- Is the positioning the same?
- Is the technique the same?

it has become commonplace for the FDA to require the image tracking database, maintained by the ICL, in order to provide proof of the audit trail.

Digitization and Processing of the Radiographs

After the films pass QC, they are digitized. Having all films digitized for evaluation has become standard practice in RA and OA clinical trials within ICLs [13, 14]. It allows for blinding of patient information, easier data transfer to readers, and easier archiving. By digitizing the films for blinded reads, loss of original data is decreased as the actual films are not transferred from reader to reader. Furthermore, multiple readers are able to review the same patient contemporaneously, thus decreasing the overall time it takes to review the data.

Digitization of hand and foot RA films should be performed at 100-μm resolution, because at this level better correlation with the gold standard (films) than films digitized at 50 μm has been demonstrated [13]. Although digitizing the films at 50-μm resolution produces higher detail, studies show that the readers "over-read" erosions because of the added detail [13]. OA knee films are routinely digitized at 150 μm.

Table 10.2 Quality control criteria for evaluating OA films

Correct rotation (based on position of patella and femoral condyles)
Correct flexion (based on tibial rim sign)
Correct placement of L and R markers (away from the joint space)
Correct exposure
Correct collimation (depicting all anatomy)
Correct center of x-ray beam (joint space centered on film)

If the images were sent by the site in digital format, they are processed the same way as the digitized films.

In preparation for the independent review, hand and foot RA images require further processing of the digital image file. The digital image files are "cropped" into smaller segments. The foot is "cropped" to display only the forefoot joints, whereas the hand is "cropped" into three smaller segments: distal interphalangeal/proximal interphalangeal (DIP/PIP) joints, metacarpophalangeal (MCP), including the thumb interphalangeal (IP) and MCP joints, and finally, the wrist (Fig. 10.3). The

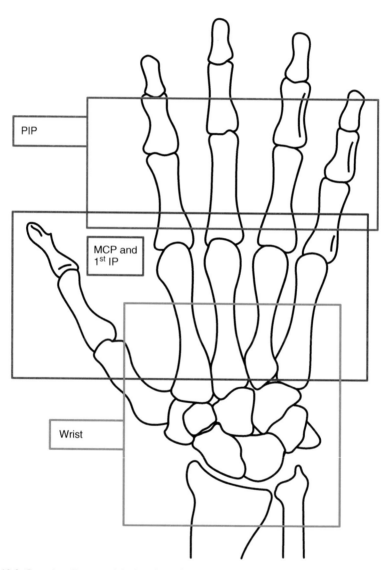

Fig. 10.3 Cropping diagram of the hand and foot

"cropping" allows for optimal window/level (brightness/contrast) settings to be made in the smaller regions. It is very difficult to adjust the window/level optimally for the wrist, without the DIP/PIP joints becoming too dark (Figs. 10.4 and 10.5).

Knee OA images do not typically require additional processing or "cropping" in preparation for the independent review. However, in addition to the qualitative review, some studies may also include semiautomated quantitative analysis methods as exploratory end points. In these instances, there may be additional processing required.

Independent Review

At the clinical site there may be a significant number of radiologists that could read the images, which allows for a large variation of the reading. Furthermore, there is

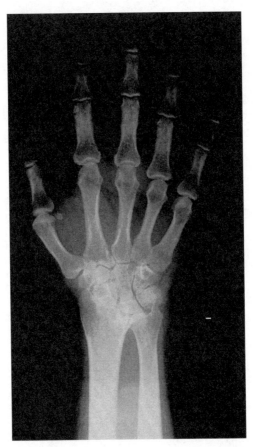

Fig. 10.4 Hand x-ray with optimal window/level settings for the wrist, displaying the inadequately dark PIP/MCP joints

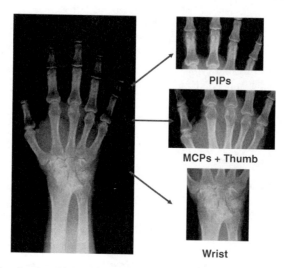

PIPs

MCPs + Thumb

Wrist

Fig. 10.5 Same hand x-ray with each segment cropped and optimal window/level settings

the influence of clinical data that may vary from time point to time point, which can lead to the radiologic interpretation of images being very subjective. Therefore, a central independent review has become a requirement when the imaging data is used as a primary or secondary end point for the study. The independent review will help to reduce the statistical noise by bringing a standardized methodology and approach in the review of the images.

It is recognized that the independent review of the image data reduces the variability. The independent review provides a true radiologist blinding and removal of the bias. When sites perform a review of the image data, the assessment of the images can vary greatly from one site to the next thus creating a great deal of variation and limiting the value of the interpretation. The FDA has accepted and understands that there will be a difference between the sites' interpretations and that of an independent review, due to many factors, including knowledge of clinical data at the site.

Selection of Independent Readers

The ICL should work with the sponsor to provide or recommend expert readers. The readers should be individuals who are truly experienced in the assessment of RA or OA images as evidenced by an individual's curriculum vitae (CV). The selection of the readers is generally subject to approval by the sponsor. In general, all readers are board-certified in musculoskeletal radiology or rheumatology. The CV should be maintained by the ICL.

Reader Training

For pivotal efficacy trials where the imaging data is the primary end point, the FDA has required all the image data to be reviewed by two readers creating two sets of independent reads.

With multiple readers, it is critical to perform reader training in order to develop consistency in the independent read results. All readers should be brought to a central location for the training.

The reader training session will serve three primary purposes:

- Ensure that the readers learn how to use the application, including both the image display and data entry functions.
- Confirm that the readers understand the assessment protocol including the definitions of any scoring or measurement system.
- Develop assessment conventions and definitions between all involved readers to optimize reader assessment agreement (or minimize inter-reader variability due to the lack of a uniform protocol definition between readers).

The ICL should develop a reading manual that will define the reading rules and interpretation plan. Sample images demonstrating the scoring system should be included. Documentation of the training session is typically maintained by the ICL with study records.

Independent Review System

The independent review system (Fig. 10.6) consists of two networked computers. The master computer serves as the data capture system and the other is the image display system. The data capture system will contain a program that displays the relevant questions and captures the readers' responses. Logic should be built into the system to control the display of the image data in the correct sequential

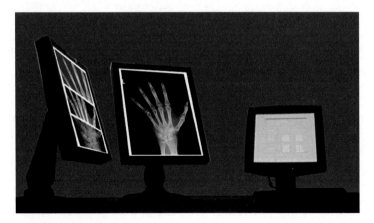

Fig. 10.6 Independent review system

or randomized order. The image display system contains image display/analysis software that allows the reader to view and interpret the images. The image display/analysis software should have standard radiologic functionality (window leveling, measurement, magnification, etc.) along with an audit trail of all the assessments in compliance with the regulatory requirements of Code of Federal Regulations (CFR) 21 Part 11. The image display system may consist of multiple monitors to display the images.

All data is captured on a real-time basis in a database. This eliminates the need to capture the readers' responses on paper case report forms (CRFs) and then the need to manually enter the results into a database.

Depending upon the read methodology and the number of read days required, the independent reads may take place at the ICL facilities or at a remote location (the readers' home or office) (Fig. 10.7).

Image Database

The FDA, in recent years, has required the electronic submission of the image data for RA studies as part of the NDA. The FDA will no longer accept hard-copy image films, and the digital image data will result in gigabytes of data. For example, a RA study of 600 subjects with three imaging time points will be of the order 60 gigabytes of image data. The FDA needs the ability to review the images quickly and efficiently as the reviewers will perform their own review of the image data to identify how the readers came to their conclusions. In addition, the reviewers can quickly search for cases based on predefined criteria and can evaluate data outliers. The image data submission should incorporate the images and independent read results and will enable the FDA reviewer to access, search, sort, and display digital image data with tools to adjust image window and level, size, and magnification.

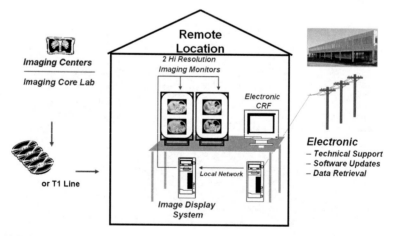

Fig. 10.7 Remote review system

Conclusion

Currently, imaging end points are one of the primary efficacy variables in RA trials and are becoming the standard for OA trials. Therefore, the requirements for the sponsor to ensure adequate quality of this vital part of the data collection has necessitated the growth of the so-called imaging core laboratory. The FDA has furthermore added to the requirements by requiring an imaging review charter prior to study start for all pivotal studies. It is interesting to note that at the time of writing, the European Agency, the Committee for Proprietary Medicinal Products (CPMP), has not followed the steps that the FDA has required, and the imaging end points can still be locally evaluated.

With careful up-front planning and introduction of a competent and experienced ICL into the protocol development at an early time frame, the imaging end points can be obtained with high quality and without excessive inertia on the study start-up activities. Obtaining study site "buy-in" and participation is important, and this is started with the acknowledgment of an ICL at the outset as principal investigators have the final drafts of the protocol and can more fully evaluate whether they wish to participate in the study.

As imaging will play a greater role in the efficacy and safety evaluation in clinical trials and will arguably become the leading biomarker in the identification of disease once the drug comes to market, the need for careful collection and evaluation of this disparate information is only enhanced.

References

1. FDA. Guidance for industry: clinical development programs for drugs, devices, and biological products for the treatment of rheumatoid arthritis (RA). Draft guidance. Bethesda, MD: U.S. FDA; February 1999.
2. Bathon JM, Martin RW, Fleischmann RM, et al. A comparison of etanercept and methotrexate in patients with early rheumatoid arthritis. N Engl J Med 2000;343(22):1586–1593.
3. Sharp JT, Strand V, Leung H, et al. Treatment with leflunomide slows radiographic progression of rheumatoid arthritis: results from three randomized controlled trials of leflunomide in patients with active rheumatoid arthritis. Am Coll Rheumatol 2000;43(3):495–505.
4. Lipsky PE, van der Heijde DM, St Clair EW, et al. Infliximab and methotrexate in the treatment of rheumatoid arthritis. N Engl J Med 2000;343(22):1594–1602.
5. van der Heijde D, Landewé R, Klareskog L, Rodríguez-Valverde V, Settas L, Pedersen R, Fatenejad S. Presentation and analysis of radiographic outcome in clinical trials: experience from the TEMPO trial. Arthritis Rheum 2005;52:49–60.
6. van Everdingen AA, Jacobs JWG, van Reesema DRS, et al. Low-dose prednisone therapy for patients with early active rheumatoid arthritis: clinical efficacy, disease-modifying properties, and side effects: a randomized, double-blind, placebo-controlled clinical trial. Ann Intern Med 2002;136:1–12.
7. FDA. Guidance for industry: clinical development programs for drugs, devices, and biological products intended for the treatment of osteoarthritis (OA). Draft guidance. Bethesda, MD: U.S. FDA; July 1999.
8. Kradjian S, Gutheil J, Baratelle A, Einstein S, Kaslow DC. Development of a charter for an endpoint assessment and adjudication committee. Drug Information J 2005;39:53–61.

9. Pearson D, Miller CG, eds. Clinical trials in osteoporosis. New York: Springer-Verlag, 2002.

10. Scott DL, Coulton BL, Popert AJ. Long term progression of joint damage in rheumatoid arthritis. Ann Rheum Dis 1986;45:373–378.

11. Dougados M. Outcome measures for clinical trials of disease modifying osteoarthritis drugs in patients with hip osteoarthritis. J Rheumatol 2004;31(Suppl 66):66–70.

12. Genant HK. Methods of assessing radiographic change in rheumatoid arthritis. Am J Med 1983;75(6A):35–47.

13. Finck BK, Weissman BNW, Rubenstein JD, et al. 100 micron digitization resolution is optimal for x-rays for a large multicenter trial in rheumatoid arthritis (RA). Arthritis Rheum 1997;40(9):S288.

14. Genant H, Jiang Y, Peterfy C, Lu Y, Redei J, Countryman P. Assessment of rheumatoid arthritis using a modified scoring method in digitized and original radiographs. Arthritis Rheum 1998;41(9):1583–1590.

Chapter 11
Biochemical Markers of Rheumatoid Arthritis and Osteoarthritis: Clinical Utility and Practical Considerations

Mario R. Ehlers and Elizabeth T. Leary

Introduction

Biochemical markers of bone and cartilage turnover and degradation are quantitative and dynamic tests that may detect early joint damage, disease progression, and response to therapy and therefore have the potential to be used to evaluate the chondroprotective activity of novel therapies for rheumatoid arthritis (RA) and osteoarthritis (OA). Inclusion of such markers in clinical development programs can provide information for their later use as adjuncts to diagnosis and treatment monitoring. The ultimate hallmark of both RA and OA is joint destruction, and there is a need for rapid, real-time markers to guide therapy.

There are now several biochemical biomarkers with emerging clinical utility and for which robust assays have been developed; these markers can be recommended for inclusion in pharmaceutical clinical trials. Markers specific for articular cartilage and synovium include peptide fragments of type II collagen and procollagen, accessory proteins present within cartilage, and products from synovial membranes. In addition, markers of bone turnover are useful in RA and OA because of the prominence of bone erosions, osteophytes, and/or subchondral sclerosis.

The inclusion of biochemical markers of joint disease in preclinical and clinical development programs for arthritis adds value by providing additional information about the mechanism of action of the investigational drug and by identifying cohorts at baseline that will progress and thus potentially identifying subgroups with a significant treatment response. Moreover, use of biomarkers can potentially differentiate novel drugs in the market after approval.

In this chapter, we provide an overview of biochemical markers currently available for use in clinical trials, including practical considerations. Readers are also directed to Chapter 16 in this volume for a more complete review of the biochemistry and clinical utility of markers for joint disease, with an emphasis on OA.

M.R. Ehlers
Chief Medical Officer, Pacific Biometrics, Inc. Seattle, WA, USA

Pathogenesis of RA and OA

Rheumatoid Arthritis

RA is a chronic systemic inflammatory disease characterized by a destructive pol-yarthritis. Although extra-articular involvement is common (e.g., vasculitis, which can be life-threatening), the ultimate hallmark of RA is joint destruction. RA is regarded as an autoimmune disease with a polygenic basis, but the precise etiology and specific precipitating events are unknown. The immuno-inflammatory process involves a T-cell activation cascade with a strong T_H1 bias, which by means of proinflammatory cytokines (such as TNF-α, IL-1, IL-6, IL-18, and IFN-γ) activates macrophages, synovial fibroblasts, osteoclasts, and chondrocytes. These activated cells degrade cartilage and bone in and around synovial joints, in part by secretion of matrix metalloproteinases (MMPs) [1].

There is a strong association between RA and several types of autoantibod-ies, the most important being rheumatoid factor (RF) but which also include anti-bodies to citrullinated proteins. Hence, B cells and autoantibodies, as well as immune complexes and complement activation, may play an important role in RA [1].

Osteoarthritis

OA is the most prevalent form of arthritis and is characterized by progressive loss of articular cartilage and by alterations of periarticular bone and synovial metabolism [2]. Although the damage to articular cartilage is progressive and appar-ently irreversible in late OA, there is evidence for increased cartilage turnover in early OA, with increased synthesis of the two main structural proteins, type II collagen and aggrecan [3, 4]. Moreover, bone may play an important role in the pathogenesis of OA, in that abnormalities in subchondral bone may result in the release of destructive factors, such as metalloproteinases, that damage the articular cartilage [2].

Role of Biomarkers in RA and OA

Rheumatoid Arthritis

The immuno-inflammatory component of the pathogenesis of RA is generally accepted, and the use of laboratory tests for markers of the activated immune and inflammatory systems is well established; for example, C-reactive protein (CRP), erythrocyte sedimentation rate (ESR), B and T cell counts, Ig levels, complement, and autoantibodies such as antinuclear antibody (ANA) and RF. Standard immunol-ogy testing will not be discussed further in this overview. Among the autoantibodies,

RF is the gold standard, but recently anti–cyclic citrullinated peptide (CCP) antibodies have emerged as highly specific for RA and as having excellent prognostic value, discussed further later.

Notably absent from routine assessments for RA diagnosis, progression, and response to therapy are biochemical markers of bone and cartilage degradation and turnover, despite the fact that the ultimate hallmark of RA is joint destruction. This can be ascribed to the fact that (a) joint involvement has traditionally been assessed by clinical and radiologic criteria, and (b) biochemical markers have not had sufficient resolution to be useful. However, in recent years there has been considerable progress in identifying relevant markers and in developing robust laboratory assays, such that these markers can now add considerable value to the clinical evaluation of novel RA therapies. These markers can provide information on joint-disease progression and treatment response more rapidly and, in some cases, with greater quantitative precision than traditional clinical and radiologic measures.

Osteoarthritis

Routine assessments for OA diagnosis, progression, and response to therapy rely on radiologic and clinical criteria, and biochemical markers of bone and cartilage degradation and turnover are not commonly used. As described for RA above, biochemical markers can provide more dynamic information about joint-disease progression and treatment response [5]. Unlike imaging techniques, which only provide a historical view of damage that has already occurred, biochemical markers can provide information about continuing or future damage [6], and hence their use in clinical trials because they demonstrate a dynamic response to therapy.

Importantly, in a substudy of the BRISK trial, radiographic progression of knee OA over 1 year was assessed in the placebo group. The results indicated that most patients showed little or no joint space loss, but that a cohort (6% to 11%) showed detectable changes [7]. This implies that in order to detect a treatment response, it will be critical to identify the cohort at baseline that will exhibit measurable joint space narrowing (JSN). Several biomarkers have been shown to predict future JSN and could therefore be used to stratify patients in the treatment groups.

Biochemical Markers of Joint Disease

Autoantibodies: Rheumatoid Factor and Anti-CCP Antibodies

The role of autoantibodies in the diagnosis and possibly also the pathogenesis of RA is well recognized. Of several autoantibody systems that have been identified, the RF system has been the most important for both RA diagnosis and prognosis and it is included in the American College of Rheumatology (ACR) classification criteria for RA [8]. Recently, the anti-CCP autoantibody system has emerged as providing additional diagnostic and prognostic information in RA. The anti-CCP autoantibody system includes a group of autoantibodies with shared reactivity for proteins containing arginine residues that have been modified to citrulline and include antiperinuclear factor (APF), antikeratin antibody (AKA), and antifilaggrin antibody (AFA) [8].

AFAs have been identified in the synovial membrane and pannus in RA, leading to the hypothesis that AFAs cross-react with citrullinated proteins in the rheumatoid synovium. CCP is a synthetic antigen but appears to be superior to natural antigens (e.g., citrullinated filaggrin) in ELISA assays, leading to the development of the current anti-CCP assays. The anti-CCP assay likely detects several of the anti-citrullinated peptide autoantibodies found in RA.

The anti-CCP assay has a remarkably high specificity for RA, of the order 98%, which is superior to that of RF [9]. More importantly for the evaluation of disease progression and treatment response, anti-CCP antibodies are predictive of progression to erosive RA and a more severe disease course. Recent studies have indicated that anti-CCP antibodies determined early in the course of RA are good predictors of radiographic joint damage [10], and that the combined analysis of anti-CCP and IgM RF provides the most accurate prediction of erosive disease [11].

Recently, anti-CCP antibodies were found to decrease significantly more than total serum Ig after B-cell depletion therapy with rituximab, and disease relapse was closely correlated with rises in anti-CCP or RF isotypes [12]. Therefore, anti-CCP, in conjunction with RF, may provide valuable information about RA disease severity, progression, and response to immune-modulating therapy.

Biochemical Markers of Bone Turnover

There is now an extensive literature on the use of biochemical markers of bone turnover in the clinical development of drugs that affect bone metabolism, such as hormone replacement therapy (HRT), selective estrogen receptor modulators (SERMs), bisphosphonates, calcitonin, parathyroid hormone (PTH), and glucocorticoids (e.g., see Refs. 13–16).

Biochemical markers of bone turnover fall into two categories: (1) markers of bone formation and (2) markers of bone resorption (degradation).

Bone formation markers include serum osteocalcin, serum bone-specific alkaline phosphatase, and serum levels of N- and C-propeptides of type I procollagen (PINP and PICP). These markers generally reflect osteoblastic activity and in the case of PINP and PICP actually reflect the synthesis of type I collagen, the major structural protein of bone.

Bone resorption markers include urinary pyridinoline (PYD) and deoxypyridinoline (DPD), urinary and serum levels of the N- and C-telopeptides of type I collagen (NTX and CTX), and serum levels of tartrate-resistant acid phosphatase 5b (TRACP-5b). These markers reflect osteoclastic activity and, except for TRACP-5b, represent degradation products of type I collagen. Of these, CTX (also referred to as CTX-I or CrossLaps, Nordic Bioscience Diagnostics A/S, Herlev, Denmark) is thought to be the most specific because the epitope is a unique cross-linked, β-isomerized peptide that is highly enriched in bone. A second marker derived from the C-telopeptide of type I collagen is ICTP, which arises from pathologic (non-osteoclastic) bone degradation and may have unique applicability in RA.

Recently, markers of bone turnover have been measured in studies involving RA patients. These studies have revealed that bone formation is broadly reduced in RA, whereas bone resorption is increased in patients with joint destruction and is positively correlated with indices of disease activity and radiologic progression [17–19]. Of particular note for drug-development programs for RA is the potential value of bone markers in predicting disease progression and in monitoring treatment response to a biologic [20, 21]. As outlined further below, the most useful markers of bone resorption are ICTP, CTX-I, and NTX; and for bone formation, PINP and osteocalcin can be recommended.

Markers of Bone Formation

Serum PINP is emerging as the single most robust and sensitive bone formation marker. During synthesis of type I procollagen in the nascent bone matrix, the N-propeptide is cleaved off and circulates in the plasma. Because bone is the major site of type I collagen synthesis, serum levels of PINP closely reflect new bone formation. Recent studies have shown that changes in serum PINP are greater than changes in serum osteocalcin (OC) or bone-specific alkaline phosphatase (BSAP) in high bone-turnover states [22, 23].

An automated assay for PINP has been developed by Roche Diagnostics (Indianapolis, IN) on the Elecsys platform. The Elecsys PINP assay has excellent precision, superior to standard immunoassays, and serum volume requirements are low. Another key consideration is stability of the analyte, and data indicate that PINP is stable for up to 21 days at 4°C and for up to 3 years at −70°C. This is often important because serum samples collected during clinical trials are not always optimally stored and transported and are sometimes exposed to repeated freeze-thaws. Therefore, analyte stability is an important consideration when selecting biomarkers for testing in clinical trials.

An alternative to PINP that could be considered is osteocalcin. Osteocalcin is also available on the Roche Elecsys platform and similarly has excellent precision. However, osteocalcin does not have the same demonstrated stability as PINP and shows a somewhat lower change in serum levels when bone turnover is elevated and in response to treatment [22, 23].

Markers of Bone Degradation

The major structural protein of bone is type I collagen and hence degradation products of type I collagen are established as useful markers of bone resorption. Osteoclast-driven degradation of type I collagen is mediated by cathepsin K and occurs at the N- and C-terminal telopeptide regions of the cross-linked triple helix, generating N- and C-telopeptide fragments referred to as NTX and CTX, respectively. In addition, non-osteoclastic (pathologic) resorption is mediated by MMPs and generates a C-telopeptide fragment referred to as ICTP [24].

In RA, bone resorption appears to be the result of both generalized osteoclastic turnover and localized pathologic degradation mediated by synovial inflammation and MMP release [25, 26]. Numerous studies have established the value of serum ICTP in monitoring bone loss and disease activity and in predicting progressive joint disease in RA [20, 25–33]. Importantly, ICTP is stable for at least 5 days at 4°C and two freeze-thaw cycles, and the commercial assay for ICTP is robust and suitable for use in clinical trials.

Alternatively, both NTX and CTX (also known as CTX-I to distinguish it from CTX-II derived from cartilage) are well established markers of bone resorption in diseases such as osteoporosis [24]. Several studies have documented that NTX levels are significantly elevated in patients with active RA versus patients with inactive RA or controls [34–36] and correlate with worsening erosion scores [37]. Similarly, changes in CTX-I have been shown to be useful in predicting disease progression and monitoring response to therapy [17, 18, 21]. However, both serum CTX-I and NTX are influenced by fasting status and time of collection and hence cannot be recommended if samples are not collected fasting and at the same time of day for every time point [38, 39]. Moreover, both NTX and CTX-I have limited stability in serum at 4°C and during repeated freeze-thaw cycles.

Biochemical Markers of Cartilage Turnover

Markers of cartilage turnover are not yet widely used in joint disease research. Nevertheless, this field has advanced substantially in recent years, and it now offers the prospect that quantitative and dynamic tests can be used to evaluate the chondroprotective potential of novel therapies for RA and OA.

Analogous to bone markers, biochemical markers of cartilage turnover fall into two categories: (1) markers of cartilage degradation and (2) markers of cartilage synthesis or turnover.

Markers of Cartilage Degradation

Articular cartilage is composed of two principal structural molecules, namely type II collagen and aggrecan, as well as several accessory proteins dispersed within the cartilage matrix, the most important being cartilage oligomeric matrix protein (COMP) and human cartilage glycoprotein 39 (HC gp-39; YKL-40). During cartilage degradation, the major structural proteins undergo proteolytic breakdown, and the resulting peptide fragments can be detected in the synovial fluid, serum, and urine. In contrast, intact COMP and YKL-40 are released from the degraded cartilage matrix and are also detected in the synovial fluid and serum. Therefore, these proteins and their fragments represent biochemical markers of cartilage degradation and turnover, and the challenge has been to develop sensitive and robust assays for their detection.

CartiLaps (CTX-II)

The urine CartiLaps assay (Nordic Bioscience Diagnostics A/S Herlev, Denmark) is emerging as an informative marker of cartilage degradation in both RA and OA. The CartiLaps assay measures the CTX-II neoepitope, a 6-amino-acid fragment from the C-telopeptide region of type II collagen that is generated by collagenases during cartilage damage. The CTX-II epitope is released from the cartilage into the synovial fluid, and the circulation and is then excreted in the urine.

Degradation of type II collagen is an important step in the progression of RA and OA, and elevated levels of degradation fragments are easily demonstrated in synovial fluid of affected joints. Moreover, because type II collagen is almost exclusively found in cartilage, this marker is highly specific for joint damage [13, 40].

Urinary CTX-II levels have been shown to be significantly increased (two- to threefold) in both RA and OA. Baseline CTX-II levels were shown to be the strongest biochemical predictor of radiologic progression in patients with early RA in the COBRA study [18]. In OA, CTX-II levels are significantly correlated with joint destruction (joint surface area and joint space width), and of the biochemical markers tested, CTX-II levels have been shown to be the most predictive of the progression of joint damage [41–43].

COMP

COMP, a member of the thrombospondin family, is a high-molecular-weight, multi-subunit protein that is abundant in cartilage but also found in tendon and other tissues, including synovium. Levels of COMP in serum and synovial fluid correlate with cartilage destruction in both RA and OA in clinical studies. Increased serum levels of COMP in OA patients correlate with extent of joint involvement and with rate of disease progression [44].

Serum COMP levels at baseline are a robust marker of radiologic progression in RA [45]. In a recent study, serum COMP levels decreased significantly in RA patients after initiation of therapy with either infliximab or etanercept, in both ACR20 responders and nonresponders [46]. In a study of postmenopausal women with RA treated with HRT, baseline COMP, ICTP, and CTX-II correlated significantly with the Larsen score, suggesting that these cartilage and bone markers provide useful tools for assessing novel treatment modalities in RA [47].

Serum COMP levels have consistently been shown to correlate with disease severity and progression in both knee and hip OA [42–44,48]. Interestingly, serum COMP levels cluster with markers of synovitis and correlate with clinical signs of joint inflammation [43], indicating that COMP is not simply a marker of cartilage degradation. The precise nature of the pathophysiologic process reflected by COMP during joint damage remains to be determined.

YKL-40

YKL-40 is a 38- to 40-kDa glycoprotein that may function as a lectin and play a role in tissue remodeling, including articular cartilage. YKL-40 is a major secretory product of chondrocytes and synovial cells but is also produced by activated macrophages, fibrotic liver cells, and bone and breast cancer cells. YKL-40 levels are low in normal human cartilage but are increased in both inflammatory and degenerative joint disease, and therefore YKL-40 may be a biomarker of cartilage turnover and synovitis [49].

Several studies have shown that serum levels of YKL-40 are significantly increased (1.5- to 3-fold) in both RA and OA patients. In RA patients treated with disease-modifying therapy, there was a significant (21%) decrease in serum YKL-40 levels among responders [49]. Interestingly, YKL-40 levels correlate with markers of systemic inflammation, such as CRP, Serum amyloid A (SAA), and ESR, but YKL-40 is more specific for joint disease and may reflect both cartilage damage and synovitis [50–52].

Measuring serum YKL-40 levels may enable stratification of patients into those with evidence of joint inflammation. This kind of analysis could be augmented further by use of a marker informative about synovitis (e.g., N-propeptide of type III collagen [PIIINP]) and a marker for systemic inflammation, such as CRP. However, it is important to note that YKL-40 is not specific for cartilage and synovium and that serum levels can change in malignancies, cirrhosis, and possibly atherosclerosis [53].

Markers of Cartilage Synthesis or Turnover

Joint diseases such as RA and OA are characterized not only by cartilage degradation but also by altered rates of turnover and new synthesis. Increased rates of turnover and synthesis are abnormal and in some cases result in the appearance of developmental epitopes and neoepitopes, which have the potential for being specific for arthritis. Examples of epitopes that reflect abnormal cartilage synthesis and turnover are N- and C-propeptides of type II procollagen and the chondroitin sulfate (CS) 846 epitope of aggrecan.

The CS-846 assay shows promise in RA [54], and based on studies in OA, both the C-propeptide (CPII assay) and the N-propeptide (PIIANP assay) have shown promise in detecting altered synthesis of type II collagen in arthritis [3, 55]. Serum PIIANP levels were found to be decreased by 53% and 35% in knee OA and RA, respectively [56]. In knee OA, there appears to an uncoupling of type II collagen synthesis and degradation, such that patients with the lowest levels of PIIANP and the highest levels of CTX-II were found to have an eightfold more rapid progression of joint damage [55]. In another study, however, type II collagen synthesis appeared to be increased in knee OA as determined by measuring CPII content in cartilage obtained postmortem [57]. This discrepancy may be related to stage of disease (late vs. early) or differences in the epitope or assay matrix. Clearly, additional studies are required to assess the role of type II collagen synthesis in OA and RA pathogenesis.

It should be noted that these assays remain experimental and the literature supporting their use for analyzing human serum samples is sparse. For example, the PIIANP assay has only recently become available from a commercial manufacturer and therefore long-term reliability and precision still need to be evaluated. Alternatively, changes in serum levels of both COMP and YKL-40 likely reflect both degradation and turnover of cartilage and therefore provide some information on this issue.

Biochemical Markers of Synovitis

In addition to bone and cartilage, the third important tissue compartment in the joint is the synovium. The critical role of synovitis and the pannus in the pathogenesis of RA has already been discussed. Moreover, although OA has long been considered a degenerative disease, recent evidence suggests a significant inflammatory component with episodic synovitis [2, 58].

A marker of synovial involvement in both RA and OA is the N-propeptide of type III collagen (PIIINP), for which a serum assay is available. In a recent cross-sectional study, PIIINP was significantly correlated with radiographic joint damage in knee OA as well as with Western Ontario and McMaster University Osteoarthritis (WOMAC) indices of pain and stiffness [41]. PIIINP correlated with pain and stiffness and was the only synovial marker that correlated significantly with radiographic parameters of joint destruction after multivariate analysis [41]. PIIINP was also found to cluster with synovitis in the hip-OA ECHODIAH cohort [43]. In a study evaluating the usefulness of PIIINP in RA, 50% of subjects were found to have elevated serum PIIINP levels, and PIIINP correlated with conventional markers of RA disease activity, such as CRP and joint swelling score [59]. In a study assessing the effects of low-dose prednisolone in early RA, serum levels of PIIINP and HA were reduced by 24% to 25% during treatment, suggesting that prednisolone reduces synovitis [60].

Type III collagen is not entirely specific for synovium, and elevated PIIINP levels have also been found in psoriatic patients with liver fibrosis after methotrexate therapy [61] and in scleroderma [62]. However, in the context of a well-controlled clinical trial for arthritis, serum PIIINP is likely to be a very useful marker of synovitis. Also important is that PIIINP is a robust marker with good stability at $4°C$, and a reliable assay is available for clinical trials.

Two additional markers that reflect synovial involvement are serum hyaluronic acid (HA) and urinary glucosyl-galactosyl pyridinoline (GGP). HA is significantly elevated in patients with knee OA [41] and, as expected, was found to cluster with markers of synovitis in hip OA [43]. However, serum HA was not found to correlate with the WOMAC index of pain and physical function or with radiologic parameters of joint damage [41]. In contrast, GGP was found to correlate significantly with both the WOMAC index and joint damage [41] and therefore appears to be an alternative to serum PIIINP in assessing synovitis. However, commercial assays for urinary GGP are not available, and the current procedure requires high-performance liquid chromatography, limiting the utility of this assay in large-scale clinical trials.

Biochemical Markers of Inflammation

Markers of systemic inflammation include CRP, fibrinogen, various cytokines, such as TNF-α and interleukins (IL-1, -2, -6, -10, etc.), and soluble adhesion molecules, such as E-selectin, intercellular adhesion molecule-1 (ICAM-1), and vascular cell adhesion molecule-1 (VCAM-1). These markers are useful for measuring the state of the inflammatory activation in RA, and the response to therapy, but changes in serum levels in these markers are not informative about specific events in the joints.

Inflammation is also becoming a recognized feature of OA, and sensitive tests for CRP are elevated [5]. It has been suggested that CRP is elevated in early knee OA and is predictive of progressive disease, whereas in established disease it is not elevated [41]. Serum CRP levels are significantly elevated in hip OA and are correlated significantly with indices of pain [43, 52]. Measurement of CRP is informative about the level of systemic inflammation and may stratify patients into those with earlier and/or rapidly progressive disease. CRP levels also add to the information obtained from tests for serum COMP, YKL-40, and PIIINP.

Practical Considerations for Measurements of Biochemical Markers

To generate useable biochemical marker data, care should be taken to consider pre-analytical and analytical factors that can impact assay values. The study objectives, logistics, and practical constraints of specific clinical trials play important roles in the selection of the most appropriate assays for each study. For example, is an 8-hour fast and a blood draw at 8 AM feasible for the study participants? This is necessary to minimize biological variability for some markers. Are biomarkers cleared by the kidneys or liver being used in subjects with compromised renal or hepatic functions? Are the personnel responsible for sample processing able or capable of adhering to the prescribed protocol (e.g., the freezer may be distant from the sample-processing station)? Are adequate sample shipping requirements available (e.g., dry-ice shipments)? The following is an overview of practical considerations when choosing a suitable biochemical marker. Table 11.1 lists the more common markers used in clinical trials in RA and OA together with a summary of key assay parameters.

Analytical Considerations

Assay Specificity

It is important to note that there is often more than one commercially available assay available for the marker of choice. These assays may involve different epitopes in different assay platforms, which result in different specificity and other performance characteristics such as sample stability. Urine and serum assays for the same biochemical marker may not be directed at the same epitope. This may be the

Table 11.1 Biochemical markers for clinical trials in RA and OA: practical considerations

Marker	Sample type	Method	Stability			Comments
			4°C	−20°C	−70°C	
Autoantibodies						
RF	Serum	ELISA	14 d	≥1 mo	≥6 mo	Gold standard for RA; moderate specificity
Anti-CCP	Serum or plasma	ELISA	1 mo	1 y	3 y	Highly specific for RA but less sensitive than RF
Markers of bone turnover						
PINP	Serum or plasma	ECLIA or RIA	21 d	3 y	>3 y	Robust and sensitive bone formation marker
OC	Serum or plasma*	ECLIA, ELISA, or RIA	5 d	3 mo	2 y	Alternative to PINP but less sensitive
ICTP	Serum or plasma	RIA or ELISA	5 d	5 y	10 y	Produced by pathologic bone degradation and increased in RA
CTX-I	Serum, plasma, or urine*	ECLIA or ELISA	8 d (1 d)†	3 y	3 y	Produced by osteoclastic bone degradation. Very sensitive but strongly affected by food intake and diurnal variation.
NTX	Serum or urine	ELISA or ECLIA	5 d	2 y	>2 y	Similar to CTX-I but less sensitive; affected by diurnal variation
Markers of cartilage turnover						
CTX-II	Urine	ELISA	1 d	2 y	> 2 y	Robust marker of cartilage degradation
COMP	Serum	ELISA	7 d	2.5 y	>2.5 y	Marker of cartilage degradation; may also reflect synovitis
YKL-40	Serum	ELISA	7 d	1 y	≥2 y	Marker of cartilage turnover and synovitis
PIIANP	Serum	ELISA	N/A	N/A	N/A	Emerging marker of cartilage synthesis

(continued)

Table 11.1 (continued)

Marker	Sample type	Method	Stability			Comments
			4°C	−20°C	−70°C	
Markers of synovitis						
PIIINP	Serum	RIA	5 d	2 y	>2 y	Robust marker of synovitis; also increased in liver fibrosis and scleroderma
GGP	Urine	HPLC	7 d	2 mo	1 y	Alternative to PIIINP but requires HPLC
Marker of inflammation						
CRP	Serum or plasma	ITM	2 mo	3 y	≥3 y	Excellent marker of systemic inflammation; reflects RA disease activity but also useful in OA

RF, rheumatoid factor; anti-CCP, anti-cyclic citrullinated peptide antibody; PINP, propeptide of type I procollagen; OC, osteocalcin; ICTP, C-telopeptide of type I collagen (MMP-generated); CTX-I, cross-linked C-telopeptide of type I collagen; NTX, N-telopeptide of type I collagen; CTX-II, C-telopeptide of type II collagen; COMP, cartilage oligomeric matrix protein; YKL-40, human cartilage glycoprotein 39; PIIANP, N-propeptide of type IIA procollagen; PIIINP, N-propeptide of type III procollagen; GGP, glucosyl-galactosyl-pyridinoline; CRP, C-reactive protein; ELISA, enzyme-linked immunosorbent assay; ECLIA, electrochemiluminescence immunoassay; RIA, radioimmunoassay; HPLC, high-performance liquid chromatography; ITM, immunoturbidimetric; N/A, not available.

*EDTA plasma preferred.

†Serum stability.

case even when both assays are produced by the same manufacturer. For example, although both the urine and serum CrossLaps (CTX-I) assays recognize the same 8-amino-acid epitope of type I collagen, the urine assay recognizes both the β-β cross-linked epitope and α-β cross-linked epitope, whereas the serum assay detects only the β-β epitope [63]. The latter is considered to be a more specific indicator of mature bone degradation. The same is true for N-telopeptide assays, in which the antibodies in the serum and urine assays are directed to slightly different antigens, resulting in possible differences in response seen with urinary and serum NTX.

Assay Precision

Precision may vary depending on the platform available (e.g., radioisotopic , ELISA, or automated EIA) and the laboratory performing the assay. Long-term precision depends on the reagent manufacturers' ability to maintain stringent lot-to-lot quality control and the laboratories' ability to maintain consistent performance and to monitor the data. Certain bone markers have been moved onto automated platforms, such as PINP, CTX, and OC onto the Elecsys (Roche Diagnostics) and urine NTX onto the Vitros ECI system (Ortho-Clinical Diagnostics, Rochester, NY). Automated assays have significantly better precision than the equivalent manual assays.

Assay Sensitivity

The low-end detection limit and dynamic range of the assays may be different among assays for the same biomarker. Reanalysis after further sample dilution is often required, usually resulting in a higher imprecision. "Loss" of patient results can occur if expected results are below the detection limit. Assay sensitivity should be reviewed based on the study patient population.

Assay Sample Stability

Assay-specific sample stability has direct practical implications for marker selection. Among-assay variability has been well studied for serum osteocalcin, for example. Much of the difference observed among assays was due to the epitope selection, as the intact osteocalcin molecule is very susceptible to cleavage of the C-terminal 43–47 fragment *in vitro*. Therefore, immunoassays that detect both the intact molecule and the main N-terminal mid-fragment are preferred [22]. Some markers are inherently unstable, and therefore a different marker that provides similar clinical information should be substituted in certain situations. For example, samples for RF isotyping do not tolerate more than one freeze-thaw cycle. However, anti-CCP antibody, which provides similar information in RA, is stable to several freeze-thaw cycles. Similarly, the bone formation marker PINP is very stable and unaffected by five freeze-thaw cycles. It may be substituted for less stable markers if meticulous specimen handling is not possible.

Batched Analysis

To minimize testing-related variation, samples collected from all visits during the clinical trial should be batched per patient and analyzed in the same test run ("patient sets"). Stability of the biomarker for the length of storage prior to analysis should be established. If interim analysis or real-time analysis is desired, appropriate quality control procedures, such as inclusion of an uncompromised baseline sample with subsequent analyses, are recommended.

Preanalytical Considerations

Biological Variation

Biological variation, such as circadian rhythm, may have a significant impact on some biomarkers levels. This is especially a source of imprecision in urinary bone degradation makers, where values at the peak and nadir over a period of 24 hours may differ as much as 50% to 70% from the mean. In general, formation markers have less variability than degradation markers, and serum markers have less variation than urine markers. Time of specimen collection should be controlled, as appropriate.

Food Effect

Some biomarkers are significantly affected by food intake. This phenomenon is well established for markers of bone resorption, such as CTX-I and, to a lesser extent, NTX, an effect that may be mediated by certain gut-derived hormones [38, 39, 64]. Therefore, only fasting samples should be used for these markers, a requirement that limits the use of CTX-I in certain clinical trials. The influence of fasting or food intake on markers of cartilage turnover has not been established. However, there have been preliminary reports of effects of exercise on cartilage markers, especially COMP [65]. In light of these uncertainties, it would seem prudent to control for fasting or eating, time of collection, and physical exercise in clinical trials that include cartilage markers.

Patient Population

Interpretation of clinical trial data may be confounded by renal or hepatic impairment in the subjects. As already discussed elsewhere in this chapter, several bone turnover markers, such as CTX-I, NTX, PINP, and osteocalcin, are cleared by the kidneys and therefore show marked increases in serum in patients with renal failure and sharp fluctuations during renal dialysis [66]. In contrast, other markers, such as BSAP and TRACP-5b, are not cleared by the kidneys and therefore provide more reliable data in patients with renal impairment [64, 66]. Therefore, depending on the study population and the clearance pathway of the biomarker, an appropriate biomarker should be selected. This issue has not been well studied for the cartilage markers and, hence, caution is advised when evaluating these markers in patients with significant renal or hepatic impairment.

Conclusion

The use of biochemical markers for diagnosis, prognosis, and treatment monitoring in RA and OA is still in its infancy, with the exception of immunologic markers in RA. The field can be compared with where biochemical markers of bone turnover were 10 to 15 years ago in the diagnosis, fracture-risk assessment, and treatment monitoring of osteoporosis. However, as has been observed for the latter field, we can expect arthritis markers to make significant inroads in the coming years because clinical assessments and imaging methods are too blunt and/or too expensive to provide dynamic information about disease progression and response to therapy for effective clinical drug development of disease-modifying drugs and their clinical use postapproval.

The ultimate hallmarks of both RA and OA are joint destruction with extensive degradation and loss of articular cartilage, periarticular bone erosions, sclerosis or remodeling, and associated synovial changes. Hence, biochemical markers informative about changes in bone and cartilage turnover and synovitis are expected to provide specific information about joint pathology. As we have shown, a variety of these markers are predictive of joint disease progression and in some cases can also provide information about response to treatment.

At present, it is unclear whether any of the current markers has sufficient robustness and dynamic range to be useful in individual patient care. Indeed, in a recent cross-sectional analysis of 10 biochemical markers of bone, cartilage, and synovium in hip OA, the authors concluded that the contribution of these markers to the interindividual variation in the clinical and radiologic findings was minor [43]. Moreover, a recent prospective trial evaluating the efficacy of risedronate in knee OA (BRISK study) revealed only a weak correlation between decreases in CTX-II and clinical and radiologic changes [67]. These and other data indicate that combinations of existing markers, as well as novel markers with greater specificity and dynamic range, will likely be required for meaningful assessments. Large, longitudinal, adequately controlled studies, preferably trials of disease-modifying drugs, are required to determine the true value of biochemical markers of RA and OA, both in clinical drug development and in individual patient care.

References

1. Smolen JS, Steiner G. Therapeutic strategies for rheumatoid arthritis. Nat Rev Drug Discov 2003;2:473–488.
2. Wieland A, Michaelis M, Kirschbaum BJ, Rudolphi KA. Osteoarthritis – an untreatable disease? Nat Rev Drug Discov 2005;4:331–344.

3. Nelson F, Dahlberg L, Laverty S, Reiner A, Pidoux I, Ionescu M, Fraser GL, Brooks E, Tanzer M, Rosenberg LC, Dieppe P, Poole AR. Evidence for altered synthesis of type II collagen in patients with osteoarthritis. J Clin Invest 1998;102:2115–2125.

4. Salminen HJ, Saamanen AM, Vankemmelbeke MN, Auho PK, Perala MP, Vuorio EI. Differential expression patterns of matrix metalloproteinases and their inhibitors during development of osteoarthritis in a transgenic mouse model. Ann Rheum Dis 2002;61:591–597.

5. Wollheim FA. Early stages of osteoarthritis: the search for sensitive predictors. Ann Rheum Dis 2003;62:1031–1032.

6. Young-Min SA, Cawston TE, Griffiths ID. Markers of joint destruction: principles, problems, and potential. Ann Rheum Dis 2001;60:545–548.

7. Buckland-Wright C, Cline G, Meyer J. Structural progression in knee osteoarthritis over 12 months. Arthritis Rheum 2003;48(9):S486.

8. Majka DS, Holers VM. Can we accurately predict the development of rheumatoid arthritis in the preclinical phase? Arthritis Rheum 2003;48:2701–2705.

9. Bizzaro N, Mazzanti G, Tonutti E, Villalta D, Tozzoli R. Diagnostic accuracy of the anti-citrulline antibody assay for rheumatoid arthritis. Clin Chem 2001;47:1089–1093.

10. Meyer O, Labarre C, Dougados M, Goupille P, Cantagrel A, Dubois A, Nicaise-Roland P, Sibilia J, Combe B. Anticitrullinated protein/peptide antibody assays in early rheumatoid arthritis for predicting five year radiographic damage. Ann Rheum Dis 2003;62:120–126.

11. Vencovsky J, Machacek S, Sedova L, Kafkova J, Gatterova J, Pesakova V, Ruzickova S. Autoantibodies can be prognostic markers of an erosive disease in early rheumatoid arthritis. Ann Rheum Dis 2003;62:427–430.

12. Cambridge G, Leandro MJ, Edwards JC, Ehrenstein MR, Salden M, Bodman-Smith M, Webster AD. Serologic changes following B lymphocyte depletion therapy for rheumatoid arthritis. Arthritis Rheum 2003;48:2146–2154.

13. Christgau S, Garnero P, Fledelius C, Moniz C, Ensig M, Gineyts E, Rosenquist C, Qvist P. Collagen type II C-telopeptide fragments as an index of cartilage degradation. Bone 2001;29:209–215.

14. Black DM, Greenspan SL, Ensrud KE, Palermo L, McGowan JA, Lang TF, Garnero P, Bouxsein ML, Bilezikian JP, Rosen CJ. The effects of parathyroid hormone and alendronate alone or in combination in postmenopausal osteoporosis. N Engl J Med 2003;349:1207–1215.

15. Eastell R, Barton I, Hannon RA, Chines A, Garnero P, Delmas PD. Relationship of early changes in bone resorption to the reduction in fracture risk with risedronate. J Bone Mineral Res 2003;18:1051–1056.

16. Ravn P, Thompson DE, Ross PD, Christiansen C. Biochemical markers for prediction of 4-year response in bone mass during bisphosphonate treatment for prevention of postmenopausal osteoporosis. Bone 2003;33:150–158.

17. Garnero P, Jouvenne P, Buchs N, Delmas PD, Miossec P. Uncoupling of bone metabolism in rheumatoid arthritis patients with or without joint destruction: assessment with serum type I collagen breakdown products. Bone 1999;24:381–385.

18. Garnero P, Landewe R, Boers M, Verhoeven A, Van Der Linden S, Christgau S, Van Der Heijde D, Boonen A, Geusens P. Association of baseline levels of markers of bone and cartilage degradation with long-term progression of joint damage in patients with early rheumatoid arthritis: the COBRA study. Arthritis Rheum 2002;46:2847–2856.

19. Verhoeven AC, Boers M, te Koppele JM, van der Laan WH, Markusse HM, Geusens P, van der Linden S. Bone turnover, joint damage and bone mineral density in early rheumatoid arthritis treated with combination therapy including high-dose prednisolone. Rheumatology 2001;40:1231–1237.

20. Aman S, Paimela L, Leirisalo-Repo M, Risteli J, Kautiainen H, Helve T, Hakala M. Prediction of disease progression in early rheumatoid arthritis by ICTP, RF and CRP. A comparative 3-year follow-up study. Rheumatology 2000;39:1009–1013.

21. Hermann J, Mueller T, Fahrleitner A, Dimai HP. Early onset and effective inhibition of bone resorption in patients with rheumatoid arthritis treated with the tumour necrosis factor alpha antibody infliximab. Clin Exp Rheumatol 2003;21:473–476.

22. Cole TG, Leary ET, Lobaugh B, Foster AP. Multi-site technical assessment of three biomarkers of bone metabolism on the Roche Elecsys® series of immunoanalyzers. Clin Chem 2004;50 (Suppl):A93.
23. Mehta N, Malootian Ar, Leary ET, et al. Six-month bone turnover marker results following daily treatment with Fortical® calcitonin nasal spray. J Bone Mineral Res 2004;19(Suppl 1):S312, SU451.
24. Ebeling PR. Potential candidates for bone turnover makers — N-telopeptide cross-links of type I collagen (NTX). In Eastell R, Baumann M, Hoyle NR, Wieczorek L, eds. Bone markers: biochemical and clinical perspectives. London: Martin Dunitz, 2001:27–38.
25. Cortet B, Guyot MH, Solau E, Pigny P, Dumoulin F, Flipo RM, Marchandise X, Delcambre B. Factors influencing bone loss in rheumatoid arthritis: a longitudinal study. Clin Exp Rheumatol 2000;18:683–690.
26. Sassi ML, Eriksen H, Risteli L, Niemei S, Mansell J, Gowen M, Risteli J. Immunochemical characterization of assay for carboxyterminal telopeptide of human type I collagen: loss of antigenicity by treatment with cathepsin K. Bone 2000;26:367–373.
27. Hakala M, Risteli L, Manelius J, Nieminen P, Risteli J. Increased type I collagen degradation correlates with disease severity in rheumatoid arthritis. Ann Rheum Dis 1993;52:866–869.
28. Hakala M, Abo K, Aman S, Luukkainen R, Kauppi M, Risteli J. Type I collagen degradation does not diminish with RA disease duration. Ann Rheum Dis 2001;60:420–422.
29. Kotaniemi A, Isomaki H, Hakala M, Risteli L, Risteli J. Increased type I collagen degradation in early rheumatoid arthritis. J Rheumatol 1994;21:1593–1596.
30. Paimela L, Leirisalo-Repo M, Risteli L, Hakala M, Helve T, Risteli J. Type I collagen degradation product in serum of patients with early rheumatoid arthritis: relationship to disease activity and radiological progression in a 3-year follow-up. Br J Rheumatol 1994;33:1012–1016.
31. Cortet B, Flipo RM, Pigny P, Duquesnoy B, Racadot A, Boersma A, Delcambre B. How useful are bone turnover markers in rheumatoid arthritis? Influence of disease activity and corticosteroid therapy. Rev Rhum Engl Ed 1997;64:153–159.
32. Jensen T, Hansen M, Madsen JC, Kollerup G, Stoltenberg M, Florescu A, Schwarz P. Serum levels of parathyroid hormone and markers of bone metabolism in patients with rheumatoid arthritis. Relationship to disease activity and glucocorticoid treatment. Scand J Clin Lab Invest 2001;61:491–501.
33. Sassi ML, Aman S, Hakala M, Luukkainen R, Risteli J. Assay for cross-linked carboxyterminal telopeptide of type I collagen (ICTP) unlike CrossLaps assay reflects increased pathological degradation of type I collagen in rheumatoid arthritis. Clin Chem Lab Med 2003;41: 1038–1044.
34. St Clair EW, Moak SA, Wilkinson WE, Sanders L, Lang T, Greenwald RA. A cross sectional analysis of 5 different markers of collagen degradation in rheumatoid arthritis. J Rheumatol 1998;25:1472–1479.
35. Al-Awadhi A, Olusi S, Al-Zaid N, Prabha K. Serum concentrations of interleukin 6, osteocalcin, intact parathyroid hormone, and markers of bone resorption in patients with rheumatoid arthritis. J Rheumatol 1999;26:1250–1256.
36. Seriolo B, Ferretti V, Sulli A, Caratto E, Fasciolo D, Cutolo M. Serum osteoclacin levels in premenopausal rheumatoid arthritis patients. Ann N Y Acad Sci 2002;966:502–507.
37. Valleala H, Laasonen L, Koivula MK, Mandelin J, Friman C, Risteli J, Konttinen YT. Two year randomized controlled trial of etidronate in rheumatoid arthritis: changes in serum aminoterminal telopeptides correlate with radiographic progression of disease. J Rheumatol 2003;30:468–473.
38. Qvist P, Christgau S, Pedersen BJ, Schlemmer A, Christainsen C. Circadian variation in the serum concentration of C-terminal telopeptide of type I collagen (serum CTx): effects of gender, age, menopausal status, posture, daylight, serum cortisol, and fasting. Bone 2002;31: 57–61.
39. Clowes JA, Hannon RA, Yap TS, Hoyle NR, Blumsohn A, Eastell R. Effect of feeding on bone turnover markers and its impact on biological variability of measurements. Bone 2002;30: 886–890.

40. Mouritzen U, Christgau S, Lehmann HJ, Tanko LB, Chritiansen C. Cartilage turnover assessed with a newly developed assay measuring collagen type II degradation products: influence of age, sex, menopause, hormone replacement therapy, and body mass index. Ann Rheum Dis 2003;62:332–336.

41. Garnero P, Piperno M, Gineyts E, Christgau S, Delmas PD, Vignon E. Cross sectional evaluation of biochemical markers of bone, cartilage, and synovial tissue metabolism in patients with knee osteoarthritis: relations with disease activity and joint damage. Ann Rheum Dis 2001;60:619–626.

42. Garnero P, Conrozier T, Christgau S, Mathieu P, Delmas PD, Vignon E. Urinary type II collagen C-telopeptide levels are increased in patients with rapidly destructive hip osteoarthritis. Ann Rheum Dis 2003;62:939–943.

43. Garnero P, Mazieres B, Gueguen A, Abbal M, Berdah L, Lequesne M, Nguyen M, Salles JP, Vignon E, Dougados M. Cross-sectional association of 10 molecular markers of bone, cartilage, and synovium with disease activity and radiological joint damage in patients with hip osteoarthritis: The ECHODIAH cohort. J Rheumatol 2005;32: 697–703.

44. Conrozier T, Saxne T, Fan CSS, Mathieu P, Tron AM, Heinegard D, Vignon E. Serum concentration of cartilage oligomeric matrix protein and bone sialoprotein in hip osteoarthritis: a one-year prospective study. Ann Rheum Dis 1998;57:527–532.

45. Den Broeder AA, Joosten LAB, Saxne T, Heinegard D, Fenner H, Miltenburg AMM, Frasa WLH, van Tits LJ, Buurman WA, van Riel PLCM, van de Putte LBA, Barrera P. Long term anti-tumour necrosis factor α monotherapy in rheumatoid arthritis: effect on radiological course and prognostic value of markers of cartilage turnover and endothelial activation. Ann Rheum Dis 2002;61:311–318.

46. Crnkic M, Mansson B, Larsson L, Geborek P, Heinegard D, Saxne T. Serum cartilage oligomeric matrix protein (COMP) decreases in rheumatoid arthritis patients treated with infliximab or etanercept. Arthritis Res Ther 2003;5:R181–R185.

47. D'Elia HF, Christgau S, Mattsson LA, Saxne T, Ohlsson C, Nordborg E, Carlsten H. Hormone replacement therapy, calcium and vitamin D_3 versus calcium and vitamin D_3 alone decreases markers of cartilage and bone metabolism in rheumatoid arthritis: a randomized controlled trial. Arthritis Res Ther 2004;6:R457–R468.

48. Sharif M, Kirwan JR, Elson CJ, Granell R, Clarke S. Suggestion of nonlinear or phasic progression of knee osteoarthritis based on measurments of serum cartilage oligomeric matrix protein levels over five years. Arthritis Rheum 2004;50(8):2479–2488.

49. Harvey S, Weisman M, O'Dell J, Scott T, Krusemeier M, Visor J, Swindlehurst C. Chondrex: new marker of joint disease. Clin Chem 1998;44:509–516.

50. Vos K, Steenbakkers P, Miltenburg AMM, Bos E, van den Heuvel MW, van Hogezand RA, de Vries RRP, Breedveld FC, Boots AMH. Raised human cartilage glycoprotein-39 plasma levels in patients with rheumatoid arthritis and other inflammatory conditions. Ann Rheum Dis 2000;59:544–548.

51. Bernardi D, Podswiadek M, Zaninotto M, Punzi L, Plebani M. YKL-40 as a marker of joint involvement in inflammatory bowel disease. Clin Chem 2003;49:1685–1688.

52. Conrozier T, Carlier MC, Mathieu P, Colson F, Debard AL, Richard S, Favret H, Bienvenu J, Vignon E. Serum levels of YKL-40 and C reactive protein in patients with hip osteoarthritis and healthy subjects: a cross sectional study. Ann Rheum Dis 2000;59: 828–831.

53. Register TC, Carlson CS, Adams MR. Serum YKL-40 is associated with osteoarthritis and atherosclerosis in nonhuman primates. Clin Chem 2001;47:2159–2161.

54. Mansson B, Carey D, Alini M, Ionescu M, Rosenberg LC, Poole AR, Heinegard D, Saxne T. Cartilage and bone metabolism in rheumatoid arthritis. Differences between rapid and slow progression of disease identified by serum markers of cartilage metabolism. J Clin Invest 1995;95:1071–1077.

55. Garnero P, Ayral X, Rousseau JC, Christgau S, Sandell LJ, Dougados M, Delmas PD. Uncoupling of type II collagen synthesis and degradation predicts progression of joint damage in patients with knee osteoarthritis. Arthritis Rheum 2002;46:2613–2624.

56. Rousseau JC, Zhu Y, Miossec P, Vignon E, Sandell LJ, Garnero P, Delmas PD. Serum levels of type IIA procollagen amino terminal propeptide (PIIANP) are decreased in patients with knee osteoarthritis and rheumatoid arthritis. Osteoarthritis Cartilage 2004;12: 440–447.

57. Squires GR, Okouneff S, Ionescu M, Poole AR. The pathogenesis of focal lesion development in aging human articular cartilage and molecular matrix changes characteristic of osteoarthritis. Arthritis Rheum 2003;48:1261–1270.

58. Sharif M, George E, Dieppe PA. Synovial fluid and serum concentrations of amino-terminal propeptide of type III procollagen in healthy volunteers and patients with joint disease. Ann Rheum Dis 1996;55:47–51.

59. Hakala M, Aman S, Luukkainen R, Risteli L, Kauppi M, Nieminen P, Risteli J. Application of markers of collagen metabolism in serum and synovial fluid for assessment of disease process in patients with rheumatoid arthritis. Ann Rheum Dis 1995;54:886–890.

60. Sharif M, Salisbury C, Taylor DJ, Kirwan JR. Changes in biochemical markers of joint tissue metabolism in a randomized controlled trial of glucocorticoid in early rheumatoid arthritis. Arthritis Rheum 1998;41:1203–1209.

61. Zachariae H, Heickendorff L, Sogaard H. The value of amino-terminal propeptide of type III procollagen in routine screening for methotrexate-induced liver fibrosis: a 10-year follow-up. Br J Dermatol 2001;144:100–103.

62. Sondergaard K, Heickendorff L, Risteli L, Risteli J, Zachariae H, Stengaard-Pedersen K, Deleuran B. Increased levels of type I and III collagen and hyaluronan in scleroderma skin. Br J Dermatol 1997;136:47–53.

63. Traba ML, Calero JA, Mendez-Davila C, Garcia-Moreno C, de la Piedra C. Different behaviors of serum and urinary CrossLaps ELISA in the assessment of bone resorption in healthy girls. Clin Chem 1999;45:682–683.

64. Hannon RA, Clowes JA, Eagleton AC, Hadari AA, Eastell R, Blumsohn A. Clinical performance of immunoreactive tartrate-resistant acid phosphatase isoform 5b as a marker of bone resorption. Bone 2004;34:187–194.

65. Mundermann A, Dyrby CO, Andriacchi TP, King KB. Serum concentration of cartilage oligomeric matrix protein (COMP) is sensitive to physiological cyclic loading in healthy adults. Osteoarthritis Cartilage 2005;13:34–38.

66. Leary ET, McLaughlin MK, Swezey D, Aggoune T, Carlson TH, Foster AP. Evaluation of serum bone turnover markers in renal dialysis patients. J Bone Mineral Res 2000;15(Suppl 1):S525.

67. Spector TD, Conaghan PG, Buckland-Wright JC, et al. Effect of risedronate on joint structure and symptoms of knee osteoarthritis: results of the BRISK randomized, controlled trial. Arthritis Res Ther 2005;7:R625–R633.

Chapter 12
Data Analysis and Presentation: Writing a Paper for Publication

Derek Pearson

Introduction

The extent to which your clinical trial will contribute to the greater scientific good will depend, to a great degree, on the quality of the presentation and dissemination of the results. Your trial is likely to be one of many that addresses the research question you have posed. In some cases, the treatment effect will be overestimated, and results, particularly from small trials, will be contradictory. The results from a number of trials will probably have to be combined in order to get a true picture of the effectiveness of a new molecular entity (NME). Ideally, the report of your trial will be of sufficient quality to be included in a meta-analysis and demonstrate the effectiveness of your intervention in the treatment of osteoarthritis (OA) or rheumatoid arthritis (RA). There are, unfortunately, a number of limitations that are common when writing up trials that lead to bias and the exclusion of studies from subsequent meta-analysis. These include [1]:

1. Use of multiple end points. (Measure 20 things on a patient—one is bound to be significant. Result: a publication).
2. Use of surrogate end points (e.g., a 20% improvement in the American College of Rheumatology [ACR] core data set—ACR20 as a surrogate for clinical outcome).
3. Too many subgroup analyses.
4. Incorrect analysis of repeated measures
5. Too many treatment groups in one study.
6. Small study numbers.

The standard of reporting of clinical trials has improved significantly over the years, but a review of the journals will reveal many of these inadequacies are still present. This is an ethical problem for investigators. For trials to provide a sound basis for effective treatment of OA/RA, they must be well designed, well executed,

D. Pearson
Clinical Director, Medical Physics, City Hospital, Nottingham, UK

D.M. Reid, C.G. Miller (eds.), *Clinical Trials in Rheumatoid Arthritis and Osteoarthritis*, 171
© Springer-Verlag London Limited 2008

and well reported. Badly executed and badly reported studies are of little benefit to patients.

The aim of this chapter is to present the results from a small study in a way that is adequate for publication. A disclaimer is needed, however: The sample data is test data and is provided so that the reader can check his sums when implementing an analysis. It does not stand up to close scrutiny against the standards laid out in this chapter, but allows calculations to be simply implemented and checked in many of the common spreadsheet and statistics packages. The chapter will also take as an example only a randomized, double-blind, controlled trial. The principles will apply to other designs of trial but the detailed statistics may not (e.g., crossover trials). A detailed description of common statistical tests (e.g., paired t tests) is not included, but analysis of variance applied to longitudinal data is covered in some detail.

The CONSORT Statement

The CONSORT statement was published in 1996 [2, 3] as a response to the "wide chasm between what a trial should report and what is actually published in the literature." It provides a checklist and flowchart that allow authors and reviewers to check that a trial is adequately reported. It provides six headings and five subheadings that can be used within a publication to allow readers to make a judgment about the trial in a standardized format (Table 12.1). The subheadings are

- Title: Make sure the title describes the type of trial (e.g., randomized, double-blind, crossover, etc.).
- Abstract: Make use of a structured format in the abstract (see the "Abstract" section later).
- Method:

  ○ Protocol: Describe the study population, together with the inclusion and exclusion criteria, the interventions and their timing, the primary and secondary outcome measures, the minimum important differences in those measures, and indicate how the proposed sample size was calculated. Describe the methods for statistical analyses and whether an intention-to-treat analysis was undertaken. If appropriate, describe any stopping rules.
  ○ Assignment: Describe the method used to assign subjects to the different treatment arms of the trial
- Blinding: Describe the methods used to blind the study, including the appearance and taste of capsules (if appropriate).

  Results:

  ○ Patient flow: Use a flowchart to show the patient flow through the trials (Fig. 12.1).
  ○ Analysis: State the effect of intervention on primary and secondary outcome measures. Remember to include confidence intervals. Always give results in

Table 12.1 The headings and content that are recommended are included by the CONSORT statement

Heading	Subheading	Description
Title		Identify the study as a randomized trial.
Abstract		Use a structured format.
Introduction		State prospectively defined hypothesis, clinical objectives, and planned subgroup or covariate analyses.
Methods	Protocol	Describe
		• Planned study population, together with inclusion/ exclusion criteria.
		• Planned interventions and their timing.
		• Primary and secondary outcome measure(s) and the minimum important difference(s), and indicate how the target sample size was projected.
		• Rationale and methods for statistical analyses, detailing main comparative analyses and whether they were completed on an intention-to-treat basis.
		• Prospectively defined stopping rules (if warranted).
	Assignment	Describe
		• Unit of randomization (e.g., individual, cluster, geographic).
		• Method used to generate the allocation schedule.
		• Method of allocation concealment and timing of assignment.
		• Method to separate the generator from the executor of assignment.
	Masking (Blinding)	Describe mechanism (e.g., capsules, tablets); similarity of treatment characteristics (e.g., appearance, taste): allocation schedule control (location of code during trial and when broken); and evidence for successful blinding among participants, person doing intervention, outcome assessors, and data analysts.
Results	Participant flow and follow-up	Provide a trial profile summarizing participant flow, numbers and timing of randomization assignment, interventions and measurements for each randomized group.
	Analysis	State estimated effect of intervention on primary and secondary outcome measures, including a point estimate and measure of precision (confidence interval).
		State results in absolute numbers when feasible (e.g., 10 of 20, not 50%).
		Present summary data and appropriate descriptive and inferential statistics in sufficient detail to permit alternative analyses and replication.
		Describe prognostic variables by treatment group and any attempt to adjust for them.
		Describe protocol deviations from the study as planned, together with the reasons.
Comment		State specific interpretation of study findings, including sources of bias and imprecision (internal validity) and discussion of external validity, including appropriate quantitative measures when possible.
		State general interpretation of the data in light of the totality of the available evidence.

Source: Reproduced with permission from *JAMA*.

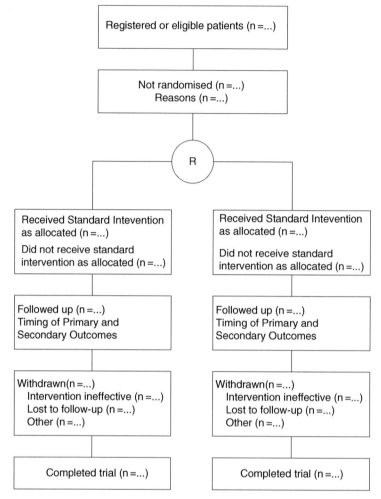

Fig. 12.1 Flowchart describing the progress of patients through a randomized trial. R, randomization. (Reproduced with permission from JAMA.)

absolute numbers where possible (e.g., "17 of 34 patients" rather than "50% of patients"). Present the summary data and statistical analysis in such a way that your results can be duplicated by someone else and the results can be used usefully in, for example, a meta-analysis.

- Comment: Present an interpretation of the study findings that is supported by the evidence (i.e., do not try and overinterpret your data). Identify any limitations and bias within your study. Put your conclusions within the context of the evidence available in the wider literature.

There is a useful bibliography in the statement that supports the inclusion of most of the descriptors. The flowchart provides information about the progress of patients through a randomized, controlled trial with two groups. An example is given in Figure 12.1. This is the most common type of trial, but the guidance in the chart can be applied to more complex trials with appropriate modification. The CONSORT statement will help you review the quality of published clinical trials and in writing the report of your trial.

The Title

The title of your report should describe, factually, the nature of the trial. In order to get a snappy title and grab the attention of readers, the title itself often introduces bias by overselling the interpretation or power of the study (known as "flashy-title" bias [4]). For example, a flashy title might be "Etanercept improves patient outcome in rheumatoid arthritis." This makes the assumption that the ACR definition of improvement is an adequate surrogate for clinical outcome. It does not mention the study population (e.g., patients with chronic RA) and so implies that it is generally applicable. The title should include the facts (if appropriate) that the trial is randomized, blinded, whether it is placebo-controlled or active comparator, and a description of the patient group. A better title for such a paper could be "A randomized, double-blind, methotrexate-controlled trial of etanercept in patients with chronic rheumatoid arthritis." Readers will immediately be able to assess the intervention, the outcome, and the study group and have some assurance that the trial was conducted in a proper manner to a proper study design. First impressions count!

The Abstract

First impressions are so important that the title and abstract of the paper are often the only part that readers ever read thoroughly. There will be a quick glance at the pictures and a scan of the conclusion. If it looks interesting, it will get photocopied and be put in the reading pile only to be moved deeper into the filing system at a later stage. It is vital, therefore, that the abstract is structured in such a way as to get across the main facts of the paper, including the magnitude of the treatment differences. This will reduce the length of time that a reader requires to make a critical appraisal of your paper and allow accurate searching of published abstracts when carrying out a structured review.

The Ad Hoc Working Group for Critical Appraisal of the Medical Literature has proposed guidelines for structured abstracts [5]. The guidelines propose dividing the abstract into seven sections. These are

1. Objective: What is the objective or question addressed in the paper?
2. Design: Describe the study design. Is it randomized, blinded, controlled? Is it a crossover trial? Is it case-controlled, a survey, cost-benefit, or cost-effectiveness analysis?

3. Setting: It is important to describe the context of the study so that the reader can assess whether it is applicable in their own circumstances. Is it primary or secondary care?

4. Patients/other participants: Describe the patient group studied, the number of participants including how many were eligible and refused to take part, the number of withdrawals, and the number completing the study. Include the number of patients withdrawn because of adverse events and summarize the nature of those events. Summarize the selection procedures (e.g., random, consecutive cases, volunteers) and major inclusion and exclusion criteria.

5. Intervention: Describe the duration and method of administration of the main intervention using generic as well as brand names of drugs used.

6. Measurements and main results: Describe the main measurements used in the study and provide an explanation of the measurement if a novel or unusual measurement is made. Describe the results. Report non-significant findings in the abstract as well to avoid bias. In a survey of three reputable journals, it was found that 70% of significant findings were reported in the abstract compared with only 25% of non-significant findings [1]. Report the statistical significance of the results quoting the actual significance level rather than an arbitrary cutoff.

7. Conclusion: The study conclusion should be supported by the main results quoted in the abstract. State if further trials are required before the NME is used in routine clinical practice for the clinical indication described in the paper.

The nonstructured abstract and structured abstract for the example study are shown in Tables 12.2 and 12.3. The structured abstract is longer than the unstructured abstract but gives the major points of the paper to allow the reader to know that this paper will be of interest. It avoids flashy-title bias and does not make unsubstantiated claims about the benefits of etanercept.

Table 12.2 Nonstructured abstract

Etanercept improves patient outcome in rheumatoid arthritis.
Seven hundred seventy-nine patients with rheumatoid arthritis were recruited to a study and treated for 12 months with etanercept (25 mg twice weekly injection) or methotrexate (20 mg oral weekly). Sharp score deteriorated less in the etanercept group ($p = 0.02$). ACR20 and nACR showed greater improvement at 4 months in the etanercept group, although by 12 months there was no significant difference between the groups. There were fewer adverse events in the etanercept group apart from the rate of reactions at the injection site. In conclusion, etanercept improves outcome in patients with rheumatoid arthritis, with a lower rate of adverse events than methotrexate.

Table 12.3 Structured abstract

A randomized, double-blind, methotrexate-controlled, multicenter trial of etanercept in patients with long-standing rheumatoid arthritis.

Study objective: To determine the efficacy and safety of etanercept in the treatment of rheumatoid arthritis.

Design: Randomized, double-blind, methotrexate-controlled trial with a 12-month treatment period.

Setting: Hospital rheumatoid arthritis clinics in 12 centers in Europe and the United States.

Patients: Seven hundred seventy-nine patients with long-standing rheumatoid arthritis were recruited to the study. Patients with at least 5 bone erosions on radiograph, at least 10 swollen joints, 15 tender or painful joints, an ESR of at least 28 mm per hour, and morning stiffness of at least 45 minutes duration were recruited to the study. Disease-modifying drugs were discontinued at least 4 weeks before the study. Eighty-four percent of patients completed 12 months of treatment. Ninety-two percent were evaluated in the intention to treat analysis.

Interventions: Twice weekly subcutaneous etanercept (25 mg) or weekly oral methotrexate (20 mg) for 12 months.

Measurements and main results: Sharp score, ACR20 and nACR, and health-related quality of life were measured every 2 months. An intention to treat analysis was undertaken. ACR20 and nACR were significantly higher in the etanercept group at 4 months (etanercept: ACR20 65%, nACR 36%; methotrexate: ACR20 52%, nACR 24%; $p < 0.05$). These differences were not maintained at 12 months (etanercept: ACR20 63%, nACR 40%; methotrexate: ACR20 59%, nACR 36%; NS). Sharp score rose by 2.4 ± 1.5 in the methotrexate group and 0.8 ± 0.7 in the etanercept group ($p = 0.02$). There were significantly more reactions at the injection site with etanercept (35% compared with 4%, $p < 0.0001$), but other adverse events were significantly lower than with methotrexate (e.g., nausea 14% compared with 32%, $p < 0.0001$).

Conclusions: Etanercept taken over 12 months is effective and safe in the control of rheumatoid arthritis. Improvement in outcome occurred sooner than with methotrexate and was maintained over 12 months. Although there were more reactions at the injection site, the number of adverse events was lower with etanercept.

What Should Be in the Introduction?

That first sentence! How we struggle over the wording of that first sentence. It is usually a warm, comforting phrase, designed to capture the readers' attention and draw them into the rest of the paper. It often introduces bias by overstating the size of the research question. "Osteoarthritis is a major cause of disability and of work-related absence in the UK." True, but your small trial is not going to solve that problem overnight. The introduction should again be factual and state the *prospectively* defined research hypothesis.

Method

The CONSORT statement discussed previously is particularly helpful in structuring the method section. In describing the protocol, the planned study population and the way in which patients were approached should be described. Was it by random selection from a general practice list? Was it by advertisement in the clinic? Were consecutive patients who met the inclusion criteria of the study approached in clinic? The method of recruitment can introduce bias, and reviewers will find life much easier if there is a clear description of the recruitment process. Describe also the inclusion and exclusion criteria in detail.

The primary outcome measure in the sample study was a numeric ACR (nACR; discussed later). Disease activity was calculated as the lowest percentage change in the number of tender joints, the number of swollen joints, and the median percentage improvement in the ACR core set measures. Describe in detail exactly how the ACR core data-set measures were obtained. Did you use Likert or visual analog scales to measure pain score and the physician's assessment? Which validated questionnaire did you use to measure self-assessed physical disability? Was erythrocyte sedimentation rate (ESR) or C-reactive protein level used to measure the acute-phase reactant value? This will allow the reader to understand the differences between your version of the ACR improvement criteria and theirs. The issues surrounding the use of nACR are discussed further later in the chapter.

The method should report the study design. In this case, the study design was based on response in previous studies involving etanercept where, at 12 months, 65% of patients reported an ACR20 response. Given that this was an active comparator equivalence trial, the clinically relevant equivalence margin was taken to be 10% following a review of previous studies. A study with 80% power of detecting a 10% difference between treatment and active comparator would require 376 patients in each arm of the study. Allowing for dropout, the study aimed to recruit 400 patients into each arm of the study.

The method should also describe the proposed statistical analysis. This should be more than the name of the statistics package used on your PC to carry out the analysis, rather a description of the statistical methods used and why they were chosen. In this case, as described later, it was planned to examine the normality of study data using the Shapiro-Francia W' test and use an analysis of variance (ANOVA) to compare the data at baseline for differences between treatment groups and centers in continuous variables. One of two possible ANOVA models was to be used to analyze the longitudinal outcome data. Where data was not normally distributed, a Kruskal-Wallis test was used to compare variables at baseline for group and center effects and at the end of the study to compare outcome. The percentage of patients with ACR20, ACR50, and ACR70 responses were compared using chi-square tests.

Intention-to-Treat Analysis and Missing Values

The treatment of missing values and whether the analysis was carried out on an intention-to-treat basis should also be included in the method. Patients leave clinical trials at all stages and for many reasons (or no reason at all), even in a well-designed and well-run trial. They may leave after randomization and before treatment when it is found that they do not meet the inclusion criteria. They may drop out of the trial for valid reasons or treatment may be stopped because of adverse events. It is important to document the number recruited, the number randomized, and the number who can be evaluated. This last category should be decided during study design and may be only patients who complete the study, those who have an acceptable number of missing values, or those who have completed a minimum number of observations. An intention-to-treat (ITT) analysis includes all patients that the investigator intended to treat but may have dropped out for a variety of reasons. Frequently in a drug trial, a modified ITT analysis is used only to include subjects who took at least one dose of study medication. The argument is that this will give a more realistic view of the treatment effect in real life, as patients will fail to comply with treatment in the clinical setting. There must be sufficient outcome data that can be evaluated to proceed with the analysis. It has to be used carefully, because the handling of missing values in the outcome data can bias the outcome and lead to an over- or underestimate of treatment effect.

Missing values can be handled in a number of ways. If it is the case, for example, that a patient was measured at 4 months posttreatment and 12 months posttreatment, but missed the 8-month visit, some form of interpolation is acceptable. Linear interpolation is the simplest model. If the missing values are at the end of the study due to patient dropout, a measurement of the primary outcome variable must be made if possible or the method of carrying forward the last observation can be used. This last method is biased if the patient dropped out because of side effects or adverse events as the treatment effect will be overestimated. If the patient drops out of the study early, carrying forward the last observation may be invalid without supporting follow-up information. For example, if much of the improvement in disease activity is the first few months of treatment, it may be valid to carry forward an 8-month observation to the end of the study. Where change is slower and over a longer period of time, the 8-month measurement may give an inadequate estimate of treatment effect. Again, judgment has to be used based on the knowledge of similar NMEs and their effect on clinical outcome. Another method of filling in missing values at the end of the study is to assign the average change in the placebo or active comparator group to the final time point. This may underestimate the treatment effect in the study drug group but may reflect the reality of clinical use of the NME. If you want to be really sophisticated, add a random error to the interpolated value, based on the standard deviation of the measurement.

Randomization and Blinding

The aim of randomization is to ensure that there is a similar distribution of baseline variables in the treatment and control groups and that unknown factors that affect the outcome of the trial are evenly spread. How has randomization been carried out? In a multicenter trial, it is often done centrally, but patients can be stratified within the randomization on the basis of center or baseline variables that may affect outcome (e.g., age, duration of disease). The details of the method used to generate the allocation to each group and the method by which the investigators are blinded to that allocation should be described. For example, in many studies, block randomization is used. The randomization codes can be generated and held by the pharmacy department on behalf of the investigators particularly if it is a single-center study. Subjects can be randomized when they attended the pharmacy to collect their medication for the first time. This allows the randomization to be blinded to both the investigator and the patient.

The mechanism of delivery of the NME and control preparations should be described (e.g., capsule, tablet, or injection) as well as the similarity in appearance between the control and the NME preparation. This may include the taste and packaging of both preparations.

Any evidence that demonstrates the quality of the blinding should be included indicating how this facet of the study blinded the subjects themselves, the investigators, and those assessing outcome (e.g., research nurse or metrologists). Many sponsors, however, insist on radiographs being analyzed by an independent imaging core laboratory to remove interpretation bias and to minimize the interpretive variation. This is presented in Chapter 8.

Other Methodological Issues

It is important to include other issues in the method section that may bias the outcome to the study. This may include a discussion of the appropriate choice of outcome measure. It is important for investigators to recognize possible bias in study design and execution and include this within a publication. There are a large number of sources of bias [4, 6], and to acknowledge them within the publication provides evidence to other investigators that the trial has been thoughtfully designed.

Many journals will not publish without there being a reference to approval by the institutional review board/independent ethics committee (IRB/IEC) and a description of the informed consent process. This, and any other ethical considerations that arise from the trial, should be included in the method section.

Issues with Outcome Measures in RA and OA

Before we move on to discussing the results, it is important to take a minor diversion and consider some of the issues relating to outcome measures in RA and OA, in particular:

- Does the definition of the outcome measure lead to inherent difficulties in interpretation?
- Are the data normally distributed?
- What are the dangers of using Likert scales?

In many RA clinical trials, the clinical outcome is measured using the ACR Definition of Improvement [7], where the outcome variable is defined as the percentage of patients who demonstrate 20% improvement in tender joint count, swollen joint count, and at least three of the five other core set measures (ACR20). The core set measures are pain, patient and physician global assessments, self-assessed physical disability, and the acute-phase reactant value (ESR or C-reactive protein level). Pain and the patient and physician global assessments are measured using a 10-cm visual analog scale (VAS) or a Likert scale. Self-assessed physical disability can be measured using a range of validated questionnaires. There are a number of problems with this as an outcome measure. First, it is binary. The patient is either a responder or a nonresponder. It does not, therefore, provide a quantitative assessment that follows the disease activity. [8]. Second, it includes visual analog and/or Likert scales. Some of the problems concerning the use of these scales will be discussed later in this section. Third, in allowing a number of different questionnaires to be used to measure self-assessed physical disability, the ACR20 cannot be compared between studies where a different questionnaire has been used. For example, the Health Assessment Questionnaire (HAQ) demonstrates a greater treatment effect than the Arthritis Impact Measurement Scale (AIMS) [9]. The HAQ is more likely to demonstrate a 20% improvement than is AIMS. Fourth, 20% improvement does not comment at all on the clinical significance of the change. A pain score improvement from 9 cm to 7 cm on a VAS may be far more clinically significant that one from 2 cm to 1.6 cm (both demonstrate an approximate 20% improvement). Which is the real responder? Finally, in using the percentage change, the researcher is dependent on the baseline value of the core set measures being precise. The minimum significant clinical difference in pain scores on a VAS is between 10 mm and 18 mm, so that a 20% decrease may not be clinically significant [10, 11]. If a patient scores on the high side at the first visit, then they may be more likely to demonstrate a 20% reduction than a patient who scores low, thus may become a responder rather than a nonresponder.

In an attempt to address some of the problems of ACR20, the numeric ACR (nACR) has been developed [8]. Disease activity is calculated as the lowest percentage change in the number of tender joints, the number of swollen joints, and the median percentage improvement in the core set measures. Where the nACR is calculated at a number of time points, the area under the curve can be calculated. Although these provide a quantitative measure of disease activity, they still depend greatly on the baseline value of the core set measures. The moral here is that the researcher should always look at the raw data as well as the composite definitions of response such as ACR20, nACR, and area under the curve to ensure that the outcome is a true reflection of the clinical significance of the changes.

A number of the outcome measures used in RA and OA are not normally distributed; for example, grip strength and walking speed in RA [12], loss of joint space in OA [13], and change in 28 swollen joint count [14]. The absolute change in disease activity score in 28 swollen and tender joints (DAS28), which also includes ESR or C-reactive protein (CRP), is normally distributed [14]. Do not, however, assume data is normal or non-normal without testing it first, because what may apply in one study population may not apply in yours.

Beware also that the mean a variable from baseline may well be dominated by a small number of patients who exhibit a large change. This has been demonstrated in the change in Sharp score in the TEMPO trial [15]. There, they plotted the cumulative probability of the change in Sharp score at 1 year. What is clear is that the majority of changes were close to 0, and it was the small number of positive extremes that had the major impact on the mean change in Sharp score. Such plots may be useful in gaining a better understanding of the data.

We have already touched on the issue of reproducibility in VAS and Likert scales. Likert scales, in particular, pose a problem in analysis. They are not continuous and should not be treated as a continuous variable in a statistical analysis. A 6-point scale (avoid Likert scales with an odd number of points as responses will always tend toward the middle) that goes from "Worst Possible Pain" to "No Pain" may not represent linear gradation of pain in the patient's mind—going from 3 to 4 may not be the same as going from 4 to 5. What is a 20% change in a Likert scale? Researchers should always look carefully at the distribution of responses to a Likert scale, as very different distributions can give the same mean and standard deviation if analyzed using parametric statistics. It may be more appropriate to use VAS, particularly the VAS version of WOMAC for assessing disease activity in OA. These can be considered as continuous variables, although they may not be normally distributed.

Results

The main problem with the presentation of results is that there are two standards:

1. The results as the statistician insists are correct, but no one understands the words between the pictures.
2. The results are generally presented in a form understood by clinicians as the *lingua franca* of arthritis trials but are not statistically correct. An example would be multiple testing of repeated measures data, comparing the change in ACR20 at 4, 8, and 12 months using multiple single sample *t* tests.

It is important that the results of the study are reported in a manner that is both statistically robust and clearly understood by the readers. The aim of this section is to attempt this using the sample data provided.

At the start of the results section, summarize the progress of patients through the study. Use the CONSORT flowchart to help you (Fig. 12.1). The inability to recruit eligible patients, for example, may indicate a problem with the complexity of the trial design.

On entry to the trial, it is important to ensure that the control and treatment groups are the same and there are no center effects in a multicenter trial. This can be achieved with an analysis of the baseline variables that describe the demographics (e.g., age, BMI), severity of disease (e.g., duration of disease, baseline Sharp score, or biochemistry). This includes critical variables that are likely to affect the response to treatment or will be used as primary or secondary outcome measures and other factors that may affect outcome (e.g., use of concomitant therapy). There is always a temptation to collect too much information rather than too little. Take care in the selection of baseline comparisons, as multiple significance testing may confound the interpretation. Use only those variables that have some rationale in relation to the study as outlined above.

Although on the one hand I have advised against using too many variables within baseline comparisons so as to avoid the problems of multiple significance testing, many of the outcome measures used in OA and RA are defined in terms of percentage change in a set of core measures. My advice would be to always look at the raw data from the core set measures as well as use the composite response scores. The problems in using such outcome variables has been discussed previously, and the issue of using variables that are measures of percentage change will be addressed later. If you want a full understanding of the data, look at each of the core set measures individually. In the same way, when using the Sharp score, always look at the erosion score and joint space narrowing score as well as total Sharp score to gain a better insight into the effects of the study drug [15].

Categorical variables can be compared using simple chi-square or Fisher's exact tests. For example, on entry to a study, compare the difference in use of NSAIDs as concomitant therapy at baseline between the treatment and control group using a chi-square test (Table 12.4).

When considering continuous variables, such as baseline Sharp score or ESR, begin with a test of the normality of data. If there are sufficient numbers, test for the normality of data within each center. There are a number of tests that can be used. Skewness (a measure of the asymmetry of the distribution) and kurtosis (a measure of how pointed a distribution is) can be used although both are susceptible to bias because of outliers. The skewness (g) divided by the standard error of skewness is distributed according to the T distribution with $n - 1$ degrees of freedom, where n is the number of patients within the group tested. These are calculated as follows:

$$g = \frac{\sum_i (x_i - \overline{x})^3}{(n - 1)\,\sigma^3}.$$ (12.1)

Table 12.4 Concomitant use of NSAIDs by group at baseline*

	Concomitant use of NSAIDs	
	Yes	No
Etanercept	140	210
Methotrexate	135	232

*There is no significant difference between etanercept and methotrexate, $\chi^2 = 0.65$, p $= 0.42$.

If the t statistic is significant, then the distribution is not normal and nonparametric statistics should be used. Kurtosis and the standard error of kurtosis are calculated as follows:

$$SE_g = \sqrt{6/n} \tag{12.2}$$

$$k = \frac{\sum_i (x_i - \bar{x})^4}{(n-1)\sigma^4} \tag{12.3}$$

$$SE_k = \sqrt{24/n}. \tag{12.4}$$

Another method is to use the Shapiro-Francia W' test [16]. This uses a plot of the normal scores against the observed data. The normal score for each data point is calculated as the standardized normal deviate for each data point. First assemble the data in ascending order. Then calculate the expected cumulative frequency of each data point:

$$P_i = \frac{(i - 3/8)}{n + 1/4}. \tag{12.5}$$

The normal score N_i is the number of standard deviations above or below the mean for a data point in a series with the expected cumulative frequency of P_i and can be found in tables or calculated in Microsoft Excel using the NORMSINV function. The correlation coefficient of N_i against x_i is calculated. W' is the square of the correlation coefficient. The closer the value of W' is to 1, the more normal the distribution. W' has been tabulated to give the probability of the null hypothesis that W' is equal to 1 [16], with small values of W' indicating that the distribution is not normal. Figure 12.2 is an example of the normal score plot for Sharp score. The W' is 0.908. From tables, the probability of the null hypothesis that W' is 1.0 is p < 0.001 and therefore the distribution is non-normal. This is confirmed by the histogram plot (Fig. 12.3) and by the t statistic calculated from skewness, 4.45 (p < 0.001).

If the data does not follow a normal distribution, then non-parametric statistics can be used. These are detailed above. Alternatively, the data can be transformed so that it follows a normal distribution. The most common transformations are a log transform or square root transform [16]. For example, Fig. 12.4 is a histogram of VAS pain score measured on a 10-cm scale. It is clearly not normal, the median pain score is 19.6, and the t statistic calculated from skewness is 10.1 (p < 0.001). After log transformation (Fig. 12.5), the data is normalized (p = 0.09).

An analysis of variance (ANOVA) on baseline variables with patient group and center as factors can be used to test for baseline differences. The model used to test this is

$$Y_{ijk} = \mu + G_i + C_k + \varepsilon_{ijk}, \tag{12.6}$$

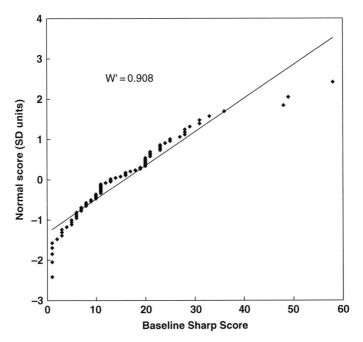

Fig. 12.2 Normal score plot of baseline Sharp score

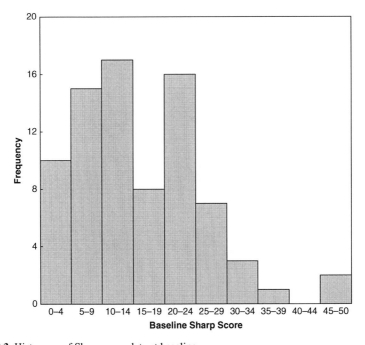

Fig. 12.3 Histogram of Sharp score data at baseline

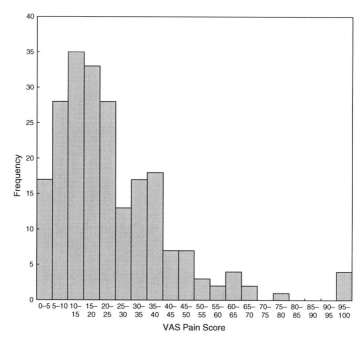

Fig. 12.4 Histogram of VAS showing skewed distribution

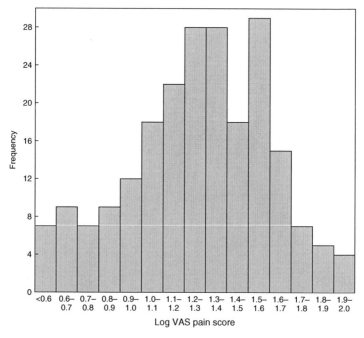

Fig. 12.5 Histogram of log-transformed VAS showing normal distribution

Table 12.5 ANOVA model used to test baseline differences

Source of variance	Sum of squares	df	Mean square	F
Group	$SSG = nm \sum_i (\bar{Y}_i - \bar{Y})^2$	$p - 1$	$MSG = \frac{SSG}{p-1}$	$\frac{MSG}{MSE}$
Center	$SSC = pm \sum_k (\bar{Y}_k - \bar{Y})^2$	$n - 1$	$MSC = \frac{SSC}{n-1}$	$\frac{MSC}{MSE}$
Residual	$SSE = SST - SSC - SSG$	$m - p - n + 1$	$MSE = -\frac{SSE}{m-p-n+1}$	
Total	$SST = \sum_i \sum_j \sum_k (Y_{ijk} - \bar{Y})^2$	$m - 1$		

where Y_{ijk} is the response of the jth subject in the ith patient group at the kth center, μ is the overall mean, G_i is the effect of ith patient group, C_k the effect of the kth center, and ε_{ijk} is the random error associated with measuring Y. Let there be p patient groups, m patients in total, and n centers. The ANOVA is given in Table 12.5.

In the example in Table 12.6, there is no significant effect of group or center on Sharp score at baseline. If there is a significant effect of either center, a post hoc range test will identify where the differences lie. There are a number of range tests that can be used including the Bonferroni method, the Scheffe method, the Tukey method, and Duncan's multiple range test [16]. They are all variations on a theme of the multiple t-test corrected for the number of comparisons made. The simplest is to calculate a t value for the comparison:

$$t = t_{p,df} \sqrt{SSE^2 \left(\frac{1}{m_1} + \frac{1}{m_2} \right)}, \tag{12.7}$$

where SSE is the residual sum of squares from the ANOVA, and $t_{p,df}$ is the t value for the desired level of significance, p, and the residual degrees of freedom, df, in the ANOVA. The level of significance is corrected for the number of possible comparisons that can be made. In this case with two groups and two centers, there are six possible comparisons. Thus, instead of using a significance level of $p = 0.05$, a significance level of $p = 0.0083$ is used. If the difference in mean WOMAC score between the control group at center A and the treatment group at center B, for example, is greater than the t value for comparison, then there is a significant difference between those two groups.

Table 12.6 ANOVA model testing for testing in differences in Sharp score at baseline between group and between center

Source of variation	Sum of squares	df	Mean square	F	Significance of F
Group	4.3	1	4.3	0.044	p = 0.835
Center	135.0	1	135.0	1.387	p = 0.244
Residual	5549.3	57	97.4		
Total	5688.6	59			

The investigator then has to consider the reason any significant difference has occurred and make a judgment about the clinical significance of the difference. Is there a difference in more than one baseline variable and is it consistent for a particular center or group? This would be a cause of concern, and the validity of the trial must be questioned. If the difference is in only one or two of the baseline variables and is not consistent between groups and centers, a judgment has to be made as to whether the analysis can continue. Most trials are robust enough to cope with small differences between the groups at baseline unless it is in one of the primary outcome variables or any variables that are likely to affect the treatment response. There is no clear-cut answer to this, but there should be a debate by the data safety monitoring committee to consider the impact on the trial.

Analysis of Outcome Data

ACR20 is one of the most common methods of assessing outcome data in RA. The limitations of this have been discussed previously. ACR20 can be compared at any time point using a simple chi-square test. For example, in an active control trial of etanercept compared with methotrexate, there was a significant difference between treatment arms 4 months into the trial that had disappeared by 12 months (Table 12.7).

The common method of analyzing and reporting longitudinal outcome data, for example Sharp score or ESR, is to report the percentage change from baseline and carry out multiple t-tests to compare outcome with baseline and treatment to control. As has already been discussed, this method is already applied to the many outcome measures that are defined as percentage change from baseline. Figure 12.6 shows a typical graph reporting the change in Sharp score and the significant differences demonstrated by using multiple t-tests. The graph shows the mean ± 1 SE. The advantage of using percentage change is that it appears to get around the problem of small differences in assessment of outcome between centers and copes with the large differences in baseline variables between patients. This allows data from multiple sites to be easily pooled. It also allows the results of a trial to be reported in clinically relevant terms that are immediately accessible to patients and clinicians [17]. There are three problems with this approach. First, the percentage changes may not be normally distributed. It has been reported that the relative change in many of the

Table 12.7 ACR20 at 4 months and 12 months*

	4 months		12 months	
	Etanercept	Methotrexate	Etanercept	Methotrexate
ACR20 (%)	65%	52%†	63%	59%‡

* More patients have achieved an ACR20 response at 4 months in the etanercept group. This is maintained at 12 months, but the methotrexate group now shows a similar outcome.
† $\chi^2 = 11.6$, p $= 0.0007$.
‡ $\chi^2 = 0.9$, p $= 0.34$.

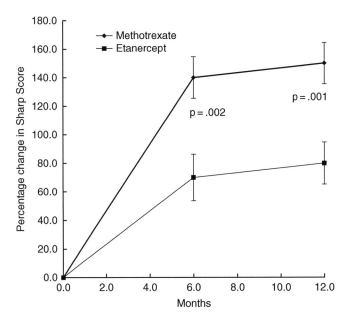

Fig. 12.6 Percentage change in Sharp score from baseline (mean ±1 SE)

ACR core set of measures is normally distributed [14], but some, such as the relative change in HAQ score or the 28 swollen joint count, are not. It is always better to describe the percentage change using medians and quartiles rather than means and SDs. Nonparametric statistics should be used. Second, percentage or relative change assumes that the change is linearly related to the baseline measurement. This should be checked if this is the chosen method of analysis. Third, and most importantly, multiple significance tests result in a greater risk of a significant difference being highlighted where one does not exist. Again, it is important to emphasize the need to look at the underlying core set measures to fully understand the data before using composite variables or percentage change.

The statistician would suggest that only the final outcome measurement needs to be analyzed to demonstrate a treatment effect. Indeed, reporting the percentage of patients with progression in Sharp score below a particular cutoff at the end of the study can be a helpful way of reporting the data. In the TEMPO study, for example, 57.1% of the methotrexate group had a change in total Sharp score of ≤ 0.5 compared with 67.9% in the etanercept group ($p < 0.01$ compared with the methotrexate group) and 79.8% in the combination therapy group ($p < 0.01$ compared with the methotrexate and etanercept groups) [15]. The clinician, however, then asks whether the changes at intermediate time points are significant, as this will affect the monitoring period for future trials and when the NME passes from the research stage into routine clinical use. An alternative is to summarize the data using the absolute change, peak change, or rate of change before analysis, but this suffers from the same problem as using the final outcome variable. There are two methods of ANOVA that come to our rescue. Both give the same answer and can be implemented in a simple spreadsheet or in many of the common statistics packages for the PC.

The main source of variation in the outcome data is the variation between subjects. The changes in outcome with time or treatment are relatively small compared with the range of the outcome variable in the patient group. In some circumstances, an outcome variable rises in the treatment group and falls or remains stable in the placebo or active comparator group. This means that the groups behave in a different way as time progresses. This is known as an interaction effect, and investigators often look to see if this interaction effect is significant. In RA/OA trials, where there is a known, effective, active comparator, it is often unlikely that the interaction effect is significant, as both NME and active comparator groups will behave in the same way. The model that accounts for the variation between subjects and for the interaction between treatment and time is

$$Y_{ijk} = \mu + T_i + P_{j(i)} + V_k + (TV)_{ik} + \varepsilon_{ijk} , \qquad (12.8)$$

where Y_{ijk} is the response of the jth subject on the ith treatment at the kth visit, μ is the overall mean, T_i is the effect of the ith treatment, $P_{j(i)}$ is the effect of the jth subject within the ith treatment (the between-subject variation), V_k the effect of the kth visit, $(TV)_{ik}$ the effect of the interaction between time and treatment, and ε_{ijk} the random error in measuring Y. The model assumes that ε_{ijk} is independent of $P_{j(i)}$ (i.e., there is no relationship between the outcome variable and the error in measuring that outcome variable). The ANOVA for this model is given in Table 12.8, and the ANOVA for Sharp score is given in Table 12.9. Note that the majority of the variation is explained by the between-subject variation (i.e., the variation in Sharp score between individual patients). The other important statistic in the table is the treatment by group interaction term. This is significant demonstrating that there is a significant treatment effect.

The alternative model is to use an analysis of variance and covariance. The analysis of covariance assumes that the score is linearly related to variables measured at baseline. These can be baseline variables that affect Sharp score (e.g., age, duration of disease) or, more simply, use the baseline Sharp Score as the covariate. The model for this analysis is

$$Y_{ijk} = \mu + T_i + \beta X_{ijk} + V_k + (TV)_{ik} + \varepsilon_{ijk} , \qquad (12.9)$$

where the components of the model are as defined in Eq. (12.8), and X_{ijk} the baseline measure of response. To calculate the ANOVA, it is necessary to calculate:

Table 12.8 ANOVA for the model in Eq. (12.8)

Source of variance	Sum of squares	df	Mean square	F
Treatment	$SST = nm \sum_i \left(\bar{Y}_i - \bar{Y}\right)^2$	$p - 1$	$MST = \frac{SST}{p-1}$	$\frac{MST}{MSP(T)}$
Patient (Treatment)	$SSP\left(T\right) = n \sum_i \sum_j \left(\bar{Y}_{ij} - \bar{Y}_i\right)^2$	$p(m - 1)$	$MSP(T) = \frac{SSP(T)}{p(m-1)}$	
Visit	$SSV = pm \sum_k \left(\bar{Y}_k - \bar{Y}\right)^2$	$n - 1$	$MSV = \frac{SSV}{n-1}$	$\frac{MSC}{MSE}$
Treatment visit	$SS\left(TV\right) = \sum_i \sum_j \sum_k \left(\bar{Y}_{ik} - \bar{Y}_i - \bar{Y}_k + \bar{Y}\right)^2$	$(p - 1)(n - 1)$	$MS(TV) = \frac{SS(TV)}{(p-1)(n-1)}$	$\frac{MS(TV)}{MSE}$
Residual	$SSE = \sum_i \sum_j \sum_k \left(Y_{ijk} - \bar{Y}_{ij} - \bar{Y}_{ik} + \bar{Y}_i\right)^2$	$p(m - 1)(n - 1)$	$MSE = \frac{SSE}{p(m-1)(n-1)}$	
Total	$SST = \sum_i \sum_j \sum_k \left(Y_{ijk} - \bar{Y}\right)^2$	$pmn - 1$		

Table 12.9 The ANOVA from Table 12.8 using the Sharp score data from the example study

Source variance	Sum of squares	df	Mean square	F	Significance of F
Treatment	2620.6	1	2620.6	5.6	p = 0.021
Patient (Treatment)	26,985.7	58	465.3		
Visit*	2467.4	3	822.5	157.9	p < 0.001
Treatment visit*	580.3	3	193.4	37.1	p < 0.001
Residual	604.2	116	5.2		
Total	21,415.8	179			

$$S_{xx} = \sum_i \sum_j \sum_k (X_{ijk} - \bar{X})^2$$

$$S_{xy} = \sum_i \sum_j \sum_k (Y_{ijk} - \bar{Y})(X_{ijk} - \bar{X})$$

$$S_{yy} = \sum_i \sum_j \sum_k (Y_{ijk} - \bar{Y})^2$$

$$T_{xx} = m \sum_i \sum_k (X_{ik} - \bar{X})^2$$

$$T_{xy} = m \sum_i \sum_k (Y_{ik} - \bar{Y})(X_{ik} - \bar{X})$$

$$T_{yy} = m \sum_i \sum_k (Y_{ik} - \bar{Y})^2$$

$$E_{xx} = S_{xx} - T_{xx}$$
$$E_{xy} = S_{xy} - T_{xy}$$
$$E_{yy} = S_{yy} - T_{yy} .$$

The slope of the regression is given by:

$$\beta = E_{xy}/E_{xx} .$$

The analysis of variance is given in Table 12.10. Many of the figures are the same for the previous model. The variance associated with the treatment is reduced because most of this is included in the regression variance. If the regression is non-significant, then the first ANOVA model should be used.

The mean Sharp score for each group at each visit can then be recalculated to take into account the regression. These are known as adjusted cells means and are calculated as:

$$\bar{Y}'_{ik} = \bar{Y}_{ik} - \beta (\bar{X} - \bar{X}_i) . \tag{12.10}$$

Table 12.10 ANOVA for the model in Eq. (12.9)

Source of variance	Sum of squares	df	Mean square	F
Treatment	$\text{SST} = nm \sum_i \left(\bar{Y}_i - \bar{Y} - \beta \left(\bar{X}_i - \bar{X} \right) \right)^2$	$p - 1$	$\text{MST} = \frac{\text{SST}}{p-1}$	$\frac{\text{MST}}{\text{MSP}(T)}$
Visit	$\text{SSV} = pm \sum_k \left(\bar{Y}_k - \bar{Y} \right)^2$	$n - 1$	$\text{MSV} = \frac{\text{SSV}}{n-1}$	$\frac{\text{MSC}}{\text{MSE}}$
Treatment visit*	$\text{SS}(TV) = \sum_i \sum_j \sum_k \left(\bar{Y}_{ik} - \bar{Y}_i - \bar{Y}_k + \bar{Y} \right)^2$	$(p-1)(n-1)$	$\text{MS}(TV) = \frac{\text{SS}(TV)}{(p-1)(n-1)}$	$\frac{\text{MS}(TV)}{\text{MSE}}$
Regression	$\text{SSR} = \frac{E_{xy}^2}{E_{xx}}$	1	$\text{MSR} = \text{SSR}$	$\frac{\text{MSR}}{\text{MSE}}$
Within plus residual	$\text{SSE} = \sum_i \sum_j \sum_j \left(Y_{ijk} - \bar{Y}_{ik} \right)^2 - \text{SRR}$	$pnm - pn - 1$	$\text{MSE} = \frac{\text{SSE}}{pnm - pn - 1}$	

Table 12.11 The ANOVA from Table 12.11 using the lumbar spine BMD data from the example study

Source of variance	Sum of squares	df	Mean square	F	Significance of F
Treatment	1948.5	1	1948.5	47.1	$p < 0.001$
Visit	2467.4	4	616.9	14.9	$p < 0.001$
Treatment visit*	580.3	4	145.1	3.5	$p = 0.008$
Regression	9412.7	1	9412.7	147.0	$p < 0.001$
Within plus residual	18,509.7	289	64.0		

Both these models assume an equal number of patients in each group and at each visit. They can be generalized to cope with unequal group sizes. The sum of squares for the treatment in Table 12.11, for example, would become:

$$\text{SST} = n \sum_i m_i \left(\bar{Y}_i - \bar{Y} \right)^2, \tag{12.11}$$

where m_i is the number of patients in the ith group. The handling of degrees of freedom is a matter for some debate. The most common method appears to be to use the harmonic mean of the numbers in each group. This is calculated as:

$$\frac{i}{\left(\sum_i \frac{1}{m_i} \right)}, \tag{12.12}$$

These ANOVA models are available in most PC-based statistics packages and can be developed within a spreadsheet if necessary. Statistics packages can generally deal with unequal numbers in each group.

Post hoc methods can then be applied to discover where the significant differences lie.

Figure 12.7 is the graphical representation of the outcome of using the second of these two ANOVA models. The baseline data plotted as mean ± 1 SD and the other data as the adjusted cell means. There is a significant treatment effect ($p < 0.001$), a significant effect of visit ($p < 0.001$), and a significant interaction term ($p = 0.008$), showing that treatment and control groups respond differently with time.

Nonparametric Statistics

The nonparametric equivalents of the ANOVAs used above can be applied to non-normal data. It is acceptable to use a Wilcoxon rank sum test to compare the control and treatment groups. In this test, the data from the control and treatment groups are combined and ranked. The ranks for each group are then summed. If m and n are

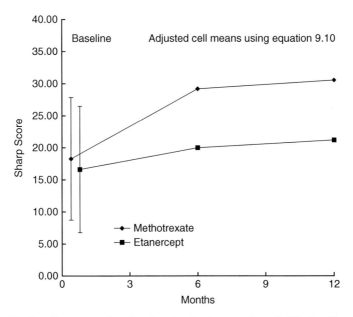

Fig. 12.7 Absolute Sharp score plotted against time for the example study. The baseline values are plotted as mean 1 ± SD and the other values as the adjusted cell means calculated using Eq. (12.10)

the number of patients in the control and treatment groups, then the sum of ranks in the treatment group is

$$r = \sum_{i=1}^{n} r_i . \tag{12.13}$$

The test statistic is the calculated as:

$$W = r - \frac{n(n+1)}{2} . \tag{12.14}$$

The acceptance region on the sum of ranks is tabulated [18] as well as methods of testing the significance of the test when the number of patients is outside the tabulated values. The W statistic is also tabulated, and the test statistic for large samples corrected for ties can also be calculated [6]. In our sample data, the baseline Sharp score has been ranked. The sum of ranks in the etanercept group is 864 and $W = 399$. The limits of acceptance of r are 769 to 1051. As r lies within these limits, there is no significant difference between control and treatment groups at baseline. The test statistic for W is

$$Z = \frac{W - nm/2}{\sqrt{\text{var}(W)}},$$

where:

$$\text{var}(W) = \frac{nm(n + m + 1)}{12}.$$

In this case, $Z = -0.75$. Z is a standardized normal deviate and is tabulated [18]. The probability of the two groups not being significantly different is 0.45. This test is available in most commercial statistics packages for the PC. The extension to this test to more than two groups is the Kruskal-Wallis test [6, 19]. In this test, the mean rank in each group is calculated and the test statistic H calculated as:

$$H = \frac{12}{N(N + 1)} \sum_{i=1}^{k} n_i (\bar{r}_i - \bar{r})^2 ,$$

where n_i is the number of subjects in the ith group, k is the total number of treatment groups, N is the total number of subjects, $\bar{r}_i$ the mean rank in the ith group, and $\bar{r}$ the overall mean rank

$$\bar{r} = \frac{N + 1}{2}.$$

If there is a significant difference between the groups, H will be greater than χ^2 for $k - 1$ degrees of freedom when there are a large number of subjects in the trial. Again, there are corrections when there are a large number of tied ranks.

Treatment Effect

It is important to be able to quantify the effect of the treatment with the control. The simplest way to calculate the treatment effect is to subtract the mean change from baseline for the control group from the mean change from baseline in the treatment group and calculate the 95% confidence interval on the difference. The significance of the treatment effect can then be tested. The difference is

$$d = \bar{Y}_t - \bar{Y}_c ,$$

where $\bar{Y}_t$ and $\bar{Y}_c$ are the mean change from baseline in the treatment and control groups. The standard deviation of the difference is

$$s = \sqrt{\frac{(n_t - 1) s_t^2 + (n_c - 1) s_c^2}{(n_t + n_c - 2)}}. \tag{12.15}$$

The confidence interval (CI) is

$$\text{CI} = s \times \sqrt{1/n_t + 1/n_c} \times t\,(0.025, n_t + n_c - 2), \tag{12.16}$$

and the significance of the treatment effect d is tested using the statistic

$$t = \frac{d}{s\sqrt{1/n_t + 1/n_c}}, \qquad (12.17)$$

with $n_t + n_c - 2$ degrees of freedom. In our example study, the mean change in Sharp score from baseline was 12.3 ± 3.4 in the control group and 4.6 ± 2.4 in the treatment group. The treatment effect was 7.7 with a standard deviation of 0.76 and confidence interval of 1.74. The t statistic is 10.2 with 58 degrees of freedom, which is highly significant.

In multicenter trials, it is important to calculate a treatment effect for each center to ensure there are no center differences.

Adverse Event Monitoring

The purpose of adverse event monitoring is to ensure that the adverse events associated with an NME are the same in the treatment and control groups (i.e., there are no significant adverse events that are due to the study drug). Normally, investigators code adverse events into four categories:

1. Probably not related to the study drug.
2. Possibly related to the study drug.
3. Probably related to the study drug.
4. Definitely related to the study drug.

It is simple, then, to compare the incidence of adverse events between the treatment and control groups in these four categories using a chi-square test. The type and severity of adverse events can also be coded and compared between treatment and control groups, as relying on the number of adverse events may be too crude a measure. It may be that, whereas the overall incidence of adverse events is the same in each group, the severity of the events differs. This may be vital evidence in an active comparator study that shows that the NME under investigation has a lower rate of side effects than the current standard treatment even if the effect on clinical outcome is the same.

For example, in a trial comparing leflunomide with placebo or methotrexate [20], gastrointestinal adverse events were more commonly reported by patients on leflunomide (60.4%) when compared with placebo (41.5%) or methotrexate (51.6%). Using a chi-square test, there is a significantly higher rate of adverse event in the leflunomide group ($\chi^2 = 9.6$, $p < 0.01$). Although there was a higher rate of allergic reaction in the leflunomide group (24.2%) compared with placebo (14.4%) or methotrexate (17.0%), this was not statistically significant ($\chi^2 = 4.5$, $p = 0.11$).

The Conclusions

The purpose of the concluding section of the publication is to put your study in the context of the available evidence surrounding its use in the treatment of RA or OA and state the interpretation of the data based on the facts presented in the results section. The conclusions of the example trial used in this book are that etanercept is a safe and effective alternative to methotrexate. It appears to improve outcome more rapidly than methotrexate as outcomes are significantly better at 4 months compared with methotrexate, although this benefit has disappeared at 12 months. Patients on etanercept have less joint space narrowing and a lower erosion score than those on methotrexate. Patients on etanercept have a lower level of adverse events than those on methotrexate apart from a reported increase in injection site reactions.

There is a danger that researchers end the conclusion with a similar general statement of the benefits of their NME that is not supported by the results of their study, particularly if the trial has a negative outcome. This should be avoided at all costs. The conclusion must be based on the facts as presented and not on speculation.

Summary

The structured reporting of clinical trials is an important part of disseminating the results from a study. The standards for structured abstracts and the CONSORT statement provide investigators with a template that is easy to follow and that also is easy to read. It allows other investigators easy access to the facts about your trial and will allow your work to be of a standard to be included in future meta-analysis. The examples used here have been simple, and trials are often far more complex in their analysis when there are many centers involved and a more complex study design. The statistics have been included, although detailed compared with the rest of this text, to help investigators and others involved in clinical trials work through the basics of testing data for normality, carry out baseline comparisons on the data, look for center effects, and analyze longitudinal data in such a way as to answer the demands of clinical colleagues while maintaining the statistical moral high ground!

References

1. Pocock SJ, Hughes MD, Lee RJ. Statistical problems in the reporting of clinical trials. A survey of three medical journals. N Engl J Med 1987;317:426–432.
2. Begg C, Cho M, Eastwood S, et al. Improving the quality of reporting of randomized controlled trials. The CONSORT statement. JAMA 1996;276:637–639.
3. Altman DG. Better reporting of randomised controlled trials: the CONSORT statement. BMJ 1996;313:570–571.
4. Jadad AR. Randomised Controlled Trials. London: BMJ Books; 1998.
5. Ad Hoc Working Group for Critical Appraisal of the Medical Literature. A proposal for more informative abstracts of clinical articles. Ann Intern Med 1987;106:598–604.

6. Chow S-C, Liu J-P. Design and Analysis of Clinical Trials. New York: John Wiley & Sons; 1998.

7. Felson DT, Anderson JJ, Boers M, et al. American College of Rheumatology. Preliminary definition of improvement in rheumatoid arthritis. Arthritis Rheum 1995;38:727–735.

8. van Riel PL, van Gestel AM. Area under the curve for the American College of Rheumatology improvement criteria: a valid addition to existing criteria in rheumatoid arthritis? Arthritis Rheum 2001;44:1719–1721.

9. Verhoeven AC, Boers M, van Der Linden S. Responsiveness of the core set, response criteria, and utilities in early rheumatoid arthritis. Ann Rheum Dis 2000;59:966–974.

10. Kelly AM. The minimum clinically significant difference in visual analogue scale pain score does not differ with severity of pain. Emerg Med J 2001;18:205–207.

11. Todd KH, Funk JP. The minimum clinically important difference in physician-assigned visual analog pain scores. Acad Emerg Med 1996;3:142–146.

12. Escalante A, Haas RW, del Rincon I. Measurement of global functional performance in patients with rheumatoid arthritis using rheumatology function tests. Arthritis Res Ther 2004;6:R315–325.

13. Buckland-Wright C, Cline G, Meyer J. Structural progression in knee osteoarthritis over 12 months. Program and abstracts of the American College of Rheumatology 67th Annual Scientific Meeting; October 2003; Orlando, FL. Abstract S1225.

14. van Vollenhoven RF, Klareskog L. Clinical responses to tumor necrosis factor alpha antagonists do not show a bimodal distribution: data from the Stockholm tumor necrosis factor alpha follow-up registry. Arthritis Rheum 2003;48:1500–1503.

15. van der Heijde D, et al. Presentation and analysis of data on radiographic outcome in clinical trials: experience from the TEMPO study. Arthritis Rheum 2005;52:49–60.

16. Atlman DG. Practical Statistics for Medical Research. London: Chapman and Hall; 1991.

17. Vickers AJ. The use of percentage change from baseline as an outcome in a controlled trial is statistically inefficient: a simulation study. BMC Med Res Methodol 2001;1:6.

18. Lentner C, ed. Geigy Scientific Tables Volume 2. 8th ed. Basle: CIBA-GEIGY Ltd.; 1982.

19. Siegel S, Castellan NJ, Nonparametric Statistics for the Behavioural Sciences. New York: McGraw-Hill; 1988.

20. Strand V, Cohen S, Schiff M, et al. Treatment of active rheumatoid arthritis with leflunomide compared with placebo and methotrexate. Leflunomide Rheumatoid Arthritis Investigators Group. Arch Intern Med 1999;159:2542–2550.

Chapter 13
Radiographic Imaging End Points in Rheumatoid Arthritis Trials

Anna M. Baratelle and Désirée van der Heijde

Introduction

The use of radiographs to quantify structural joint damage in RA was initially proposed by Steinbrocker in 1949 [1] then further developed by Sharp [2] and Larsen [3]. Dr. Sharp, a pioneer in developing radiographic scoring methods, published his methodology in 1971, stating, "the method should contribute to the ease of designing an objective analysis of a therapeutic agent since the x-rays can be read randomly, blindfold and independent by multiple observers" [2]. Many clinical trials have reviewed serial (annual) hand and/or foot radiographs—some by analog film and more recently through digitized radiographs. Images must be standardized to reduce the variability in the presentation and consequently improve the validity of the blinded reading of the images. Posteroanterior (PA) views of the hands and anteroposterior (AP) views of the feet, commonly affected by rheumatoid arthritis (RA), are easily reproducible across patients at follow-up time points. The most important feature in clinical trials is change over time. Consequently, all efforts should be directed to good reliability of change scores more so than for status scores. Other imaging modalities such as magnetic resonance imaging (MRI) and ultrasonography display useful features in RA but will likely not replace standard radiographs in clinical trials to assess structural damage in the foreseeable future [4, 5].

Radiographic Acquisition

It is critical that the imaging protocol generates images that demonstrate features of the disease and can be followed by multiple centers. All sites participating in the clinical trial should receive the same instructions for positioning the patient's hand/foot. The hand and wrist must be positioned flat on the x-ray cassette, with the fingers slightly spread, aligning the index finger and radius (Fig. 13.1). The central beam is directed between the second and third metacarpophalangeal (MCP) joint. Although many clinical practices permit both hands to be exposed simultaneously,

A.M. Baratelle
Centocor Malvern, PA USA

D.M. Reid, C.G. Miller (eds.), *Clinical Trials in Rheumatoid Arthritis and Osteoarthritis*, 201
© Springer-Verlag London Limited 2008

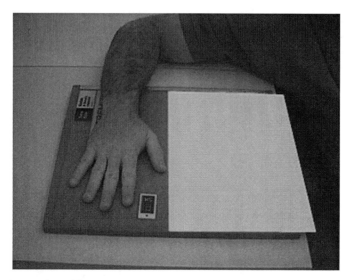

Fig. 13.1 A properly positioned hand and a sample trace film

this is not recommended for clinical trial images for two reasons: First, bilateral exposure means a divergence of the beam toward the outer phalanges, causing inhomogeneous exposure in increased parallax errors. Furthermore, when trying to expose both hands simultaneously, it is almost impossible for a healthy person, let alone a patient with RA, to comfortably position both hands flat, with the index finger and radius aligned on each hand within the confines of the x-ray plate. The result of bilateral exposure is imperfect positioning—overlapping of joints and ulnar deviation, thus creating a nonevaluable portion of the hand image for radiographic scoring. The methodology described of imaging each hand independently ensures much greater reproducibility of acquisition.

To improve reproducibility further, it is recommended, at the initial protocol time point visit, to place a piece of clear acetate on top of the x-ray cassette, before positioning the patient; after positioning the hand, but prior to exposure, trace the patient's hand outline with a permanent marker. This piece of acetate will not affect the radiograph and can be retained with the patient's study records for retrieval at follow-up visits. When the patient returns, the acetate can once again be placed on the x-ray cassette and the patient positioned according to their personalized "template" (Fig. 13.2).

Scoring Methods of Radiographs

The scoring method used to assess the efficacy of drugs on retarding structural damage must be valid, reliable, sensitive, and feasible. Although there are a number of automated software tools that measure joint spaces to quantitate structural damage [6], current standard technique is to assess disease progression in RA clinical trials by qualitatively "scoring" serial radiographs. There are many validated, so-called semiquantitative methods for scoring radiographs; however, the

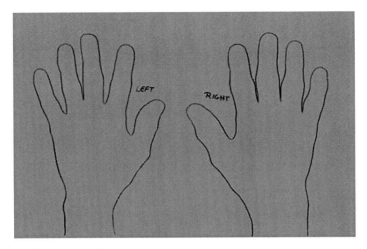

Fig. 13.2 A reference/trace film

two primary methods used are Sharp [2] and Larsen [3] and modifications of each. Several modifications have been made to both Sharp [7, 8] and Larsen [9, 10], but at the time of writing, the Sharp scoring method, albeit modified, has become the most widely used method in clinical trials and, by default, for submissions to the regulatory authorities [11–15].

This chapter will describe the various scoring methods, both global and detailed, in chronological order by the published date.

Steinbrocker Index (1949)

The Steinbrocker method is a global assessment for the patient as a whole, based primarily on radiographic findings but also on physical exam and functional status. The scoring is a four-level staging for the patient; the joint with the worst score determines the stage for the entire patient [1].

Kellgren's Method (1957)

Kellgren developed a standard set of radiographs that could be used to grade joints of the hands and wrists. The scoring was a global score, ranging from 0 to 4 [16–18]. The grade was applied to the entire hand and wrist, not to the individual joints. One grade was given as a summary of abnormalities of all the joints in the hands and wrists.

Sharp Scoring Method (1971)

The Sharp method is a detailed scoring of erosive disease and joint space narrowing, both scored separately (Table 13.1; Fig. 13.3). The original Sharp scoring

Table 13.1 Sharp scoring method

Erosion scoring (Maximum score = 290)	Joint space narrowing scoring (Maximum score = 216)
0 = No erosions	0 = No narrowing
1 = One discrete erosion	1 = Focal narrowing—narrowing on one side of the joint space with a normal space on the other side
2 = Two discrete erosions	2 = Diffuse narrowing with loss of <50% of the original space
3 = Three discrete erosions	3 = Narrowing with loss of >50% of the normal space
4 = Four discrete erosions	4 = Absence of a joint space, ankylosis
5 = Extensive destruction	

Joints Scored (Erosions red and Joint Space Narrowing green)

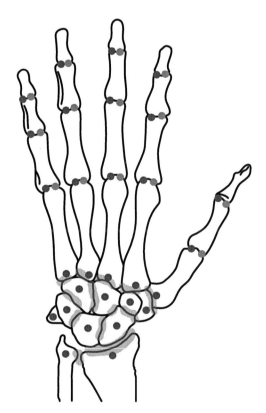

Fig. 13.3 Original Sharp scoring method

method [2] scored 29 bones of each hand-wrist for erosions (14 finger joints, 5 metacarpal bases, 8 carpal bones, the radius and ulna) and 27 joints of each hand-wrist for joint space narrowing (14 finger joints, 5 carpometacarpal, and the trapezium-navicular, navicular-lunate, lunate-triquetrum, triquetrum-hamate, hamate-capitate, capitate-navicular-lunate, radiocarpals, and radioulnar joints).

Larsen Scoring (1977)

The Larsen method was developed by Larsen, Dale, and Eek [3] (Table 13.2; Fig. 13.4). It has been modified several times by the authors [19–22]. It is a 6-point global scoring of joints, based primarily on erosive damage. However, grade 1 can be based on soft tissue joint swelling only, which is not a real sign of structural damage and is also difficult to assess reliably. The method can be applied to many joints but is primarily used for the hands and wrists and also for the feet. The original Larsen method evaluates 11 areas in each hand-wrist: interphalangeal (IP) of digit 1; proximal interphalangeal (PIP) joints 2 to 5; MCP joints 1 to 5; and the wrist as a single joint. In the feet, the five metatarsal phalangeal joints (MTPs) are evaluated. This gives a total of 32 joints to evaluate, for a maximum score of 160. Larsen produced a set of standard reference films to compare the grading of the joints.

Table 13.2 Larsen scoring

Maximum score = 160

0 = Normal conditions. Abnormalities not related to arthritis, such as marginal bone deposition may be present.

1 = Slight abnormality. One or more of the following lesions are present: slight joint space narrowing; periarticular soft tissue swelling and periarticular osteoporosis should only be scored if they represent a major feature.

2 = Definite abnormality. Small erosions are present in the finger and toe joints. JSN is not obligatory in these joints. In the large joints, JSN must be present, erosions being not obligatory.

3 = Marked abnormality. Erosion and joint space narrowing must be present.

4 = Severe abnormality. The original articular surfaces are still partially preserved.

5 = Mutilating abnormality. The original articular surfaces have disappeared. Gross bone deformation is present. Dislocation and bony ankylosis, being late and secondary, should not be considered in the grading; if present, the grading should be made according to the concomitant bone destruction or deformation.

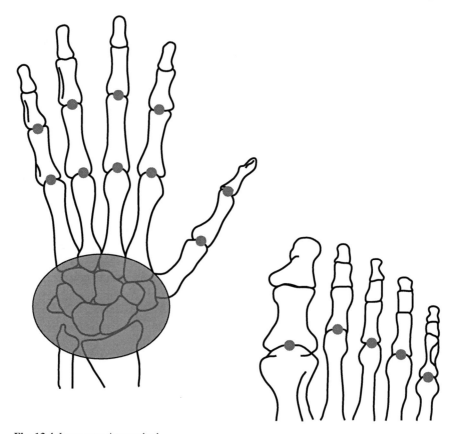

Fig. 13.4 Larsen scoring method

Genant Scoring Method (1983)

Similar to Sharp's method, Genant [8] scored erosions and joint space narrowing separately (Table 13.3; Fig. 13.5). However, the major difference with the original Sharp method is that a 5-point grading system is used for joint space narrowing and for erosions ranging from normal to severe. Sixteen areas are scored for erosions in the hand and six in the foot: IP of digit 1; PIP of digits 2 to 5, MCP of digits 1 to 5; mid-navicular, radius (styloid and ulnar), and ulna (radial, styloid and outer aspect). In the foot, the IP and five MTP joints are scored. Eleven joints in the hand are scored for joint space narrowing and six in the foot: IP of digit 1; PIP of digits 2 to 5; MCP of digits 1 to 5; and radiocarpal joint. The joints in the foot are the IP and five MTP joints.

Table 13.3 Genant scoring method

Erosion scoring (Maximum score = 176)	Joint space narrowing scoring (Maximum score = 136)
0 = Normal	0 = Normal
1 = Questionable	1 = Questionable
2 = Definite, but mild	2 = Definite, but mild
3 = Moderate	3 = Moderate
4 = Severe	4 = Severe

Erosions red and Joint Space Narrowing green

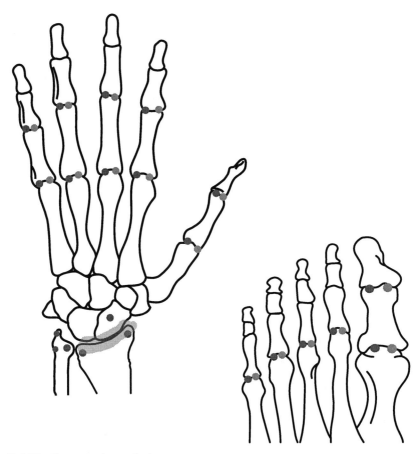

Fig. 13.5 The Genant scoring method

Modified Sharp (1985)

Sharp et al. further defined which joints to score based on the frequency of RA involvement (Table 13.4; Fig. 13.6). They decreased the number of joints of each

Table 13.4 Modified Sharp scoring method

Erosion scoring (Maximum score = 170)	Joint space narrowing scoring (Maximum score = 144)
0 = No erosions	0 = No narrowing
1 = One discrete erosion	1 = Focal narrowing
2 = Two discrete erosions	2 = Diffuse narrowing of less than 50% of the original space
3 = Three discrete erosions	3 = Definite narrowing with loss of more than 50% of the normal space
4 = Four discrete erosions	
5 = Extensive destruction—more than 50% bone loss of either articular bone	4 = Absence of a joint space, presumptive evidence of ankylosis

Joints Scored (Erosions red and Joint Space Narrowing green) – Note: The multangular bones are now scored as one unit, along with the triquetrum and pisiform as one unit.

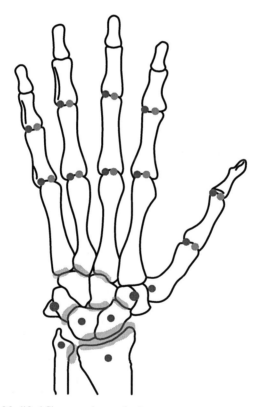

Fig. 13.6 Modified Sharp scoring method

hand/wrist to 17 for erosions and 18 for JSN [23]. Erosions are counted when discrete, and surface erosions are scored according to the surface area involved [18, 23]. The maximum erosion score, per joint, remains 5. When either articulating bone in an MCP, PIP, or carpal bone is eroded more than half, the erosion score for that joint is scored as 5. Joint space narrowing is scored 1 if it is focal, 2 if the narrowing is less than 50% of the original joint space, 3 if more than 50% of the joint space, and 4 if the joint is ankylosed. If a joint is subluxed, it is not scored.

Kaye (1987)

Kaye et al. [24] combined and modified the methods described by Genant [8] and Sharp et al. [23] (Table 13.5; Fig. 13.7). In this method, (mal)alignment is scored in addition to erosions and joint space narrowing. Some of the joints that were evaluated in the Genant and Sharp methods were excluded and/or combined. The joints evaluated for each category are demonstrated in Figure 13.5. Joints with prior articular surgery were assigned erosion and joint space narrowing (JSN) scores of 4. Sites were considered inevaluable if they were missing from the radiograph or if they had flexion deformity. Inevaluable joints were not scored and were therefore excluded from analysis. The score of 1 was not used to avoid equivocal scores. The ultimate score is calculated by the sum of the absolute score divided by the number of joints evaluated.

The Sharp/van der Heijde Scoring Method (1989)

The most noticeable difference in the van der Heijde modification is the addition of the joints of the forefoot (Table 13.6; Fig. 13.8). Another change was the decreased number of joints in each hand-wrist scored [7]. The addition of the joints in the forefoot was done because the joints in the feet show disease earlier and more severe than the hand, especially in the earlier stages of the disease. The deleted joints from the hands-wrists were joints that were difficult to assess in a reliable fashion, mainly due to superimposition. Erosions are evaluated in 6 joints of each foot and 16 joints in each hand-wrist. Joint space narrowing is scored in 6 joints of each foot and 15 joints of each hand-wrist. When scoring erosions in the forefoot, both sites (tarsal

Table 13.5 Kaye scoring

Erosion scoring (Maximum score = 88)	Joint space narrowing scoring (Maximum score = 140)	Alignment (Maximum score = 120)
0 = Normal	0 = Normal	0 = Normal
2 = Mild	2 = Mild	2 = Subluxation
3 = Moderate	3 = Moderate	4 = Dislocation
4 = Severe	4 = Severe	
	5 = Bone ankylosis	

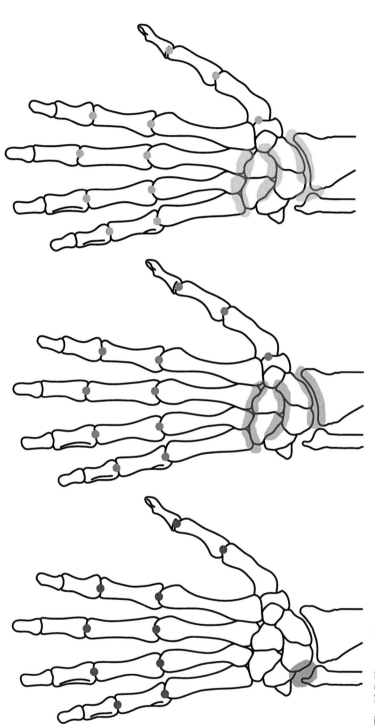

Erosions red / Joint Space Narrowing green/ Alignment violet

Fig. 13.7 Kaye scoring

Table 13.6 Sharp/van der Heijde scoring method

Erosion scoring (Maximum score = 280)	Joint space narrowing scoring (Maximum score = 168)
0 = No erosions	0 = Normal
1 = One discreet erosion	1 = Focal or doubtful
2 to 4 = Dependent on the surface area affected	2 = Generalized, >50% of the original joint space left
5 = Complete collapse of bone	3 = Generalized, <50% of the original joint space left or subluxation
	4 = Bony ankylosis or complete luxation

Erosions red and Joint Space Narrowing green

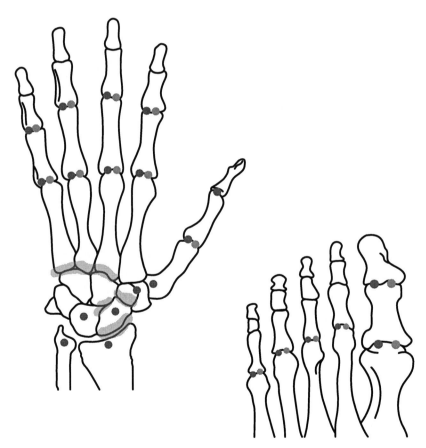

Fig. 13.8 The Sharp/van der Heijde scoring method

Table 13.7 Scott/Larsen scoring method

Maximum score = 200

0 = Normal conditions. Abnormalities not related to arthritis, such as marginal bone deposition may be present.

1 = Periarticular osteoporosis/joint swelling if these are major features, or if suggested erosions/cysts at two sites in joint are less than 1 mm, score 1.

2 = If one or more erosions greater than 1 mm are present with a break in the cortical margin.

3 = If erosions at both sides of joint are of significant size with preservation of some joint surface.

4 = If subluxation is present.

5 = Mutilating abnormality. The original articular surfaces have disappeared. Gross bone deformation is present. Dislocation and bony ankylosis, being late and secondary, should not be considered in the grading; if present, the grading should be made according to the concomitant bone destruction or deformation.

site and phalangeal site) are scored 0 to 5, allowing for a maximum score per joint of 10. Another point of interest with this modification is that erosions are scored, regardless if they are caused by the rheumatoid process or osteoarthritic lesions, as this is frequently difficult to differentiate. Joint space narrowing was modified to incorporate (sub)luxation in the score.

Scott/Larsen Scoring Method (1995)

Scott's proposal to modify the Larsen method consisted of a change to the definitions of the grades [9, 25] (Table 13.7). The same joints as Larsen [3] are evaluated. The wrist score is multiplied by 5 in order to give extra weighting to the wrist, thus allowing for a maximum score of 200. Also, the definition of grade 1 was modified, leading to an improved inter-reader agreement.

Modified Larsen Score According to Rau and Herborn (1995)

Rau and Herborn [10] suggested a modification to Larsen's method to further define the different stages (Table 13.8; Fig. 13.9). The original 32 regions evaluated by Larsen [3] are evaluated, however, the grading definitions are modified. The modifications were made in order to perform the scoring in a more quantitative manner.

Table 13.8 Rau and Herborn modified Larsen method

Maximum score = 160

0 = Normal

1 = Soft tissue swelling and/or joint space narrowing/subchondral osteoporosis

2 = Erosions with destruction of the joint surface (DJS) of <25%

3 = DJS 26% to 50%

4 = DJS 51% to 75%

5 = DJS >75%

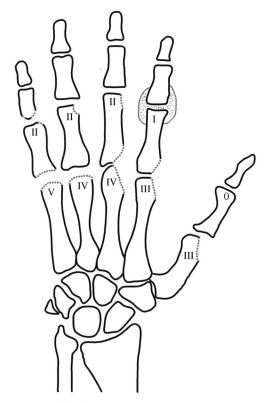

Fig. 13.9 Rau and Herborn modified larsen

However, the authors modified this method a few years later and do recommend use of the modification.

Larsen's 1995 Modification

Larsen's modification in 1995 [22] was written to evaluate radiographs in long-term studies (Table 13.9; Fig. 13.10). Larsen gives several reasons for these modifications. First, multicenter studies introduce variability in the quality of radiographs,

Table 13.9 Modified Larsen 1995

Maximum score = 160	
Grade 0	Intact bony outlines and normal joint space.
Grade 1	Erosions less than 1 mm in diameter or joint space narrowing.
Grade 2	One or several small erosions (diameter more than 1 mm).
Grade 3	Marked erosions.
Grade 4	Severe erosions. There is usually no joint space left; the original bony outlines are partly preserved.
Grade 5	Mutilating changes: The original bony outlines have been destroyed.

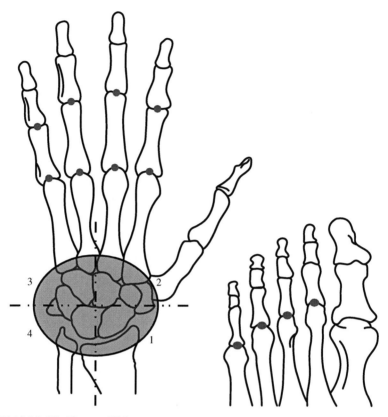

Fig. 13.10 Modified Larsen 1995

which makes soft tissue and osteoporosis scoring difficult and also gives variable resolution of erosions. Second, in long-term follow-up, the soft tissue swelling diminishes and the incidence of osteoporosis remains constant during the course of RA. As a result, these features are less relevant in long-term follow-up studies. The opinion is that erosions are the most important long-term variable because bone is affected earlier than cartilage. This modification impacts which sites are evaluated along with the definitions of the grading. The main differences in the sites evaluated are the exclusion of the thumbs and the first MTPs, along with the subdivision of the wrist into four regions. The most striking difference in the grading is the deletion of soft tissue swelling and osteoporosis and the distinction between erosions less than 1 mm and greater than 1 mm in size.

Modified Genant Scoring Method (1998)

Genant et al. modified their method in 1998 [26] (Table 13.10; Fig. 13.11). Fourteen areas are scored for erosions on an 8-point scale, with 0.5 increments: IP of thumb;

Table 13.10 Modified Genant scoring method

Erosion scoring (Maximum score = 98)	Joint space narrowing scoring (Maximum score = 104)
0 = Normal	0 = Normal
0+ = Questionable or subtle change	0+ = Questionable or subtle change
1 = Mild	1 = Mild
1+ = Mild worse	1+ = Mild worse
2 = Moderate	2 = Moderate
2+ = Moderate worse	2+ = Moderate worse
3 = Severe	3 = Severe
3+ = Severe worse	3+ = Severe worse
	4 = Ankylosis or dislocation

+ = 0.5.

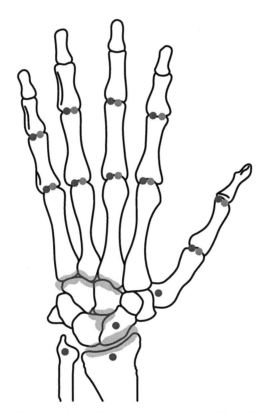

Fig. 13.11 Modified Genant scoring method (erosions red and Joint Space Narrowing green)

PIP of digits 2 to 5; MCP of digits 1 to 5; CMC of digit 1; scaphoid, distal radius, and distal ulna. Thirteen joints are scored for joint space narrowing on a 9-point scale, also with 0.5 increments: IP of thumb, PIP of digits 2 to 5; MCP of digits 1 to 5; combination of carpometavarpal joint (CMC) joints of digits 3 to 5; combination of capitate-scaphoid-lunate, and radiocarpal joint.

Ratingen Score (1998)

Rau et al. developed a new method, derived from the Larsen score (Table 13.11; Fig. 13.12). The Ratingen [27] method redefines the grading by restricting the scoring of a joint to definite change of erosion and joint destruction. How far the erosion extends into the bone is not taken into consideration. Instead, the amount of joint surface destruction (JSD) is defined by the length of the clearly visible interruption of the cortical plate as it relates to the total joint surface. The following joints

Table 13.11 Ratingen score

Maximum score = 190
0 = Normal
1 = One or more several, definite erosions totaling destruction of up to 20% of the total surface
2 = JSD 21% to 40%
3 = JSD 41% to 60%
4 = JSD 61% to 80%
5 = JSD >80%

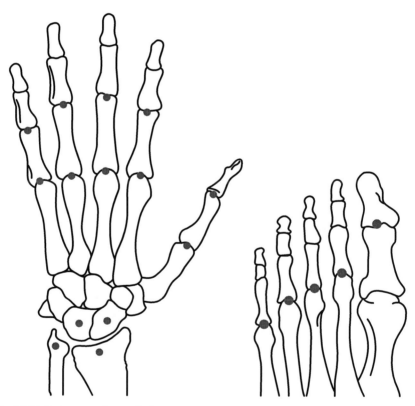

Fig. 13.12 Ratingen scoring method

Table 13.12 SENS

Erosion scoring (Maximum score = 44)	Joint space narrowing scoring (Maximum score = 42)
0 = No erosions	0 = No narrowing
1 = Erosions	1 = Narrowed

are scored: all PIPs and MCPs, four sites in the wrists (naviculum, lunatum, distal radius, and distal ulna), IP of the great toe, and MTP2-5.

Simple Erosion Narrowing Score (1999)

van der Heijde et al. [28] simplified the Sharp/van der Heijde method for the purpose of clinical practice, not clinical trials. The method, abbreviated as SENS (Table 13.12), scores the same joints as the 1989 van der Heijde modification of the Sharp method, however, the "score" is determined by the number of eroded and number of narrowed joints without taking into account the amount of damage.

Short Erosion Scale (2000)

Wolfe et al. [29] further modified the Larsen scoring system to score only three areas in both hands (MCP 2, 3, and 5) and three sites in both wrists (three of four quadrants: medial-proximal, medial-distal, and lateral-proximal). These areas are scored for erosions only. This reduction in number of sites to score was based on statistical methods to ensure that all information was kept. The method has never been applied in a study.

Comparison of Scoring Methods

Depending on which method or modification used, the range of scores of the Sharp methods is usually from 0 to 314 up to 448 for the van der Heijde modification, and the Larsen methods range is from 0 to 150 up to 200. All the methods listed have been tested to show good reliability. There is some evidence that the Sharp methods show increased sensitivity to change [30–32]. The advantage of the Sharp methods is that separate information on erosions and joint space narrowing is obtained, allowing for assessing a possible differential effect on bone and cartilage.

Reviewing Radiographs for a Clinical Trial

U.S. Food and Drug Administration (FDA) guidance [33, 34] suggests that clinical trials seeking approval for prevention of structural damage should have radiographs obtained at baseline and follow-up and be at least 1 year in duration, although it has been shown that a 3-month follow-up period is already sufficient to show sufficient progression in a sufficient number of patients to be useful to test the effect of a new compound on structural damage [35]. It is also recommended that all patients have images obtained at all time points, regardless of withdrawal from the trial. The radiographs should be read by at least two independent reviewers providing scores for at least two readers for each film.

Recent clinical trials scored serial radiographs, utilizing modified Sharp methods, in random time-point order, and demonstrated statistically significant results. Bruynesteyn et al. [36] suggest that knowing the sequence of serial radiographs increases the detection of relevant changes, but the argument against this is the radiologist recognizes change and interpolates to the final assessment. Blinded sequence removes this bias but on the other hand does increase variability.

Especially to assess repair of damage, it is essential to score radiographs in random order [37]. Together with the fact that agencies request random-order time order makes that almost all clinical trials are scored with time sequence blinded.

Scoring Radiographs for Repair

At the moment, there is also interest in repair of structural damage. For a long time, it was considered as being a very rare phenomenon and occurring in isolated cases. However, in recent trials it has been shown that negative progression scores occur in a substantial number of patients. However, a negative progression score in an individual patient is not equal to repair of damage, though it has been suggested that repair on a group level exists if the mean progression score with the entire 95% confidence interval is below zero [37]. A group of experts within outcome measures in rheumatology clinical trials (OMERACT) interested in radiographic scoring performed several exercises showing that repair of damage can indeed be picked up by experts although they are unable to link specific features such as recortication, sclerosis, and "filling in" to differentiate between progression and repair. Negative scores in the Sharp/van der Heijde score did in fact reflect repair as judged by the expert panel in a large number of cases. Special scoring methods for repair of structural damage do not seem necessary [37–42].

Analyzing and Reporting the Scores from Trials

As a result of the new treatments available in RA, several meetings between the FDA and opinion leaders have been held to discuss different outcome measures for new drugs/agents in RA. It is recommended that hands and feet radiographs be obtained in trials of at least 1 year, that both erosions and joint space narrowing are important features, and the smallest detectable difference (SDD) based on the 95% limits of agreement of the observers should be reported as a form of quality control.

More recently, it has been advised to use the smallest detectable change (SDC) as a cutoff to determine progression in individual patients. Two readers should review the films and their scores averaged for analyses. The intraclass correlation coefficient (ICC) assessing interreader reliability of progression scores should be presented [43]. Reporting of the various radiographic scores has proved difficult to compare.

Analysis of radiographic results of a clinical trial is a challenging task. Missing films and/or missing patients are more difficult to handle compared with clinical results. The main reason is that in principle, radiographic damage shows progression, whereas clinical data can fluctuate in two directions. Another important factor is that data on structural damage are highly skewed (a minority of patients show major progression). The best strategy is to perform several types of sensitivity analyses to handle missing films and/or patients with various statistical tests. This has been presented with the results of a clinical trial as an example [44]. This paper also provides recommendations on the presentation of the data. The use of so-called probability plots is a useful aid in presenting and understanding the data in a trial [45].

Conclusion

Most end points used in RA clinical trials are encompassed by clinical evaluation, signs, and symptoms. Radiographs play an important role in RA clinical trials as a surrogate end point, which has clinical relevance because of the relationship with outcomes such as mortality, work disability, and functional loss.

Using a validated scoring method is required to show radiographic changes, and there are many methods available. However, a decision as to which methodology to employ needs to be decided prior to the study start and the study appropriately powered for that end point.

References

1. Steinbrocker O, Traeger CH, Batterman RC. (1949). Therapeutic criteria in rheumatoid arthritis. JAMA 140(8):659–662.
2. Sharp JT, Lidsky MD, Collins LS, Moreland J. (1971). Methods of scoring radiologic changes in rheumatoid arthritis: correlation of radiologic, clinical and laboratory abnormalities. Arthritis Rheuma 14:706–720.
3. Larsen A, Dale K, Eek M. (1977). Radiographic evaluation of rheumatoid arthritis and related conditions by standard reference films. Acta Radiol Diagn 18:481–491.
4. Boers M. (2000). Value of magnetic resonance imaging in rheumatoid arthritis? Lancet 356:1458–1459.
5. Lassere MND, Bird P. (2001). Measurement of rheumatoid arthritis disease activity and damage using magnetic resonance imaging. Truth and discrimination: does MRI make the grade? J Rheumatol 28:1151–1157.
6. Angwin A, Heald G, Lloyd A, Howland K, Davy M, James M. (2001). Reliability and sensitivity of joint space measurements in hand radiographs using computerized image analysis. J Rheumatol 28:1825–1836.

7. van der Heijde DM. (1989). Effects of hydroxychloroquine and sulfasalazine on progression of joint damage in rheumatoid arthritis. Lancet 1:1036–1038.
8. Genant H (1983). Methods of assessing radiographic change in rheumatoid arthritis. Am J Med 75:35–47.
9. Scott DL, Houssien DA, Laasonen L. (1995). Proposed modification to Larsen's scoring methods for hand and wrist radiographs. Br J Rheumatol 34:56.
10. Rau R, Herborn G. (1995). A modified version of Larsen's scoring method to assess radiologic changes in rheumatoid arthritis. J Rheumatol 22:1976–1982.
11. Bathon JM, Martin RW, Fleischmann RM, et al. (2000). A comparison of etanercept and methotrexate in patients with early rheumatoid arthritis. N Engl J Med 343(22): 1586–1593.
12. Sharp JT, Strand V, Leung H, et al. (2000). Treatment with leflunomide slows radiographic progression of rheumatoid arthiritis: results from three randomized controlled trials of leflunomide in patients with active rheumatoid arthritis. Am Coll Rheumatol 43(3):495–505.
13. Lipsky P, van der Heijde DMFM, St Clair EW, et al. (2000). Infliximab and methotrexate in the treatment of rheumatoid arthritis. N Engl J Med 343(22):1594–1602.
14. van der Heijde D, Landewé R, Klareskog L, Rodríguez-Valverde V, Settas L, Pedersen R, Fatenejad S. (2005). Presentation and analysis of radiographic outcome in clinical trials: experience from the TEMPO trial. Arthritis Rheum 52:49–60.
15. van Everdingen AA, Jacobs JWG, van Reesema DRS, et al. (2002). Low-dose prednisone therapy for patients with early active rheumatoid arthritis: clinical efficacy, disease-modifying properties, and side effects: a randomized, double-blind, placebo-controlled clinical trial. Ann Intern Med 136:1–12.
16. Kellgren JH, Lawrence JS. (1957). Radiological assessment of rheumatoid arthritis. Ann Rheum Dis 16:485–493.
17. Kellgren JH, Jeffrey MR, Ball J. (1963). The epidemiology of chronic rheumatism. In: Atlas of Standard Radiographs of Arthritis. Vol. II. Oxford: Blackwell, pp. 22–32.
18. van der Heijde DM. (1996). Plain X-rays in rheumatoid arthritis: overview of scoring methods, their reliability and applicability. Baillieres Clin Rheumatol 10(3):435–453.
19. Larsen A, Dale K. (1977). Standardized radiological evaluation of rheumatoid arthritis in therapeutic trials. In: Dumonde DC, Jasani JK, eds. Recognition of Anti-Rheumatic Drugs. Lancaster, PA: MTP Press, pp. 285–292.
20. Larsen A, Horton J, Howland C. (1984). The effects of auranofin and parenteral gold in the treatment of rheumatoid arthritis: an X-ray analysis. Clin Rheumatol 3(Suppl 1):97–104.
21. Larsen A, Thoen J. (1987). Hand radiography of 200 patients with rheumatoid arthritis after an interval of one year. Scand J Rheumatol 16:395–401.
22. Larsen A. (1995). How to apply Larsen score in evaluating radiographs of rheumatoid arthritis in long-term studies. J Rheumatol 22:1974–1975.
23. Sharp JT, Young DY, Bluhm GB, et al. (1985). How many joints in the hands and wrists should be included in a score of radiologic abnormalities used to assess rheumatoid arthritis? Arthritis Rheum 28:1326–1335.
24. Kaye JJ, Callahan LF, Nance EP, et al. (1987). Rheumatoid arthritis: explanatory power of specific radiographic findings for clinical status. Radiology 1987;165:753–758.
25. Boini S, Guillemin F. (2001). Radiographic scoring methods as outcome measures in rheumatoid arthritis: properties and advantages. Ann Rheum Dis 60:817–827.
26. Genant H, Jiang, Y, Peterfy C, Lu Y, Redei J, Countryman P. (1998). Assessment of rheumatoid arthritis using a modified scoring method in digitized and original radiographs. Arthritis Rheum 41(9):1583–1590.
27. Rau R, Wassenberg S, Herborn G, Stucki G, Gebler A. (1998). A new method of scoring radiographic change in rheumatoid arthritis. J Rheumatol 25:2094–2107.
28. van der Heijde DM, Dankert T, Nieman F, Rau R, Boers M. (1999). Reliability and sensitivity to change of a simplification of the Sharp/van der Heijde radiological assessment in rheumatoid arthritis. Rheumatology 38:941–947.

29. Wolfe F, van der Heijde DM, Larsen A. (2000). Assessing radiographic status of rheumatoid arthritis: introduction of a short erosion scale. J Rheumatol 27:2090–2099.
30. Lassere M, Boers M, van der Heijde D, et al. (1999). Smallest detectable difference in radiological progression. J Rheumatol 26:731–739.
31. Scott DL. (2004). Radiological progression in established rheumatoid arthritis. J Rheumatol 31(Suppl 69):55–65.
32. Bruynesteyn K, van der Heijde D, Boers M, et al. (2004). The Sharp/van der Heijde method out-performed the Larsen/Scott method on the individual patient level in assessing radiographs in early rheumatoid arthritis. J Clin Epidemiol 57(5):502–512.
33. FDA. (1999, February). Guidance for Industry. Clinical development programs for drugs, devices, and biological products for the treatment of rheumatoid arthritis (RA). Bethesda, MD: U.S. FDA.
34. FDA. (2000, July). Briefing Document for Arthritis Advisory Committee. Discussion and consideration of proposed radiographic outcome measures for investigational agents for the treatment of rheumatoid arthritis. Available at http://www.fda.gov/ohrms/dockets/ac/00/questions/3623q2.pdf. Accessed January 20, 2003.
35. Bruynesteyn K, Landewé R, van der Linden S, van der Heijde D. (2004). Radiography as primary outcome in rheumatoid arthritis: acceptable sample sizes for trials with 3 months' follow- up. Ann Rheum Dis 63(11):1413–1418.
36. Bruynesteyn K, van der Heijde D, Boers M, et al. (2002). Detecting radiological changes in rheumatoid arthritis that are considered important by clinical experts: influence of reading with or without known sequence. J Rheumatol 29:2306–2312.
37. van der Heijde D, Landewe R. (2003). Imaging: do erosions heal? Ann Rheum Dis 62(Suppl 2):ii10–12.
38. Rau R, Wassenberg S, Herborn G, Perschel W, Freitag G. (2001). Identification of radiological healing phenomenon in patients with rheumatoid arthritis. J Rheumatol 28:2608–2615.
39. Sharp J, van der Heijde D, Boers M, et al., for the Subcommittee on Healing of Erosions of the OMERACT Imaging Committee. (2003). Repair of erosions in rheumatoid arthritis does occur. Results from two studies by the OMERACT subcommittee on healing of erosions. J Rheumatol 30(5):1102–1107.
40. van der Heijde D, Sharp J, Rau R, Strand V, on behalf of subcommittee on healing of erosions of the OMERACT imaging committee. (2003). OMERACT Workshop: repair of structural damage in rheumatoid arthritis. J Rheumatol 30(5):1108–1109.
41. van der Heijde D, Landewé R, Winalski C, Weissman B, Wassenberg S, Rau R, Herborn G, Einstein E, Boonen A, Sharp JT. (2004). Erosion repair in RA is recognised by expert readers but cannot be distinguished from progression by specific features. Arthritis Rheum 50(9 Suppl):S167.
42. Landewé R, van der Heijde D, Boonen A, Einstein E, Herborn G, Rau R, Wassenberg S, Weissman B,Winalski C, Sharp JT. (2004). Providing readers with films of the entire hand or foot compared to single joints does not improve discrimination between progression and repair in RA. Arthritis Rheum 50(9 Suppl):S174.
43. van der Heijde DM, Simon L, Smolen J, et al. (2002). How to report radiographic data in randomized clinical trials in rheumatoid arthritis: guidelines from a roundtable discussion. Arthritis Rheum 47:215–218.
44. van der Heijde D, Landewé R, Klareskog L, et al. (2005). Presentation and analysis of radiographic outcome in clinical trials: experience from the TEMPO trial. Arthritis Rheum 52: 49–60.
45. Landewé R, van der Heijde D. (2004). Radiographic progression depicted by probability plots: presenting data with optimal use of individual values. Arthritis Rheum 50(3):699–706.

Chapter 14
Radiography in Clinical Trials Investigating Osteoarthritis

Cornelis van Kuijk

Introduction

Osteoarthritis (OA) is a disease of joints characterized by cartilage loss and bone remodeling due to the changing biomechanical demands as the function of the cartilage as a cushion is slowly lost. The bone surrounding the joint is reacting in an attempt to enforce itself. This leads to (subchondral) sclerosis and the formation of osteophytes. These bony changes, secondary to the disease, are well depicted on conventional radiographs of arthritic joints. The loss of cartilage cannot be seen with conventional radiography. However, joint space narrowing (JSN) is an indirect and surrogate measure of cartilage loss.

In clinical trials investigating drugs that are hypothesized to stop or slow down the disease, radiographs are used to investigate the progression of OA. Several methods have been developed to grade or measure the extent and severity of the disease. These methods can be divided into two groups: quantitative and semiquantitative methods. Joint space width can be measured, and as such this is a quantitative measure of joint space changes. These measurements can be done manually or automated using computerized image analysis methods. Grading the disease by visual expert assessment gives a semiquantitative measure. Several grading schemes have been published, some more refined and elaborate than others.

These quantitative and semiquantitative methods have been published for hand, hip, and knee joints. However, most of the work has been conducted concerning grading and measuring OA of the knee. The accurate and reproducible acquisition of radiographs is a key issue when radiographs are used to monitor osteoarthritis and the pharmaceutical interventions intended to halt the disease.

In this chapter, the use of radiographs in clinical trials studying OA is discussed. The acquisition of radiographs and the analysis methods for quantifying or grading OA are also discussed.

C. van Kuijk
Department of Radiology, VU University Medical Center, Amsterdam, The Netherlands

D.M. Reid, C.G. Miller (eds.), *Clinical Trials in Rheumatoid Arthritis and Osteoarthritis*, 223

The Acquisition of Radiographs

As there is an abundance of literature concerning the acquisition of radiographs in knee OA, we will review some of the key elements [1–11] (Table 14.1).

Standardization and rigid quality control of methods used are mandatory in clinical trials. This holds true also for radiographs used to produce primary or secondary outcome parameters in clinical trials. First, one should establish an imaging protocol that ensures a high reproducibility in a multicenter environment and that also provides images that can be used to measure or grade the disease or features of the disease with high precision. As OA is a slowly progressing disease entity in which

Table 14.1 Imaging techniques to study knee OA

Standing AP view (Fig. 14.1)	Film cassette against posterior knee. No flexion of knee. Horizontal x-ray beam. AP view.
Fluoroscopic-guided semiflexed AP view (Fig. 14.2)	Patient in front of and close to film cassette. Knees are flexed under fluoroscopic control. Image made when medial joint space is visualized with superimposing anterior and posterior margins with horizontal x-ray beam. Feet can be rotated to center the tibial spines in the femoral notch. AP view.
Fluoroscopic-guided Lyon Schuss view (Fig. 14.3)	Film cassette against anterior knee. Upper legs against x-ray unit. The x-ray beam is angled under fluoroscopic control until the anterior and posterior margins of the medial joint space are superimposed and image is made. Feet can be rotated to center the tibial spines in the femoral notch. PA view.
Semiflexed metatarsophalangeal view (Fig. 14.4)	Film cassette against anterior knee. MTP joints vertically aligned with cassette. Knees are flexed (10 degrees). Horizontal x-ray beam. Feet rotated externally (15 degrees). PA view.
Fixed-flexion PA view (Fig. 14.5)	Film cassette against anterior knee. Upper legs against x-ray unit. The x-ray beam is angled 10 degrees downward. Feet rotated externally (10 degrees). PA view.

AP, anteroposterior; PA, posteroanterior; MTP, metatarsophalangeal.

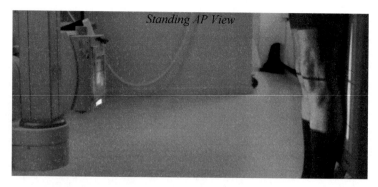
Standing AP View

Fig. 14.1 Film cassette against posterior knee. No flexion of knee. Horizontal x-ray beam. AP view

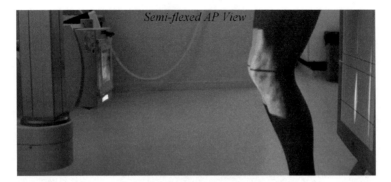

Fig. 14.2 Patient in front of and close to film cassette. Knees are flexed under fluoroscopic control. Image made when medial joint space is visualized with superimposing anterior and posterior margins with horizontal x-ray beam. Feet can be rotated to center the tibial spines in the femoral notch. AP view

joint space and surrounding bone is changing very slowly over years, very small changes have to be picked up significantly in a study population that can be handled both logistically and economically to prove the efficacy of the treatment under study. This requires methodology that is highly precise.

In clinical, day-to-day practice, standardized radiographs are made for knee OA. However, it has been argued and been shown that the standing anteroposterior (AP) view that is routinely made does not fit the requirements set for clinical trials. Several other imaging protocols have therefore been published. Some authors argue that the radiographs should be made under fluoroscopic control as is done for the

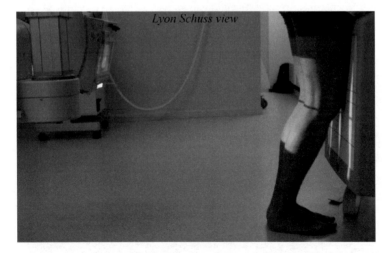

Fig. 14.3 Film cassette against anterior knee. Upper legs against x-ray unit. The x-ray beam is angled under fluoroscopic control until the anterior and posterior margins of the medial joint space are superimposed and image is made. Feet can be rotated to center the tibial spines in the femoral notch. PA view

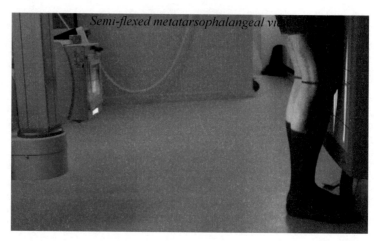

Fig. 14.4 Film cassette against anterior knee. MTP joints vertically aligned with cassette. Knees are flexed (10 degrees). Horizontal x-ray beam. Feet rotated externally (15 degrees). PA view

semiflexed AP view and the Lyon Schuss view. Others argue that this is unpractical and that other views such as the semiflexed metatarsophalangeal (MTP) view and the fixed-flexion posteroanterior (PA) view has preference. This has led to considerable debate between experts that still is unresolved. No consensus has been reached between experts what the best imaging protocol is. A recent review by Mazzuca and Brandt [12] discusses all these different imaging methods in terms of reproducibility and use in clinical trials. They show that these specific imaging methods all have a short-term high precision in strictly controlled environments with some advantage for the fluoroscopic techniques. However, most clinical trials in OA are

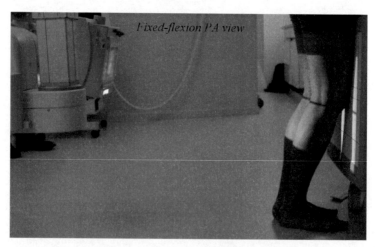

Fig. 14.5 Film cassette against anterior knee. Upper legs against x-ray unit. The x-ray beam is angled 10 degrees downward. Feet rotated externally (10 degrees). PA view

long-term multicenter trials that are subjected to considerable dangers, both due to those that happen over time such as changes of equipment and those due to technologist turnover and intercenter differences both in terms of reliability and experience with the demands of clinical trials.

In all cases, the film technique (kVp, mAs, film-focus distance, tube-angulation, and patient positioning) should be well described and standardized.

Measuring Joint Space Width

Joint space narrowing is a key feature of OA. The measurement of joint space width (JSW) over time is therefore a potential surrogate outcome measure to evaluate drug efficacy in preserving cartilage integrity. Under the assumption that we have optimally standardized image acquisition, the next step is to find the best technique to measure JSW. JSW can be measured manually with rulers and callipers or in a more sophisticated way with computerized techniques. Digital images of radiographs of arthritic joints and image analysis techniques that can detect the borders of the joints and derive distances between those borders are used to measure JSN. Automated techniques are preferred over manual techniques because of the higher precision. Furthermore, these measurements are time consuming and very labor intensive, even for highly trained staff, when done manually. Automated techniques have been published for the joints in the hand, the hip, and the knee. Again it is the knee that is usually studied in clinical trials, and several analysis algorithms have been published for measuring JSN but also for osteophyte size (Fig. 14.6).

Mazzuca [13] showed that the effect of measurement error on sample size in a disease-modifying OA drug trial is considerable. Automated measurements on radiographs with the semiflexed technique compared with manual measurements on radiographs with the standing AP view would decrease the sample size by approximately 44%.

A study by Ravaud et al. [14] compared four different manual measuring instruments (ruler, calliper, graduated magnifying glass, and digitized measurement with an electric grid) for measuring JSW on standardized knee radiographs. It was concluded that the ruler and digitized assessment had a better reliability. Semiautomated and true automated measurements on digitized films were published by Dacre and Huskisson [15], Lynch et al. [16], Duryea et al. [17], and Duryea et al. [18]. The latter study showed that a reproducibility of less than 0.2 mm for the medial compartment of the knee could be achieved.

Techniques for measuring JSW in the hip have been described [19–22]. However, the joint space itself is rather small to begin with, and although high reproducibility of fully automated measurements can be achieved, the sensitivity to detecting change in normal or pathologic hip joints has not been studied adequately with the fully automated techniques.

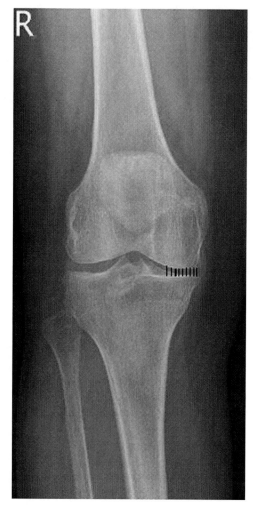

Fig. 14.6 Finding minimal JSW. Manual or computerized methods are used to measure JSN

Grading Disease Severity

Again, an abundance of literature is available discussing several grading schemes for assessing disease severity. Some of them score overall disease severity taking into account the complete picture of all the radiographic features of OA. One of these is the well-known method published by Kellgren and Lawrence [23]. More sophisticated techniques grade the different features of OA independently. JSN, subchondral sclerosis, and other features such as osteophytosis can all be graded separately. Usually a four-level grading scheme is used; 0 being normal; 1, or mild disease being abnormal 1% to 33%; 2, or moderate disease being abnormal 34% to 66%; 3, or severe disease being abnormal 67% to 100%. A comprehensive list of grading schemes was published by Gunther and Sun [24]. There is quite a difference between the different scoring schemes in number of grades and the weight that is given to certain features of OA. Figures 14.7 to 14.10 show some examples of knee films from normal to severe OA.

These gradings are subjective visual assessments and subject to interobserver and intraobserver variability depending on the experience of the readers. Usually in clinical trials, a limited number of readers is used, who, before the study starts, are trained in the grading scheme and have done a number of consensus readings to decrease the interobserver variability. This inter-reader and intrareader variability is usually worse for the initial grading at baseline than for the grading of disease progression.

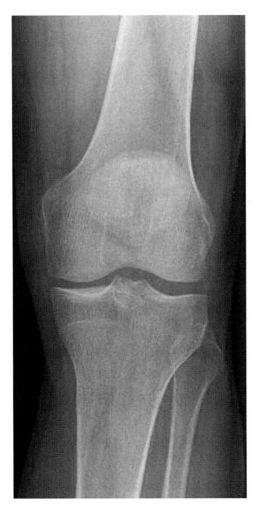

Fig. 14.7 Normal knee

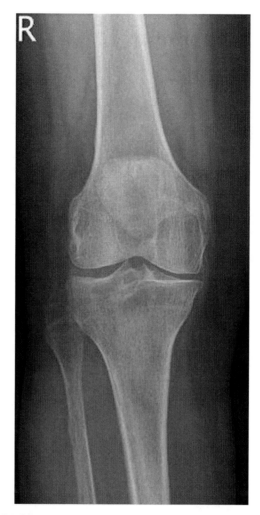

Fig. 14.8 Mild medial OA

Grading is facilitated by atlases that have been published that provide example images to compare with. One of these is the "Radiographic atlas for osteoarthritis of the hand, hip and knee" published by the Osteoarthritis Research Society (*Osteoarthritis and Cartilage* 1995;3[Suppl A]) in which an atlas of individual radiographic features in OA is described by Altman et al. [25]. For the hand, marginal osteophytes, JSN, malalignment, subchondral erosions, and sclerosis are graded in several joints. For the hip, JSN, marginal osteophytes, femoral buttressing, and subchondral lucencies and sclerosis are graded for acetabular and femoral changes. For the tibiofemoral knee joint, JSN, marginal osteophytes, and subchondral sclerosis are graded in the medial and lateral compartment at the femoral and the tibial sites; malalignment and the hypertrophy of tibial spinous processes is noted.

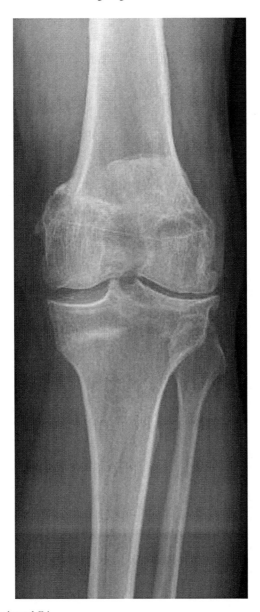

Fig. 14.9 Moderate lateral OA

For the patellofemoral knee joint, JSN, marginal osteophytes, patellar subchondral sclerosis, and subluxation are graded.

The inter-reader reliability expressed as percentage of agreement in this type of detailed grading schemes is between 70% and 95% with an intraclass correlation coefficient (ICCS) between 0.6 and 0.8. For intrareader reliability, this is between

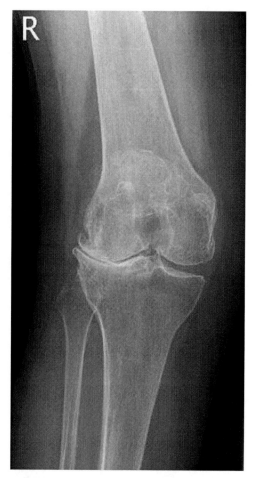

Fig. 14.10 Severe lateral OA

80% and 100% (percentage of agreement) and between 0.8 and 0.95 (ICCS). For the overall grading schemes, the inter-reader reliability is around 50% agreement and 0.7 ICCS, and the intrareader reliability is around 65% agreement and 0.9 ICCS [26].

Data from Clinical Trials

In the previous paragraphs, we have discussed the image acquisition, the measurement of JSN as surrogate measure of OA disease, and the semiquantitative grading of the disease using radiographs. But how does this all work out in clinical trials? In a paper by Mazzuca and Brandt [27], a nice review is given about the use of plain radiography as an outcome measure in clinical trials studying knee osteoarthritis. They reported the effect of technical quality of the x-ray films on the measurement of minimum JSW in the medial compartment of knees that were imaged twice. They showed that the standard error of measurement increased to 0.4 mm in poor-quality films with a percentage coefficient of variation (CV) of 10% compared with good-quality films with a standard error of 0.25 mm and a CV of 7%, thus showing the need for strict quality control procedures. Furthermore, they showed that sample size and duration of studies investigating the potential disease-modifying efficacy of drugs increase dramatically when the standard error of the measurement increases. Thereby, the authors demonstrated the need for using the optimal imaging acquisition protocol as well as the need for highly precise measurements.

Ravaud et al. [28] followed 55 patient with knee OA for 1 year and evaluated quantitative methods and grading schemes to assess longitudinal reproducibility. They suggested that measuring JSW should be preferred as outcome measure for clinical trials.

Reginster et al. [29] showed that JSN was halted in a 3-year study in patients treated with glucosamine sulfate compared with placebo controls. Mean joint space loss was 0.3 mm (CI, 0.5 to 0.1) in 106 placebo controls after 3 years and was not significant in patients treated. As the natural disease progression of OA is rather slow, the best reproducibility of measurements and/or use of grading schemes is mandatory if study sample size and length of study is to be kept within manageable limits.

References

1. Buckland-Wright JC, MacFarlane DG, Lynch JA, Jasani MK. Quantitative microfocal radiography detects changes in OA knee joint space width in patients in placebo controlled trial of NSAID therapy. J Rheumatol 1995;22(5):937–943.
2. Piperno M, Hellio Le Graverand MP, Conrozier T, Bochu M, Mathieu P, Vignon E. Quantitative evaluation of joint space width in femorotibial osteoarthritis: comparison of three radiographic views. Osteoarthritis Cartilage 1998;6(4):252–259.
3. Ravaud P, Giraudeau B, Auleley GR, Drape JL, Rousselin B, Paolozzi L, Chastang C, Dougados M. Variability in knee radiographing: implication for definition of radiological progression in medial knee osteoarthritis. Ann Rheum Dis 1998;57(10):624–629.
4. Buckland-Wright JC, Wolfe F, Ward RJ, Flowers N, Hayne C. Substantial superiority of semiflexed (MTP) views in knee osteoarthritis: a comparative radiographic study, without fluoroscopy, of standing extended, semiflexed (MTP), and schuss views. J Rheumatol 1999;26(12):2664–2674.
5. Mazzuca SA, Brandt KD, Dieppe PA, Doherty M, Katz BP, Lane KA. Effect of alignment of the medial tibial plateau and x-ray beam on apparent progression of osteoarthritis in the standing anteroposterior knee radiograph. Arthritis Rheum 2001;44(8):1786–1794.
6. Inoue S, Nagamine R, Miura H, Urabe K, Matsuda S, Sakaki K, Iwamoto Y. Anteroposterior weight-bearing radiography of the knee with both knees in semiflexion, using new equipment. J Orthop Sci 2001;6(6):475–480.
7. Mazzuca SA, Brandt KD, Buckwalter KA, Lane KA, Katz BP. Field test of the reproducibility of the semiflexed metatarsophalangeal view in repeated radiographic examinations of subjects with osteoarthritis of the knee. Arthritis Rheum 2002;46(1):109–113.
8. Wolfe F, Lane NE, Buckland-Wright C. Radiographic methods in knee osteoarthritis: a further comparison of semiflexed (MTP), schuss-tunnel, and weight-bearing anteroposterior views for joint space narrowing and osteophytes. J Rheumatol 2002;29(12):2597–2601.

9. Yamanaka N, Takahashi T, Ichikawa N, Yamamoto H. Posterior-anterior weight-bearing radiograph in 15 degree knee flexion in medial osteoarthritis. Skeletal Radiol 2003;32(1):28–34.

10. Peterfy C, Li J, Zaim S, Duryea J, Lynch J, Miaux Y, Yu W, Genant HK. Comparison of fixed-flexion positioning with fluoroscopic semi-flexed positioning for quantifying radiographic joint-space width in the knee: test-retest reproducibility. Skeletal Radiol 2003;32(3):128–132.

11. Mazzuca SA, Brandt KD, Buckwalter KA. Detection of radiographic joint space narrowing in subjects with knee osteoarthritis: longitudinal comparison of the metatarsophalangeal and semiflexed anteroposterior views. Arthritis Rheum 2003;48(2):385–390.

12. Mazzuca SA, Brandt KD. Is knee radiography useful for studying the efficacy of a disease-modifying osteoarthritis drug in humans? Rheum Dis Clin North Am 2003;29(4):819–830.

13. Mazzuca S. Plain radiography in the evaluation of knee osteoarthritis. Curr Opin Rheumatol 1997;9(3):263–267.

14. Ravaud P, Chastang C, Auleley GR, Giraudeau B, Royant V, Amor B, Genant HK, Dougados M. Assessment of joint space width in patients with osteoarthritis of the knee: a comparison of 4 measuring instruments. J Rheumatol 1996;23(10):1749–1755.

15. Dacre JE, Huskisson EC. The automatic assessment of knee radiographs in osteoarthritis using digital image analysis. Br J Rheumatol 1989;28(6):506–510.

16. Lynch et al. Osteoarthritis Cartilage 1993;1:209–218.

17. Duryea J, Li J, Peterfy CG, Gordon C, Genant HK. Trainable rule-based algorithm for the measurement of joint space width in digital radiographic images of the knee. Med Phys 2000;27(3):580–591.

18. Duryea J, Zaim S, Genant HK. New radiographic-based surrogate outcome measures for osteoarthritis of the knee. Osteoarthritis Cartilage 2003;11(2):102–110.

19. Gordon CL, Wu C, Peterfy CG, Li J, Duryea J, Klifa C, Genant HK. Automated measurement of radiographic hip joint-space width. Med Phys 2001;28(2):267–277.

20. Conrozier T, Lequesne M, Favret H, Taccoen A, Mazieres B, Dougados M, Vignon M, Vignon E. Measurement of the radiological hip joint space width. An evaluation of various methods of measurement. Osteoarthritis Cartilage 2001;9(3):281–286.

21. Auleley GR, Duche A, Drape JL, Dougados M, Ravaud P. Measurement of joint space width in hip osteoarthritis: influence of joint positioning and radiographic procedure. Rheumatology (Oxford) 2001;40(4):414–419.

22. Hilliquin P, Pessis E, Coste J, Mauget D, Azria A, Chevrot A, Menkes CJ, Kahan A. Quantitative assessment of joint space width with an electronic caliper. Osteoarthritis Cartilage 2002;10(7):542–546.

23. Kellgren JH, Lawrence JS. Radiological assessment of osteo-arthrosis. Ann Rheum Dis 1957;16(4):494–502.

24. Gunther KP, Sun Y. Reliability of radiographic assessment in hip and knee osteoarthritis. Osteoarthritis Cartilage 1999;7(2):239–246.

25. Altman RD, Hochberg M, Murphy WA Jr, Wolfe F, Lequesne M. Atlas of individual radiographic features in osteoarthritis. Osteoarthritis Cartilage 1995;3(Suppl A):3–70.

26. Scott WW Jr, Lethbridge-Cejku M, Reichle R, Wigley FM, Tobin JD, Hochberg MC. Reliability of grading scales for individual radiographic features of osteoarthritis of the knee. The Baltimore longitudinal study of aging atlas of knee osteoarthritis. Invest Radiol 1993;28(6):497–501.

27. Mazzuca SA, Brandt KD. Plain radiography as an outcome measure in clinical trials involving patients with knee osteoarthritis. Rheum Dis Clin North Am 1999;25(2):467–480.

28. Ravaud P, Giraudeau B, Auleley GR, Chastang C, Poiraudeau S, Ayral X, Dougados M. Radiographic assessment of knee osteoarthritis: reproducibility and sensitivity to change. J Rheumatol 1996;23(10):1756–1764.

29. Reginster JY, Deroisy R, Rovati LC, Lee RL, Lejeune E, Bruyere O, Giacovelli G, Henrotin Y, Dacre JE, Gossett C. Long-term effects of glucosamine sulphate on osteoarthritis progression: a randomised, placebo-controlled clinical trial. Lancet 2001;357(9252):251–256.

Chapter 15
Use of Quantitative Magnetic Resonance Imaging in the Cross-Sectional and Longitudinal Evaluation of Structural Changes in Knee Osteoarthritis Patients

Jean-Pierre Raynauld, Johanne Martel-Pelletier, François Abram, and Jean-Pierre Pelletier

Introduction

Assessment of structural damage of the articular cartilage is important for monitoring the progression of osteoarthritis (OA) and evaluating therapeutic response. For many years, clinical studies of drug interventions on symptomatic knee OA have focused mainly on clinical parameters, such as pain and joint function, using self-administered questionnaires but without assessing the effect of treatment on structural changes caused by the disease and the role of treatment in preventing cartilage degradation. Recently, such attempts were made to evaluate cartilage damage and its progression in OA. Serial radiographs of affected joints have appeared as a logical means of documenting the progression of OA over time, providing that a validated, reliable, and easily reproducible technique is used [1]. Improvements in the standardization and interpretation of radiographs have enhanced the reliability of the measurement of the joint space width (JSW) and the evaluation of the joint space narrowing (JSN) [2, 3]. However, the sensitivity to change of this measurement is such that a minimum follow-up of 2 to 3 years and more and large numbers of patients (at least 1500 for a two-arm study) is necessary to establish an effect of pharmacological interventions on OA progression. Moreover, measurement of JSW does not capture information on the cartilage changes alone but is also dependent on the integrity of surrounding tissues, especially the meniscus and the subchondral bone. For instance, enucleation of the knee medial meniscus, which may occur during longitudinal studies, can dramatically change the JSW and affect the reliability of such measurement [4], potentially impairing its use in the assessment of cartilage degradation over time. Finally, the JSW progression provides only one measurement

J-P. Raynauld

Osteoarthritis Research Unit, Notre-Dame Hospital, University of Montreal Hospital Center (CHUM), Montreal, Canada

D.M. Reid, C.G. Miller (eds.), *Clinical Trials in Rheumatoid Arthritis and Osteoarthritis*,   235
© Springer-Verlag London Limited 2008

point, which considerably restricts the statistical power of this technique and gives no indication of the real cartilage volume. The use of arthroscopy to assess cartilage appears reliable and sensitive to change at 1 year [5]. However, only the cartilage surface can be evaluated, and the method is semiquantitative and, above all, invasive. Large studies are, therefore, difficult to conduct. Magnetic resonance imaging (MRI) allows precise visualization and assessment of joint structures such as cartilage, bone, synovium, ligaments, and menisci and their pathologic changes. Magnetic resonance (MR) acquisitions are noninvasive and nonradiant, providing a clear advantage over arthroscopy and fluoroscopy.

Clinical Practice for MRI Acquisition of the Knee

The use of a 1.5 T or 3.0 T magnet is nowadays mandatory for quantitative evaluation of the cartilage volume. The MRI acquisition of the knee is performed with a knee antenna, also called an extremity antenna because most are compatible with ankle acquisition. This kind of antenna entirely surrounds the knee, providing a more homogeneous signal for a better image quality. The patient lies down on the table in supine position and is inserted feet first in the magnet. The antenna is not centered in the magnet; it is rather shifted to the side of the pathologic knee for better patient comfort. Because of the height of the antenna, the knee angle is between 10 and 20 degrees. Sagittal slices of 1 mm to 1.5 mm are best for cartilage quantification. Over any longitudinal study, the field of view is constant to preserve the pixel resolution and is fixed at 16 cm. The phase chosen to be anteroposterior (AP) and the field-of-view ratio adjusted to include the entire leg width contribute to avoiding wrapping artifacts. To allow the best quality, a 512×512 phase oversampling matrix is used for a final 0.31×0.31 mm^2 image resolution [6]. Fast imaging acquisition technique preserving short repetition time (TR) is used to ensure an acceptable acquisition time (see next section). The phase oversampling (typically set at 80%) is adjusted to decrease the duration of the acquisition. If the protocol is correctly set up, the main cause of artifact is the movement of the patient, which can result in the sequence being rejected at quality control (QC) time. A proper immobilization of the knee in the antenna is a major key to avoid patient movement.

Recent advances in MRI technology have led to significant improvement in spatial resolution and contrast, enabling researchers to evaluate anatomic damage of all these joint structures across both cross-sectional and longitudinal planes (Fig. 15.1). The types of MR sequences that have been most commonly used for cartilage quantification over recent years have been T1-weighted spoiled GE (gradient echo) sequences, FLASH (fast low angle shot), spoiled GRASS (gradient recalled acquisition at steady state), SPGR (spoiled gradient recalled), or the T1-weighted fat suppressed FISP (fast imaging at steady-state precession) sequence (Table 15.1). All these sequences are very similar, with a reasonable acquisition time (between 10 and 30 minutes) and are available on most clinical MRI systems at ≥ 1.5 T field strength. All of these GRE sequences use fat suppression to better delineate the bone-cartilage

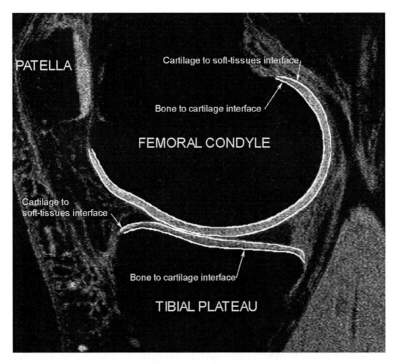

Fig. 15.1 Human knee cartilage in sagittal view acquired with 1.5 T magnet using FISP acquisition with fat suppression. This sequence acquisition produces maps with the highest cartilage contrast. Cartilage interfaces are delineated

margin. This is accomplished either by spectral fat-saturation using a prepulse tuned to the resonant frequency of fat or, more recently, by frequency-selective water excitation (WE). Fat suppression (FS) is required to provide a sufficient dynamic range to the image contrast to delineate the cartilage but also to eliminate chemical-shift artifacts, which arise at the cartilage-bone interface. Acquisition times are generally

Table 15.1 Samples of parameters for MRI acquisition protocol on two different instruments

Siemens: 3D FISP WE	GE: 3D SPGR FS
Slice thickness = 1.5 mm	Slice thickness = 1.5 mm
Repetition time = 22 ms	Repetition time = 42 ms
Echo time = 9 ms	Echo time = 7 ms
Fat suppress = water excitation	Fat suppress = normal
Field of view = 16 cm	Field of view = 16 cm
Percent sampling = 100%	Percent sampling = 100%
Percent phase = 87.5%	Percent phase = 87.5%
Flip angle = 14 degrees	Flip angle = 20 degrees
(Duration 10 to 15 minutes)	(Duration 20 to 30 minutes)

shorter for selective water-excitation protocols than for those using spectral fat suppression, as the latter requires an additional pulse at the beginning of the sequence.

MRI Acquisition Sequences to Identify Macromolecules Content in Articular Cartilage

The concentration of glycosaminoglycan (GAG) in articular cartilage is also known to be an important determinant of tissue mechanical properties based on numerous studies. This cartilage property can now be explored by using delayed gadolinium-enhanced MRI of cartilage (dGEMRIC). In a recent study [7], tibial plateaus from patients undergoing total knee arthroplasty were imaged by dGEMRIC. At different test locations for each tibial plateau, the load response to focal indentation was measured as an index of cartilage stiffness. Overall, a high correlation was found between the dGEMRIC index ($T1_{Gd}$) and local stiffness (Pearson correlation coefficients r = 0.90, 0.64, 0.81; p < 0.0001) when the GAG at each test location was averaged over a depth of tissue comparable with that affected by the indentation. These results demonstrate the importance of MRI in yielding spatial localization of GAG concentration in the evaluation of cartilage mechanical properties and suggest the possibility that the evaluation of mechanical properties may be improved further by adding other MRI parameters sensitive to the collagen component of cartilage.

Recently however, the FDA issued a warning regarding important safety information about gadolinium-containing contrast agents and a disease known as Nephrogenic Systemic Fibrosis or Nephrogenic Fibrosing Dermopathy (NSF/NFD) that occurs in patients with kidney failure. Therefore, the impact of this warning on future research on cartilage imaging techniques using a contrast agent is unknown.

In this context, Regatte et al. [8] have explored a noninvasive technology which enables the assessment of cartilage degeneration through the measurement of GAG content with the same efficiency as the dGEMRIC. This method used a spin-lock pulse sequence allowing evaluation by $T1\rho$ parameter, comparable with the T1 or $T1_{Gd}$.

Another MR acquisition technique, a transverse relaxation time (T2)-mapping, detecting changes in cartilage water content was reviewed by Mosher et al. [10], which discussed the relationship between cartilage T2 and water content, proteoglycan concentration, collagen concentration, or tissue anisotropy. Using this sequence, Liess et al. [9] demonstrated on 20 healthy volunteers that reducing the water content of the patellar cartilage by repetitive knee bending can be quantified. Hence, the detection of small physiologic changes in water content may help in the early diagnosis of OA.

The quality of the cartilage is dependent on the structural organization of the collagen, and the transverse relaxation time (T2) appears also relevant for collagen variation assessment. Alternatively, the MR diffusion tensor imaging (DTI) could also be used for analyzing the internal anisotropy of tissues, being very helpful to detect early changes in collagen fiber alignment. Beyond the conventional MR diffusion-weighted imaging (DWI) used to assess the apparent diffusion coefficient of water in tissues, diffusion tensor MRI allows determination of the degree of diffusion anisotropy and the direction of local diffusion in tissues. By using DWI technology a study [11] conducted with a 9.4 T magnet field was able to identify the orientation of collagen fibers in the patella.

Precision and Reliability of Knee Cartilage Quantification

Although structural cartilage changes can be seen with acquisition sequences like the SPGR or FISP, quantification of these changes has been the real challenge for many years. Initial attempts at quantitative measurement of cartilage were performed only in healthy subjects [12] or in animal models [13]. The recent improvement in image analysis has led to reliable quantitative measurement of cartilage volume and thickness of normal but also OA conditions. Methods for measuring cartilage volume for the complete knee joint (femur and tibia) are now used for determining the volume of the cartilage over time [14] (Fig. 15.2). Research teams are now using the specific MRI acquisitions (SPGR, FISP) combined with a computer software to obtain valuable information on cartilage volume in normal and OA patients [15–18]. Moreover, standard cartilage views can be anatomically segmented, allowing evaluation of cartilage volume and thickness in anatomical subregions and specific focal defects [19].

The reliability and precision of quantitative MRI assessments of any given radiology center are first established with the use of phantoms, mimicking human tissue interfaces. Several acquisitions of these over short periods of time are used to assess the precision of both image acquisition and data extraction. These phantoms are also useful to assess any drift of the MR signal over a long time period combined with periodical machine maintenance. The principal issue is the assessment of distortion of the MRI equipment. Thus, enabling the evaluation of any abnormal shift of the acquisition.

There have been demonstrations of the precision and reliability of MRI technology for the assessment of change in cartilage volume of the knee over time in OA patients. For example, Eckstein et al. [20] published a study on precision errors in healthy volunteers under short-term imaging conditions (acquisitions immediately following each other with joint repositioning), long-term imaging conditions (acquisitions taken approximately over 9 months, but postprocessed immediately after each other), and resegmentation (postprocessing) of the same data sets spaced over 12 months. They found that long-term precision errors (1.9 to 3.9 CV% coefficient of variation %) were not significantly larger than short-term acquisition conditions (2 to 3.6 CV%). Also, no systematic drift was observed, suggesting that scanner conditions had remained stable throughout this period. However, resegmentation errors were somewhat higher over time suggesting that digital postprocessing of the MRI in longitudinal studies should be performed upon completion of studies in one session. Our group [17] looked at the inter-reader and intra-reader reliability of

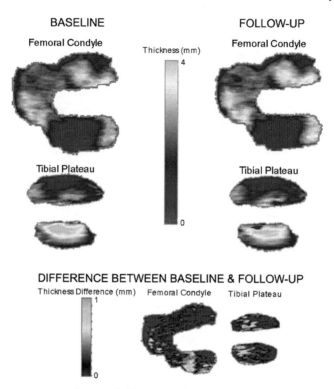

Fig. 15.2 Representation of gray-coded images of human osteoarthritic knee cartilage volume. Cartilage thickness was defined as the Euclidian distance between the bone-cartilage interface defined by the baseline image and the cartilage surrounding tissue interface. Each thickness value was measured. A typical data set provides approximately 60,000 reading measurement points for the femoral condyle and 40,000 for the tibial plateau. Elementary volume is defined as volume between the bone-cartilage interface offset map and its corresponding cartilage-synovium offset map. Change in knee cartilage volume is obtained by subtracting follow-up cartilage volume from baseline volume. Maps showing difference between baseline and 1-year acquisition are displayed for femoral condyles and tibial plateaus

the technology using similar combinations of MRI acquisitions and a software to quantify cartilage volume in patients with knee OA. The objectives were to assess measurement reliability by determining the differences between readings of the same image made by the same reader 2 weeks apart (test-retest reliability), determining the differences between the readings of the same image made by different readers (between-reader agreement), and determining the differences between the cartilage volume readings obtained from two MR images of the same knee acquired a few hours apart (patient positioning reliability). Forty-eight MRI examinations of the knee from normal subjects, patients with different stages of symptomatic knee OA, and a subset of duplicate images were independently and blindly quantified by three readers using the imaging system. Between-reader agreement of measurements was excellent, as shown by intraclass correlation (ICC) coefficients ranging from 0.958 to 0.997 for global cartilage, 0.974 to 0.998 for the compartments, and 0.943 to 0.999 for the femoral condyles. Test-retest reliability of within-reader data was also excellent, with Pearson correlation coefficients ranging from 0.978 to 0.999. Patient positioning reliability was also excellent, with Pearson correlation coefficients ranging from 0.978 to 0.999.

Cross-sectional Quantitative Cartilage Measurements

Estimates of cartilage thinning during normal aging (in the absence of OA) have been derived from cross-sectional data obtained in healthy elderly subjects without history of knee joint symptoms, trauma, or surgery (50 to 78 years; 11 men, 12 women) relative to a cohort of young, healthy subjects that met the same criteria (20 to 30 years; 49 men, 46 women). The authors [21] reported an estimated 0.3% to 0.5% reduction of cartilage thickness per annum for all knee compartments. In the patella, women displayed a higher estimated loss than men, but no gender difference was found for other compartments of the knee. Burgkart et al. [15] determined cartilage volume in 8 OA patients prior to total knee replacement and estimated the loss by comparison with a group of 28 healthy volunteers. They reported a difference of approximately 1300 mm^3 in the medial tibia in patients with varus OA, and differences of approximately 1800 mm^3 in the lateral tibia in patients with valgus or bicompartmental OA. These values were found to exceed the precision error in the tibia of healthy volunteers and OA patients by a factor of >20:1. Recently, however, larger age- and gender-specific reference data on normal volunteers have been published [21, 22] and provide T- and Z-scores for the OA population, as currently used in the diagnosis of osteoporosis. One problem with this approach, however, is the relatively large intersubject variability of cartilage volume in healthy individuals. Because of a weak correlation of cartilage volume with body height and weight but a much larger one with bone size [23], it has been suggested that cartilage volume should be normalized to the original bone interface area (before the onset of disease) to achieve better discrimination between OA patients and healthy subjects.

Optimization of cross-sectional analysis is particularly important for patient selection into longitudinal trials. It has been shown that patients with a JSW less than 4 mm in semiflexed weight-bearing radiographs are more likely to progress over the years and that these may therefore be more suitable candidates for disease-modifying osteoarthritis drug (DMOAD) trials. Small cartilage volume alone is not a suitable selection criterion, because this would include subjects with small bone size rather than subjects with reduced cartilage thickness. This is particularly relevant because cartilage thickness and joint size have been shown to be not highly correlated [23].

Quantitative Cartilage Measurements in Longitudinal Studies

Data on changes in cartilage volume from longitudinal studies have recently become available. Wluka et al. [18] have quantified the changes in cartilage volume in the medial and lateral tibia of 123 patients (52 men, 71 women; age 63.1 ± 10.6 years) with symptomatic and radiographic evidence of knee OA over a period of approximately 2 years. The mean loss of tibial articular cartilage was 5.3% per year. The initial cartilage volume was the most significant determinant of loss of tibial cartilage. Age and body mass index (BMI) were also found to be weakly associated with cartilage (tibia) loss. The authors found no significant difference in the amount of relative (%) cartilage loss between women and men and only a relatively low correlation between changes in the medial and lateral tibia. Cicuttini et al. analyzed patellar cartilage changes in 110 patients from the same cohort [24]. The rate of relative (%) cartilage loss was significantly higher in women (5.3%) compared with men (3.5%), and there was no significant association between change in the patella and both the medial and lateral tibia, the latter suggesting different OA pathogenetic mechanisms. Subjects with higher baseline pain scores displayed higher loss than those with lower pain scores, as did those with high BMI.

Another recently published study examined the progression of cartilage volume loss on 32 patients with symptomatic knee OA over 2 years. The MRI acquisitions were done at baseline, 6, 12, 18, and 24 months [25]. Knee OA progression (cartilage volume loss expressed as percent of loss compared with the baseline value for each patient) computed at all the follow-up points was statistically significant: a mean of 3.8% of global cartilage loss (femoral condyle and tibial plateau) and 4.3% for the medial compartment (femoral condyle and tibial plateau) at 6 months; 3.6% and 4.2% loss at 12 months; and 6.1% and 7.6% loss at 24 months. Using discriminatory function analysis, two groups were identified: 21 subjects progressed slowly over the 24-month period of observation (<2% of global cartilage loss) and 11 progressed rapidly (>15% of global cartilage loss). The risk factors that were identified to be associated with a fast progression of the disease were female gender, high BMI, reduced range of movement of the study knee, greater knee circumference, and higher knee pain and stiffness as assessed by the Western Ontario and McMaster Universities Osteoarthritis Index (WOMAC) questionnaire.

A second study by Raynauld et al. [26] using a larger number of OA patients ($n = 107$) further explored the changes in knee cartilage volume over 24 months using qMRI. These findings were contrasted with demographic, clinical, and biochemical variables and other MRI anatomic features of disease progression. In this study, three different populations were identified according to cartilage volume loss: fast ($n = 11$ patients), intermediate ($n = 48$), and slow ($n = 48$) progressors, with 13.2%, 7.2%, and 2.3% of mean loss of global cartilage, respectively, at 24 months.

Comparing MRI Measurements with Joint Space Width and Narrowing on Standardized Knee Radiographs

Few studies have directly compared change of cartilage volume from MRI to quantitative measurements of JSN in radiographs, and these have produced contradictory results. A cross-sectional study by Cicuttini et al. [22] compared tibial cartilage volume measured by MRI to radiologic grade (osteophytes and JSN) of 252 subjects. This study revealed that JSN was inversely correlated with tibial cartilage volume as assessed by MRI. Such inverse relationship was even stronger while adjusting for age, sex, and BMI. Gandy et al. [27] studied 11 patients with knee OA over a 3-year period and demonstrated narrowing of JSW in weight-bearing extended radiographs of −0.21 mm, but no significant change in cartilage volume was found in any of the knee compartments. They argued that radiography may be more sensitive than analysis of total cartilage plates by MRI, because in radiographs measurements are obtained in the central portion of the joint surface, where most of the change may occur. However, it should also be kept in mind that the cohort was relatively small and that, in contrast with most other studies, the authors used a 1.0 T (rather than 1.5 T) magnet for their study with associated precision errors relatively high. In contrast, Raynauld et al. [25] described no significant change in weight-bearing semiflexed radiographs positioned in 32 patients with OA over 2 years but reported a highly significant change in cartilage volume from MRI both in the medial and lateral compartments (femoral condyles and tibial plateaus together). These findings were further reinforced from a larger cohort of 107 patients with knee OA, followed for 2 years, which had simultaneously qMRI and standardized radiographs [26]. Although significant changes in cartilage volume were demonstrated, no significant correlation with JSW was found in these patients. However, in a recent study [19], a correlation was found between JSN and the loss of cartilage but only in the central area of the medial femoral condyle and, to a lesser extent, in the medial central tibial plateau. These regions are in close accordance with patient knee positioning during X-ray exams, and data suggested that the latter technique assessed only the focal loss of cartilage. Therefore, MRI appears to be significantly more sensitive at detecting volume change in the global and subregions of articular cartilage, whereas JSW is an indirect measurement, which could be subject to a number of artifacts related to factors such as positioning, image acquisition, and changes in joint structure other than cartilage.

Influence of Other Knee Structure Changes on OA Cartilage Loss

Other advantages of MRI compared with conventional imaging technologies are its ability to globally assess all major joint structures, including the cartilage, meniscus, bone marrow alteration (Fig. 15.3), synovial tissue, and ligaments.

For example, cartilage loss can be dependent on other structural damage such as meniscal damage or joint misalignment. The menisci transmit 50% to 90% of load over the knee joint, depending on knee flexion angle, femoral translation and rotation. The meniscus also contributes to knee joint proprioception and probably also to joint stability [28]. Cicuttini et al. [29] studied patients who underwent a surgical meniscectomy and controls and looked at articular cartilage volume loss assessed by qMRI with an average 28 months of follow-up. The study suggests that there is more cartilage loss over time in patients who underwent partial meniscectomy. The results suggest the strong role of the meniscal apparatus in protecting cartilage, especially in older subjects, or those suffering from obesity or joint instability. A

MENISCAL PATHOLOGY

Tear   Extrusion

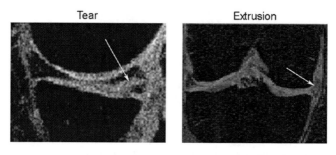

BONE MARROW HYPERSIGNAL

Edema   Cyst

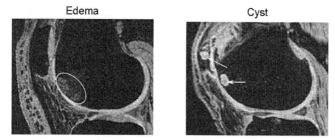

Fig. 15.3 Representative knee meniscal pathologies (tear and extrusion) and bone marrow hyper-signal in human OA knee, as seen by MRI acquisition with fat-suppressed FISP sequence

study by Biswal et al. [30] also looked at the risk factors for progressive cartilage loss in knee OA patients using MRI. Baseline and follow-up MRIs of the knees (minimum time interval of 1 year, mean 1.8 years, range 52 to 285 weeks) were done, and cartilage loss was graded semiquantitatively in the anterior, central, and posterior regions of the medial and lateral knee compartments. The results of this study revealed that meniscal and anterior cruciate ligament tears were associated with more rapid cartilage loss. Moreover, this study also demonstrated that the central portion of the medial compartment showed more rapid progression of cartilage loss than the anterior or posterior portions. These data are a clear indication that cartilage loss in OA is not evenly distributed in the knee.

Another MRI study done by Berthiaume et al. evaluating the impact of meniscal damage [31] on cartilage volume loss assessed by MRI showed a strong and highly statistically significant association ($p < 0.002$) between the global cartilage (condyle and plateau) volume loss and the presence of a severe medial meniscal extrusion. An even greater association was found between the medial meniscal extrusion and the loss of cartilage in the medial compartment ($p < 0.0001$). Similarly, a major correlation was found between the presence of a medial meniscal extrusion and loss of cartilage in the medial compartment ($p < 0.001$). These data revealed that meniscal tear and extrusion are among the most significant risk factors associated with the progression of knee OA.

The importance of other structural changes such as bone marrow hypersignal (Fig. 15.3) in assessing knee OA was demonstrated by Felson et al. [32]. In this study, patients with knee OA had baseline assessments including MRI and fluoroscopically positioned radiography and were followed for 30 months. Progression was defined as a decrease over follow-up in medial or lateral joint space, based on a semiquantitative grading. Knees with medial bone marrow lesions showed a higher incidence of medial progression versus knees without lesions (odds ratio for progression, 6.5 [95% CI, 3.0 to 14.0]). These findings were in agreement with the recent studies of Raynauld et al. in knee OA [26, 33], which provide additional arguments to support the relationship between the cartilage volume loss and other anatomic knee changes. In the first study [26], data showed that the strongest predictors of cartilage loss in knee OA patients were the presence of severe meniscal extrusion, severe medial tear, medial and/or lateral bone hypersignal along with clinical variables such as high BMI progressors), weight and age. In the second study [33], it was demonstrated that bone lesions such as edema and cysts, which are extremely prevalent in knee OA (more than 75 %) showed strong correlation between the increase in the edema size in the medial compartment and the cyst in the medial femoral condyle over time (2 years) and a greater loss of cartilage volume in these areas, underlining the likelihood of a role for subchondral bone lesions in OA pathophysiology.

Redefining "Primary" OA

What is not known at this time is whether the population of patients at very high risk (fast progressors) would benefit the most or the least from DMOAD agents (treatment that may slow down cartilage degradation). The implications of the MRI findings in OA patients about the cartilage and the surrounding tissues may also impact the definition of "primary" OA in the future. The American College of Rheumatology criteria of primary OA of the knee [34] are actually based on clinical and/or radiologic findings. Because the cartilage is not vascularized nor innerved, the pain experienced in OA is likely to originate from bone, synovial, capsule, or ligament alterations. The "pure" anatomic cartilage loss over time, if chosen to define primary OA, may not be reflected, at first, by changes in symptoms, precede considerably the radiologic changes, and may be accelerated by unsuspected concomitant meniscal damage and bone leisons.

Conclusion

The main reasons for the quantitative assessment of cartilage thickness and volume and other structural changes in OA are to objectively evaluate the disease course and to evaluate treatment that may slow down cartilage degradation: the so-called DMOAD agents. However, to be practical, problems faced by clinical research necessitate that such MR technology be based on readily available MR acquisition parameters that are easily reproducible in most available apparatus. As a result, the technology could be exportable to other centers with comparable MR facilities and be used in multicenter trials.

Moreover, because of the state of the patients and the symptoms they experience, image acquisition should be performed in a time-wise fashion without compromising image quality. This is particularly critical when one wishes to proceed to the quantification of disease progression over time. The future of OA research pertaining to prevention or repair of structural damage can be compared to some extent with the evolution experienced in the field of osteoporosis in the past few decades. In the beginning, a significant bone loss was necessary to diagnose osteoporosis on plain radiographs. With the advent of osteodensitometry, relatively small changes in bone mass can be detected and early diagnosis can be established. This outcome tool opened the door to clinical research on new therapies to slow or prevent bone mass loss. Everyone knows the impact of these medications on the outcome of osteoporosis today. Similarly, quantification of cartilage loss and the other structural changes seen in OA over time will improve the monitoring of OA and possibly help to develop new interventions to prevent the evolution of this extremely prevalent disease.

References

1. Altman RD, Fries JF, Bloch DA, Carstens J, Cooke TD, Genant H, et al. Radiographic assessment of progression in osteoarthritis. Arthritis Rheum 1987;30:1214–1225.
2. Buckland-Wright JC. Quantitative radiography of osteoarthritis. Ann Rheum Dis 1994; 53:268–275.
3. Lequesne M, Glimet T, Masse JP, Orvain J. Speed of the joint narrowing in primary medical osteoarthritis of the knee over 3–5 years. Osteoarthritis Cartilage 1998;1:23.
4. Adams JG, McAlindon T, Dimasi M, Carey J, Eustace S. Contribution of meniscal extrusion and cartilage loss to joint space narrowing in osteoarthritis. Clin Radiol 1999;54: 502–506.
5. Ayral X, Gueguen A, Ike RW, Bonvarlet JP, Frizziero L, Kalunian K, et al. Inter-observer reliability of the arthroscopic quantification of chondropathy of the knee. Osteoarthritis Cartilage 1998;6:160–166.
6. Hargreaves BA, Gold GE, Beaulieu CF, Vasanawala SS, Nishimura DG, Pauly JM: Comparison of new sequences for high-resolution cartilage imaging. Magn Reson Med 2003;49: 700–709.
7. Samosky JT, Burstein D, Eric Grimson W, Howe R, Martin S, Gray ML. Spatially-localized correlation of dGEMRIC-measured GAG distribution and mechanical stiffness in the human tibial plateau. J Orthop Res 2005;23:93–101.
8. Regatte RR, Akella SV, Wheaton AJ, Lech G, Borthakur A, Kneeland JB, et al. 3D-T1rho-relaxation mapping of articular cartilage: in vivo assessment of early degenerative changes in symptomatic osteoarthritic subjects. Acad Radiol 2004;11:741–749.
9. Liess C, Lusse S, Karger N, Heller M, Gluer CC: Detection of changes in cartilage water content using MRI T2-mapping in vivo. Osteoarthritis Cartilage 2002;10:907–913.
10. Mosher TJ, Dardzinski BJ. Cartilage MRI T2 relaxation time mapping: overview and applications. Semin Musculoskelet Radiol 2004;8:355–368.

11. Filidoro L, Dietrich O, Weber J, Rauch E, Oerther T, Wick M, et al. High-resolution diffusion tensor imaging of human patellar cartilage: feasibility and preliminary findings. Magn Reson Med 2005;53:993–998.
12. Eckstein F, Westhoff J, Sittek H, Maag KP, Haubner M, Faber S, et al. In vivo reproducibility of three-dimensional cartilage volume and thickness measurements with MR imaging. AJR Am J Roentgenol 1998;170:593–597.
13. Calvo E, Palacios I, Delgado E, Ruiz-Cabello J, Hernandez P, Sanchez-Pernaute O, et al. High-resolution MRI detects cartilage swelling at the early stages of experimental osteoarthritis. Osteoarthritis Cartilage 2001;9:463–472.
14. Kauffmann C, Gravel P, Godbout B, Gravel A, Beaudoin G, Raynauld JP, et al. Computer-aided method for quantification of cartilage thickness and volume changes using MRI: validation study using a synthetic model. IEEE Trans Biomed Eng 2003;50:978–988.
15. Burgkart R, Glaser C, Hyhlik-Durr A, Englmeier KH, Reiser M, Eckstein F: Magnetic resonance imaging-based assessment of cartilage loss in severe osteoarthritis: accuracy, precision, and diagnostic value. Arthritis Rheum 2001;44:2072–2077.
16. Peterfy CG, van Dijke CF, Janzen DL, Gluer CC, Namba R, Majumdar S, et al. Quantification of articular cartilage in the knee with pulsed saturation transfer subtraction and fat-suppressed MR imaging: optimization and validation. Radiology 1994;192:485–491.
17. Raynauld JP, Kauffmann C, Beaudoin G, Berthiaume MJ, de Guise JA, Bloch DA, et al. Reliability of a quantification imaging system using magnetic resonance images to measure cartilage thickness and volume in human normal and osteoarthritic knees. Osteoarthritis Cartilage 2003;11:351–360.
18. Wluka AE, Stuckey S, Snaddon J, Cicuttini FM. The determinants of change in tibial cartilage volume in osteoarthritic knees. Arthritis Rheum 2002;46:2065–2072.
19. Pelletier JP, Raynauld JP, Berthiaume MJ, Abram F, Choquette D, Haraoui B, et al. Risk factors associated with the loss of cartilage volume on weight bearing areas in knee osteoarthritis patients assessed by quantitative MRI: a longitudinal study. Arthritis Res Ther 2007;9:R74.
20. Eckstein F, Heudorfer L, Faber SC, Burgkart R, Englmeier KH, Reiser M. Long-term and resegmentation precision of quantitative cartilage MR imaging (qMRI). Osteoarthritis Cartilage 2002;10:922–928.
21. Hudelmaier M, Glaser C, Hohe J, Englmeier KH, Reiser M, Putz R, et al. Age-related changes in the morphology and deformational behavior of knee joint cartilage. Arthritis Rheum 2001;44:2556–2561.
22. Cicuttini FM, Wluka AE, Forbes A, Wolfe R. Comparison of tibial cartilage volume and radiologic grade of the tibiofemoral joint. Arthritis Rheum 2003;48:682–688.
23. Eckstein F, Winzheimer M, Hohe J, Englmeier KH, Reiser M. Interindividual variability and correlation among morphological parameters of knee joint cartilage plates: analysis with three-dimensional MR imaging. Osteoarthritis Cartilage 2001;9:101–111.
24. Cicuttini F, Wluka A, Wang Y, Stuckey S. The determinants of change in patella cartilage volume in osteoarthritic knees. J Rheumatol 2002;29:2615–2619.
25. Raynauld JP, Martel-Pelletier J, Berthiaume MJ, Labonté F, Beaudoin G, de Guise JA, et al. Quantitative magnetic resonance imaging evaluation of knee osteoarthritis progression over two years and correlation with clinical symptoms and radiologic changes. Arthritis Rheum 2004;50:476–487.
26. Raynauld JP, Martel-Pelletier J, Berthiaume MJ, Beaudoin G, Choquette D, Haraoui B, et al. Long term evaluation of disease progression through the quantitative magnetic resonance imaging of symptomatic knee osteoarthritis patients: correlation with clinical symptoms and radiographic changes. Arthritis Res Ther 2006;8:R21.
27. Gandy SJ, Dieppe PA, Keen MC, Maciewicz RA, Watt I, Waterton JC. No loss of cartilage volume over three years in patients with knee osteoarthritis as assessed by magnetic resonance imaging. Osteoarthritis Cartilage 2002;10:929–937.
28. Aagaard H, Verdonk R. Function of the normal meniscus and consequences of meniscal resection. Scand J Med Sci Sports 1999;9:134–140.

29. Cicuttini FM, Forbes A, Yuanyuan W, Rush G, Stuckey SL. Rate of knee cartilage loss after partial meniscectomy. J Rheumatol 2002;29:1954–1956.
30. Biswal S, Hastie T, Andriacchi TP, Bergman GA, Dillingham MF, Lang P. Risk factors for progressive cartilage loss in the knee: a longitudinal magnetic resonance imaging study in forty-three patients. Arthritis Rheum 2002;46:2884–2892.
31. Berthiaume MJ, Raynauld JP, Martel-Pelletier J, Labonté F, Beaudoin G, Bloch DA, et al. Meniscal tear and extrusion are strongly associated with the progresion of knee osteoarthritis as assessed by quantitative magnetic resonance imaging. Ann Rheum Dis 2005;64: 556–563.
32. Felson DT, Chaisson CE, Hill CL, Totterman SM, Gale ME, Skinner KM, et al. The association of bone marrow lesions with pain in knee osteoarthritis. Ann Intern Med 2001;134: 541–549.
33. Raynauld J, Martel-Pelletier J, Berthiaume MJ, Abram F, Choquette D, Haraoui B, et al. Correlation between bone lesion changes and cartilage volume loss in knee osteoarthritis patients as assessed by quantitative MRI over a 24 month period. Ann Rheum Dis 2007:(In press; published online first doi: 10.1136/ard.2007.073023).
34. Altman RD, Asch E, Bloch DA, Bole G, Borenstein D, Brandt KD, et al. Development of criteria for the classification and reporting of osteoarthritis. Classification of osteoarthritis of the knee. Arthritis Rheum 1986;29:1039–1049.

Chapter 16
Biochemical Markers as Surrogate End Points of Joint Disease

L. Stefan Lohmander and David R. Eyre

Introduction

This chapter will discuss the potential for biochemical markers as surrogate end points for clinical outcome in drug trials and management of joint diseases. The focus of the chapter is on osteoarthritis (OA), but the basic aspects of biomarker development and validation and their qualification as surrogate outcomes apply to both OA and other joint diseases such as rheumatoid arthritis (RA).

Osteoarthritis: The Disease and the Needs

OA is most common in the hands, knees, hips, and spine. A single joint may be involved, but most individuals have several affected joints at different stages of disease development. OA is steeply age-related. Most people over the age of 70 years have some radiologic evidence of OA in some of their joints. As our populations age, degenerative skeletal disorders impose an increasing burden in health care costs and lost life quality. Today there are 600 million people over 60 years of age on the planet. This will double by 2025 and double again by 2050 according to the World Health Organization (WHO).

OA is by far the most common type of arthritis and is a leading cause of chronic disability [1]. Disease burden due to OA is on the top 10 list based on the DALY score of all chronic and acute conditions.[1] For women in Europe, the proportion of total disease burden is greater than 6% and for men 3% of total DALYs. Although OA is often regarded as a disease of the elderly, it is of note that the peak of OA

L.S. Lohmander
Institute of Clinical Sciences, Department of Orthopaedics, Lund University Hospital, Lund, Sweden

[1] DALY (Disease Adjusted Life Year) is an integrated measure of mortality and disability, combining mortality and morbidity in a single measure. One DALY can be thought of as one lost year of "healthy" life, and the burden of disease as a measurement of the gap between current health status and an ideal situation where everyone lives into old age free of disease and disability.

D.M. Reid, C.G. Miller (eds.), *Clinical Trials in Rheumatoid Arthritis and Osteoarthritis*,   249
© Springer-Verlag London Limited 2008

disease burden occurs around age 60 (variable in different world regions) and is very significant already in the age group 30 to 44 years [1].

A recent report from the WHO characterized two conditions as "high burden diseases with no curative treatments": OA and Alzheimer's disease [1]. The report further stated that currently available treatment is inadequate and that "Both are common and increasing among the elderly, and available treatment is ineffective in reversing disease progression. A major challenge for both diseases is the absence of biomarkers which could be used to diagnose and monitor the progression of disease or the effect of treatment. Continued support is needed for basic research on these diseases. Pharmaceutical companies invest heavily in research on both of these diseases but there are major biological challenges in understanding and then reversing these progressive diseases."

Treatments for OA are available that mitigate pain and improve function, but there are at present none that can cure, reverse, or halt OA disease progression (disease modification). New compounds are under development in the pharmaceutical industry for treatment of OA-related symptoms and for disease modification. However, considerable challenges exist in identifying and selecting the most promising treatment targets and in monitoring the efficacy of a particular compound against a target in early-stage drug development. This represents an important area of use for future OA biomarkers. Biomarkers may have further public health benefits in that they may make it possible to reduce the numbers of patients needed in early-stage drug development, speeding drug development and testing and reducing the number of persons exposed to new compounds where understanding side effects is yet limited. As with treatment of any other chronic disease, long-term safety issues are a major concern and may require large-scale clinical studies to assess in the relevant populations. Surgical treatment of advanced OA with severe symptoms is an effective treatment but is only relevant for a minority of all patients with OA.

OA develops as focal areas of damage to the articular cartilage, typically in the load-bearing areas, associated with new bone formation at the joint margins (osteophytes), changes in menisci, ligaments, and in the subchondral bone, variable degrees of usually mild synovitis, and thickening of the joint capsule. When these pathologic features are advanced, they are recognizable on plain radiographs as joint space narrowing, osteophytes, and sometimes changes in the subchondral bone. Magnetic resonance imaging (MRI) of joints is a rapidly developing technique with the potential to identify and monitor these features of joint pathology at much earlier stages than plain radiographs (see Chapters 14 and 15).

The patient-relevant problems associated with these pathologic and radiographic changes include all or some of the following: joint pain in use and sometimes at rest, short-lasting inactivity stiffness of joints, restricted range of movement, and instability and lack of confidence in joint function. Pain is particularly important, and OA may be the most significant cause of the great prevalence of regional joint pain in older people. However, the correlation between radiographic evidence (whether by x-ray or by MRI) of OA and the symptomatic disease is rather weak. This raises issues relating to the definition of the "OA disease" and the extent to which our efforts should be directed toward the treatment of the pathology of joint damage or the causes of pain and physical disability [2].

OA is a multifactorial disease involving endogenous factors, such as age, sex, and genes, as well as exogenous environmental factors such as joint load and trauma. Convergence of these risk factors leads to the initiation of the disease state (Fig. 16.1). Whether the factors that lead to disease initiation are the same that drive the disease from its initiation to any of its various outcomes, such as osteophyte formation, cartilage loss, inflammation, or pain, is unclear. To monitor OA incidence, a group of at-risk individuals are followed along a continuum progressing from a more or less normal state to a disease state. At some point, the individual crosses a borderline between what is recognized as absence of OA to presence of OA. The distinction between incident cases of OA and progression of prevalent cases depends on where along the continuum patients are considered to have overt OA.

Publications on the natural history of OA remain sparse, but OA is considered a progressive condition. Whereas this view may be correct on the group and population level, it may be less so on the level of the individual. Several recent studies suggest that the group mean rate of progression of joint damage reported in earlier studies is affected by a small number of fast-progressing individuals. These observations are accompanied by other reports that describe a similar heterogeneity in the progression of OA symptoms in a susceptible population. It also appears likely that even when there is disease progression, it is intermittent. We may thus ask whether we can identify early on either those patients who will experience rapid progression

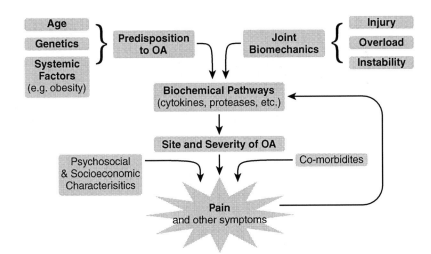

Fig. 16.1 Pathogenic mechanisms of OA. Endogenous factors such as age, genetics, and obesity interact with environmental factors influencing joint biomechanics and load. Factors that drive changes in joint structure are not necessarily the same factors that drive symptoms and pain. Joint pain is possibly enhanced by inflammation, and pain may drive inflammation. (Modified from Dieppe PA, Lohmander LS. Pathogenesis and management of pain in osteoarthritis. Lancet 2005, 365:965–973.)

of disease or, equally important, those patients who will not. Clearly, patients at risk for rapid progression should be at the focus of our current and future efforts to slow or stop disease progression in OA. These patients also, in consequence, serve as a population of interest for clinical trials of new disease-modifying drugs for OA, while a natural history study should be representative of the whole population [3] (Fig. 16.2).

Studies of OA indicate that obesity, number of joints affected, ligament and meniscus integrity, and genetics are associated with progression of structural joint changes. Limb malalignment, both static and dynamic, is another potent risk factor for progression of structural change in knee OA. Evaluations of the relationship between pain severity and OA disease progression (structure and or symptoms) have produced variable results. Other factors reported to be linked to an increased risk of progression of radiographic signs of OA and loss of joint cartilage include low vitamin D levels, low vitamin C intake, serum testosterone in men, and low bone density.

Elements making up a high-risk profile would thus likely include demographics, signs and symptoms, structural changes, and family history (genetic background). Some recent results suggest that OA biomarkers may now begin to contribute to the risk profile (see further discussion below).

Development of a high-risk patient profile is still complex, however, because we do not yet fully understand the interactions between different risk factors for OA.

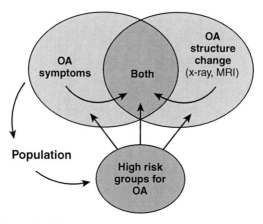

Fig. 16.2 What subjects should be selected for OA studies? A study could examine a random sample of the entire population or subjects with or without OA. Should the subjects selected for study of potential disease modification or prevention be those who are asymptomatic and do not yet have radiographic changes but who, for some reason, are at high risk of developing OA in the future (corresponding to the bottom center circle)? Or should we select subgroups of subjects who have symptoms of OA but no radiographic changes, or those who have radiographic changes but no symptoms? We do not know how many persons fit into each of these categories or what is the "conversion rate" to "OA classic" ("Both"). What proportion will convert in a given time period? The choice of study population determines the conclusions possible to draw from a biomarker validation study. (Modified from Dieppe PA, Lohmander LS. Pathogenesis and management of pain in osteoarthritis. Lancet 2005, 365:965–973.)

For example, if we assume a "background" rate of progression (or incidence) of OA in the population, what is the effect of adding a specific risk factor? Does the proportion of individuals entering the "OA pathway" increase? Does the rate of disease progression remain the same or does it change in the presence of the added risk factor? Do certain risk factors for OA become active only in certain environments and in the presence of other factors, within a "permissive environment"? Large-scale investigations such as the Osteoarthritis Initiative are under way to generate such information [4]. OA may thus serve as a "case study" of a high-burden disease lacking curative treatment and where biomarkers would have significant utility.

Clinical Assessment and Biomarkers: Definitions and Classifications

There are several ways by which OA outcomes can be assessed: (a) patient-related measures of joint pain, impairment, and disability (scores such as WOMAC [5] or KOOS [6], and others [7]); (b) measurements of the structural (anatomic) changes in the affected joints (plain radiographs [8], MRI [9], arthroscopy [10], high-frequency ultrasound [11]); or (c) measurements of the disease process exemplified by changes in metabolism or functional properties of the articular cartilage, subchondral bone, or other joint tissues (biochemical markers of cartilage and bone metabolism, bone scintigraphy, measurement of cartilage compression resistance).

These different dimensions of outcome are related to the concept of defining an end point for use in measuring OA disease development or for use in a clinical trial when comparing two different treatments. In the greater context of treatment of a medical condition such as OA, how a patient feels, functions, or survives is the most relevant outcome. Other measures and end points may be relevant as well but need to be validated against this gold standard for their long-term value to be established and be classified as surrogate outcome measures.

As exemplified in the previous section of this chapter, there is a recognized need for biomarkers in OA. Examples of potential uses include but are not limited to exploring disease mechanisms and dynamics, identifying molecular targets for treatment, identifying patients-at-risk for rapid disease progression, monitoring effects of disease-monitoring therapy and predicting clinical response, and to tailor treatment to response. The need for biomarkers is particularly acute in the proof-of-concept stages of drug development of disease-modifying OA therapy. It may further be speculated that access to useful biomarkers in OA could have public health benefits in that the number of patients that would need to be exposed to a new drug in development might be decreased. Biomarkers could help speed drug development and allow testing of more alternatives in this complex disease area. Further rationale for continued OA biomarker research is provided by the increasing awareness of the severe limitations of plain radiography as a method to monitor OA outcome.

A *biomarker* may be defined as a structural or physical measure, or a cellular, molecular, or genetic change or feature by which alterations in a biologic process can be identified and monitored. A biomarker may thereby have diagnostic or prognostic utility. Biomarkers, in order to be useful, must be reliably and reproducibly measured by standardized, published methods in several laboratories and validated to prove that they are indeed measuring the intended analyte and/or process with sufficient specificity.

A *surrogate marker* or *end point*, on the other hand, is a measurement or biomarker that can serve as a substitute for a clinically meaningful outcome or end point. A surrogate marker might thus also serve to predict the effect of a clinical intervention.

A *clinical end point* may be defined as a characteristic or variable that measures how a *patient* feels, functions, or survives. It follows from these definitions that even in the best of cases, only some biomarkers of OA may serve as surrogate end points for OA. In order for the biomarker to be validated as a surrogate end point, it must be shown that its measurement can serve as a reliable substitute for, or predict, a clinically meaningful end point [12, 13].

A significant challenge in the validation of a surrogate marker is that its measurement may not take into account adverse events, as the processes associated with an adverse event may not be monitored by the marker. Such adverse events may null all or some of the treatment benefit and require identification of biomarkers specific for such events. Further, a surrogate marker may not register all beneficial effects of treatment if these are not in the marker pathway. Although a biomarker may have good face validity as a surrogate outcome, changes in its measurement may not monitor the intended molecular or cellular process in the tissue it is thought to, leading to erroneous conclusions.

Biomarkers may have several different potential uses, and a general classification has been proposed [14]. According to this framework, a natural history marker is defined as a marker of disease severity that reflects underlying pathogenic mechanisms and predicts clinical outcome independent of treatment. Such biomarkers, *type 0*, are identified as prognostic in longitudinal history studies of the disease. Type 0 markers can be used for baseline stratification in clinical trials and as milestones of disease progression in the natural history of the disease. A next suggested stage in marker development is to assess the influence of treatment on a promising prognostic type 0 marker. Such a *type I* biological activity marker is defined as one that responds to therapy. A type I biomarker would likely be evaluated in early stage clinical trials with the aim of providing proof-of-concept that a new treatment has promising activity related to its suggested mode of action. Possibly, a type I biomarker could be used to help estimate optimal drug dosing. Finally, a *type II* biomarker (or a composite of several markers) may be defined as one that predicts a subsequent favorable clinical outcome and thereby accounts for the clinical efficacy of an agent or treatment. Such a biomarker would be defined as a surrogate marker of therapeutic efficacy. It is more likely, however, that any surrogate marker will explain only a part of the clinical efficacy, the proportion of treatment effect explained (PTE) [15]. As discussed [14], a correct interpretation of the PTE requires a thorough understanding of the underlying mechanisms of disease and drug activity. Only if it is known that the agent operates primarily through its action on the marker and the marker is directly in the causal pathway of the disease can marker results be interpreted reliably. Conclusive proof of this remains a challenge for many currently explored biochemical markers of OA.

Validation of a biomarker for its intended use (type 0, I, or II) should follow a stepwise approach, beginning with an initial hypothesis on pathogenesis. Early studies are usually descriptive and cross-sectional cohort studies of limited size. Subsequent validation stages need to expand significantly in size and be longitudinal, initially retrospective, and later prospective. For biomarkers of type I or type II, access to an active intervention is required. The continued absence of a drug or treatment with an unambiguous disease-modifying activity in OA (however defined, see above) makes any attempt to validate a type II biomarker for OA problematic at this time. Current biomarker work in OA is therefore largely limited to a search for type 0 and type I biomarkers.

For a disease-modifying therapy in OA, it may be argued that a clinically meaningful outcome should combine evidence of joint structure (or joint survival) benefit with more direct patient-relevant benefit relating to pain, function, or joint-related quality-of-life. This clinical outcome would then serve as the gold standard against which any biomarker aspiring to be defined as a surrogate OA marker (type II) needs to be validated. Investigators in the field need to agree on a standard clinical end point to be used for each proposed use of a biomarker or surrogate marker. If a biochemical marker is validated against "structural" joint outcome only, it will serve as a case of one biomarker being related to another, and not against a clinical outcome. However, this does not necessarily mean that a biomarker not fully validated as a surrogate outcome is not useful. It may indeed be so, in that it may be able to support the identification of a treatment target, to monitor *in vivo* or *in vitro* a specific cellular or molecular process of interest in drug development, and so forth. Biomarker validation is not all or none, but a process of gradual strengthening of evidence. In validating an OA biomarker, studies will need to account for interactions generated by which joint(s) are studied, disease stage, comorbidities and medications, ethnicity, sex, age, body mass, and yet other factors.

The Status of OA Biomarkers: Strengths and Limitations

OA and other joint diseases such as RA are associated with a loss of the normal balance between synthesis and degradation of the structural components of the extracellular matrix. These components are necessary to provide articular cartilage, menisci, ligaments, and bone with their normal biomechanical and functional properties. Concomitantly, synovitis develops, which is usually much less pronounced in OA than in RA. These processes result in the destruction of joint cartilage, menisci and ligaments, with extensive remodeling of subchondral bone. The active processes in the joint, involving changes in both synthesis and degradation, result in the altered release of matrix molecules, proteolytic molecular fragments, and other molecules involved in their altered metabolism such as proteases, cytokines, chemokines, growth factors, and so forth. For the synovial joint, the joint fluid is a likely first and most proximal compartment where these potential biomarkers, intact or fragmented, may be present. Products released into the synovial compartment may be removed from there by capillary and lymphatic flow to appear in the blood circulation, and in some cases they may survive metabolism and appear in the urine after further processing by the kidneys.

The Quantitative Relationship Between Biomarker and Tissue Turnover

Although simple in principle, the relationship between changes in biomarker concentrations in a body fluid compartment and changes in joint tissue metabolism is complex and not fully understood (Fig. 16.3). To use joint cartilage as an example: the concentration of a marker of cartilage matrix degradation in joint fluid will depend not only on the rate of degradation of hyaline joint cartilage matrix but also on the clearance rate of the molecule or fragment in question from the joint fluid compartment [16], and the amount of cartilage matrix remaining in the joint [17]. Because the clearance of macromolecules from the joint fluid compartment to the lymphatics or directly to capillaries may be increased by inflammation [16], differences in the rates of release of markers from joint cartilage into joint fluid between control joints and diseased joints with inflammation may actually be underesti-

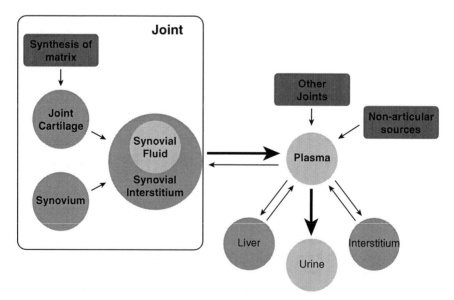

Fig. 16.3 Biomarker concentrations in body fluid compartments are influenced by many processes. (Modified from Simkin PA, Bassett JE. Cartilage matrix molecules in serum and synovial fluid. Curr Opin Rheumatol 1995, 7:346–51.)

mated. The contribution of biomarker release into systemic circulation from other joints with OA or from normal joints adds complexity, as may contributions from other hyaline cartilage structures in the body. For example, articular cartilage makes up only 8% of the total hyaline cartilage of a young dog, so this is not a trivial hurdle [18]. In monoarticular disease, any markers released from the affected joint are thus mixed with markers released from normal cartilages. Hence, determinations of cartilage markers in serum or urine may be of more use in polyarticular or systemic disease and may be less likely to be useful in monoarticular disease where measurement of joint fluid may provide a more accurate insight into the local pathology.

Quantitatively, type II collagen is the most abundant component of joint cartilage and its destruction is a central, irreversible feature of joint failure, so it presents an attractive target as a biomarker. However, in skeletally mature adults, type II collagen is found in articular cartilages, fibrocartilages (intervertebral disks, menisci, etc.), respiratory tract cartilages, rib cartilages, and the insertion sites of tendons and ligaments into bone. Small amounts also occur concentrated in tissues of the inner ear and the eye. The source of any collagen II fragments found in body fluids therefore cannot be assumed to be primarily from joint cartilages without any further data on the source and a likely mechanism of generation. In relation to type I collagen and in the body as a whole, collagen type II probably represents of the order 1%. On the other hand, the turnover rate of type II collagen in adult cartilage will normally be very low compared with bone type I collagen, for example, so elevated degradation and synthesis in even a single joint might be expected to raise systemic levels of fragments significantly.

Reported estimates from MRI studies of the volume loss of articular cartilage in knee OA are in the range 200 to 500 mm^3 per joint per year [19]. If representative, this corresponds with 40 to 100 mg of type II collagen per year or about 0.1 to 0.3 mg (0.3 to 1 nmol) per day. Such levels are in a range that a sensitive immunoassay can quantify if diluted into the blood or excreted into urine.

Inflammation, OA, and Biomarkers

Hyaluronan concentrations are high in joint fluid, and hyaluronan is synthesized by cells of the synovium as well as by cells of other connective tissues. Increased hyaluronan concentrations in serum correlated with OA joint space width and disease progression in some studies, but not in others [20–23]. Synovitis in OA has a significant effect on serum cartilage oligomeric matrix protein (COMP), suggesting that COMP levels may relate to joint inflammation in OA [24]. Both chondrocytes and synovial cells produce MMP-3 (matrix metalloproteinase-3), but the cell number and rates of synthesis in synovial tissue may be higher in the inflamed synovium than in cartilage, so that a significant proportion of the MMP-3 detected in joint fluid, plasma, or serum originates in the synovium. High concentrations of MMP-1, MMP-3, and TIMP-1 (tissue inhibitor of metalloproteinases-1) protein are found in joint fluid shortly after injury, perhaps as a reflection of synovial activation and inflammation [25, 26]. Interestingly, plasma levels of MMP-3 were shown to be predictive of knee joint space narrowing over 16 months in a prospective, longitudinal OA clinical trial [27]. Reports on a possible relationship between serum C-reactive protein (CRP) and OA have been variable, with some suggesting a relationship and others failing to find one [28–31]. Several studies suggest that serum CRP, like several other OA biomarkers, is influenced by obesity, body mass index, and comorbidities, which is likely to confound interpretation of results.

The results of these studies, using a variety of biomarkers, suggest that inflammation is a feature of at least some phases of OA. This view is consistent with recent reports showing increased levels in synovial fluid and serum of OA patients of several different cytokines and chemokines [32, 33]. It is likely that in some phases of the OA disease process, inflammation may be a relevant pathogenic driver and relevant treatment target in OA [34–36].

Neoepitopes Add Specificity

Even if specific for the particular structure (epitope) detected, as well as for its target molecule, many of the currently used biomarker assays lack specificity for the metabolic process generating them. In contrast, immunoassays that rely on the detection of a neoepitope generated through specific proteolytic substrate cleavage can provide information on the activity of that specific proteolytic pathway [37]. Such information is particularly valuable for the monitoring of disease-modifying therapy of OA and any other joint diseases for which proteolytic inhibitors are now being developed. Type II collagen and aggrecan may serve as examples of the role of neoepitope-specific biomarker assays.

Lessons from Studies of Degradation of Collagen in Bone and Cartilage

The evolution of collagen degradation products as biomarkers of bone resorption in the osteoporosis field may be informative for OA biomarker research. Pyridinoline cross-links (hydroxylysylpyridinoline [HP] and lysylpridinoline [LP]) and peptides containing them are present in blood and urine from tissue collagen degradation (Fig. 16.4). Because there is no mechanism for their metabolism, these residues give an index of collagen breakdown. Urinary pyridinolines (HP and particularly LP) measured by HPLC give a more accurate index than hydroxyproline, a traditional marker of systemic bone resorption.

Even more specific are assays for telopeptide fragments containing the cross-linking residues [38, 39]. The cross-linked telopeptides of bone collagen (N-telopeptide-to-helix [NTx] and C-telopeptide-to-helix [CTx]) (Fig. 16.5) survive into blood and urine and can be isolated from urine as a discrete low-molecular-weight peptide pool (<2 kDa) [38, 40, 41]. Antibodies raised that recognize them as proteolytic neoepitopes have formed the basis of immunoassays developed to

Proteolytic pathways of collagen degradation: Bone resorption

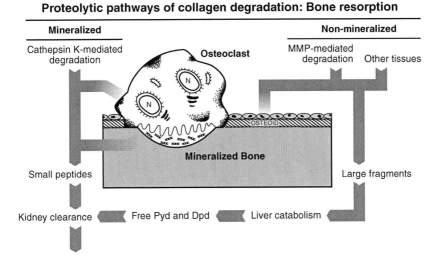

Fig. 16.4 The cross-linking amino acids, pyridinoline (Pyd) and especially deoxypyridinoline (Dpd), in urine were found to be more effective markers of bone resorption than hydroxyproline. In the past decade, the small telopeptide fragments NTx and CTx, measured by immunoassay, have proved to be even more sensitive and convenient markers of bone resorption. Their release from bone and excretion by the kidney is believed to depend on the osteoclastic degradation of bone collagen directly to low-molecular-weight peptides as shown in the cathepsin-K–mediated path on the left

quantify NTx and CTx fragments as biomarkers of bone resorption. The NTx epitope was shown to be generated during osteoclastic degradation of bone collagen through the action of cathepsin K [42, 43] and so is a marker of the process of degradation as well as specific to type I collagen (Fig. 16.5).

Although bone collagen is the principal source of the pyridinoline cross-links in urine, other tissues also contribute, notably cartilage type II collagen in growing children [44]. A C-telopeptide fragment containing HP from type II collagen was identified [41, 45]. From the sequence of a collagen type II C-telopeptide fragment identified in human urine [45], a monoclonal antibody, 2B4, was prepared that recognizes the cross-linked structure [46] (Fig. 16.5). An ELISA assay based on this antibody was able to monitor culture medium for collagen II breakdown products from IL-1–stimulated cartilage explants *in vitro* [47], increased urinary excretion in OA patients [48] and higher levels in knee synovial fluid of patients after joint injury [49], in dogs after anterior cruciate ligament (ACL) section [50], and in rabbits after meniscectomy [51]. The same 2B4 assay applied to urine was also used to compare cartilage collagen degradation with bone resorption (NTx assay) in high-performance college athletes in three different sports: crew (rowing), cross-country, and swimming [112]. Interestingly, bone resorption was highest in the crew and lowest in the swimmers, whereas cartilage degradation was highest in the runners and lowest in the swimmers. Each group showed statistically significant differences in each marker from the other.

Type I Collagen (bone resorption)

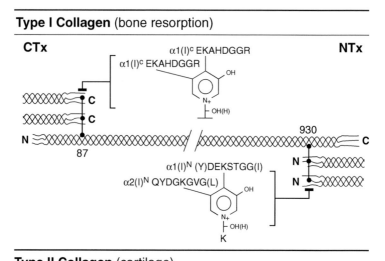

Type II Collagen (cartilage)

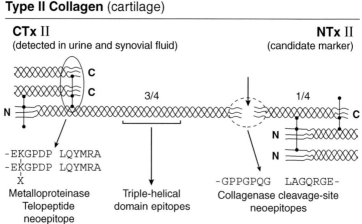

Fig. 16.5 Collagen peptide epitopes as biomarkers of bone and cartilage degradation. In measuring bone resorption, the cross-linked telopeptide markers NTx and CTx, from osteoclastic breakdown of type I collagen, can be assayed in urine. Similarly, CTx II, a cross-linked C-telopeptide from type II collagen, can be assayed in urine. It probably represents an index of mineralized type II degraded by osteoclasts [44]. The type II collagen telopeptide, NTx II, is theoretically another marker of type II collagen breakdown in the same category. In addition, antibodies and assays against the neoepitopes created by collagenase are in use

From our unpublished results, we know there is not a simple correlation between urine, serum, and synovial fluid in collagen II CTx epitope levels. As with the bone telopeptide markers NTx and CTx (see below), there is a need to determine the origin and fate of the proteolytic epitope (2B4) in the body fluid compartments. We suspect that in synovial fluid, large molecular fragments of type II collagen from articular cartilage are the source of the immunoassay signal, whereas in urine the peptides carrying the signal are small and less than 2 kDa in size. The antibody will detect the neoepitope, whether on the end of the whole molecule or at the end of a short peptide. The peptides in urine probably originate mostly from osteoclast-degraded mineralized type II collagen as do type I collagen NTx and CTx [41]. We suggest that larger cross-linked fragments that originate from matrix metalloproteinase–driven mechanisms are degraded to free pyridinolines in the liver. This concept is supported compellingly in the recessive skeletal disorder pycnodysostosis caused by a homozygous null cathepsin K gene. Type I NTx, type I CTx [52], and type II CTx epitope levels are very low in urine in pycnodysostosis compared with age-matched normals, yet total urinary HP and LP are normal (unpublished). This can be explained if HP- and LP-containing products of collagen degradation are fully degraded to the free cross-links, which are then excreted (Fig. 16.4). Without cathepsin K, resorbing osteoclasts demineralize bone but cannot degrade the collagen, which is removed by macrophages or other phagocytic cells [53]. Based on this information, we suggest that type II CTx fragments in urine may reflect primarily the breakdown and remodeling by osteoclasts of mineralized cartilage collagen [50].

Urine levels of type II collagen CTx fragments have been reported to correlate with arthritis severity, joint disease load, and to predict OA progression [54]. However, although this may fulfill the requirements for a type 0 biomarker, the results discussed above suggest that CTxII may not necessarily be a suitable type I biomarker showing therapeutic response related to a potential treatment effect on hyaline joint cartilage. CTxII levels in urine were shown to be suppressed markedly by the bisphosphonate risedronate in a phase III trial of this compound for slowing the progression of knee osteoarthritis [55]. Though the marker had good face validity (assessing collagen type II destruction) and responded as anticipated for chondroprotection with marked suppression, the trial end point of radiographic assessment of joint space narrowing or symptoms showed no risedronate benefit over the placebo-controlled arm. From animal studies, we already knew that bisphosphonates suppressed the CTxII analyte in growing guinea pigs [56] and presumed this was a result of the inhibition of osteoclastic resorption of mineralized cartilage by active growth plates. Based on the predicted route of small cross-linked telopeptides to urine from osteoclast activity, it seems likely that the main source of urinary CTxII is type II collagen in mineralized tissue, perhaps from joint remodeling that involves osteophytes and the tidemark cartilage interface with mineralized cartilage and bone, but also perhaps from skeletal sources other than joints. This illustrates the complexities and pitfalls inherent in using a type 0 biomarker as a type I biomarker without a thorough evaluation and understanding of the underlying metabolism.

Biomarkers of Aggrecan Degradation and Turnover

Aggrecan degradation and loss has significant consequences for the resilience of joint cartilage, and experiments with cartilage explants even suggest that aggrecan loss is a prerequisite for collagen loss [57]. Although several assays have been developed to monitor aggrecan fragment levels in body fluids, they lack the specificity to detect activity of specific proteolytic cleavages of this molecule [58–60]. Several lines of evidence indicate that aggrecanases, primarily ADAMTS-4-5, play an important role in aggrecan degradation in human joint disease [61–65]. However, a role for matrix metalloproteinases or other proteases in some phases of aggrecan turnover in the human joint is difficult to exclude [66], and there is little or no information on possible variations in proteolytic activity associated with the individual, with disease stage, or with specific joint disease (Fig. 16.6). For these reasons, assays that detect only aggrecan fragments resulting from specific protease activity would be helpful in understanding the relative roles of different proteases and for monitoring efficacy in early compound screening and clinical development.

Other Matrix Components of Joint Cartilage

Cartilage oligomeric matrix protein (COMP) is an oligomeric pentameric glyco-protein present in cartilage, tendon, meniscus, ligament, and some other connective tissues and may serve as yet another example of a matrix molecule released into body fluids in joint disease. Fragments of this molecule have been detected in synovial fluid and serum in OA and other joint diseases. The enzyme(s) responsible for COMP degradation *in vivo* have yet to be identified, and the fragment population present in body fluids is heterogeneous [67, 68]. Several investigators have identified COMP in serum as a predictor of OA disease state and progression, suggesting that serum COMP may serve as a type 0 biomarker for OA [69–73]. In addition to the

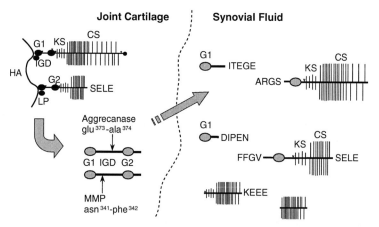

Fig. 16.6 Aggrecan degradation and generation of neoepitopes. Several assays exist for the detection of aggrecan fragments in body fluids. However, so far they lack specificity for the different possible proteolytic pathways degrading aggrecan. For example, assays that rely on dye precipitation will detect all fragments containing chondroitin sulfate or keratan sulfate (CS, KS), irrespective of the proteolytic cleavage site. The availability of assays specific for the proteolytic neoepitopes indicated (ARGS, ITEGE, FFGV, DIPEN, SELE, KEEE), or others, would make it possible to monitor specifically the activity of, for example, the aggrecanase or matrix metalloproteinase pathways

examples provided here in the form of type II collagen, aggrecan, and COMP, other proteins in cartilage and joint tissues may serve as sources of OA biomarkers [74].

Identifying the Source of the Biomarker

Molecules or molecular fragments that are present in joint fluid and that we know are normally resident in, for example, joint cartilage may be generated primarily from the cartilage of the joint (Fig. 16.3). However, this assumption relies on the molecule being significantly more abundant in healthy or arthritic cartilage than in any other joint tissue, or that its metabolic rate in cartilage is much higher than in other joint tissues. Comparisons within patients of joint fluid versus serum concentrations of a marker may help in determining the source. COMP, an OA biomarker of continued interest, may serve as an example: the total mass of COMP in the menisci of the knee may approach that in the joint cartilage of the knee [75], and COMP is also present in other joint tissues [76]. COMP is produced in increased amounts in OA cartilage [74, 77] but it is also synthesized by synovial cells exposed to interleukin-1, and serum levels are related to synovitis in OA [24]. Therefore, while being of considerable interest as an OA biomarker, its significance as a marker of a specific event or process in a specific joint tissue remains unclear. The source of the molecule or molecular fragment of interest may thus not always be evident and is often more complex than originally proposed.

The process of production or source of a molecular fragment needs to be considered even when the biomarker is the product of a specific proteolytic event. For example, fragments could result from the degradation of a newly synthesized matrix molecule that has not yet been incorporated into a functional matrix, a molecule recently incorporated into cell-associated matrix, or be derived from a resident matrix molecule that is a critical functional part of the mature matrix (Fig. 16.7). The consequences for cartilage function may differ. In general, markers are not specific for these processes, perhaps with the exception of some collagen II and aggrecan biomarkers. Specific neoepitope-containing degradation fragments containing collagen cross-links are likely specific for the degradation and loss of "mature," cross-linked, functional type II collagen from the tissue matrix [41, 49, 78, 79]. In contrast, other type II collagen fragments not containing cross-links may result from degradation of newly synthesized or mature collagen.

Poole and colleagues have developed antibodies and assays that recognize terminal sequences released when tissue collagenases have cleaved type II collagen chains [80–82]. These antibodies have been particularly useful in detecting sites of collagen degradation in tissue sections from animal and human joints. Immunoassays based on such antibodies have also been applied to synovial fluid [50] and other body fluids [81]. A sandwich (two-site) assay that targets the collagenase neoepitope from type II collagen has also been reported that, applied to urine, could distinguish OA patients from controls [79]. Body fluid assays based on antibodies recognizing other epitopes in the collagen II triple-helical domain have also been described, including a recent report of immunoassays for a site of tyrosine nitration as a marker of the side-products of inflammation [83].

Cartilage Matrix Turnover

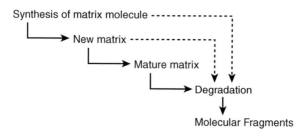

Fig. 16.7 Fragments of matrix molecules may be generated by degradation of: newly synthesized molecules that are never incorporated into the functional matrix, molecules that have recently been incorporated into a functional matrix, and molecules that have been long-time members of the "resident" functional matrix. It is not always possible to distinguish these different sources of fragments. Another source of heterogeneity is the origin of fragments from pericellular, territorial, and interterritorial matrix, as well as from superficial and deep layers of the joint cartilage. (Modified from Lohmander LS, Poole AR. Defining and validating the clinical role of molecular markers in osteoarthritis. In Osteoarthritis, 2nd ed. Edited by Brandt KD, Doherty M, Lohmander LS. Oxford University Press, Oxford, 2003, pp. 468–77.)

Assay of low-abundance epitopes associated with altered sulfation of chondroitin sulfate on aggrecan may help to identify newly synthesized aggrecan molecules, and assay of the C-terminal type II collagen propeptide may reflect type II collagen synthesis [60, 84, 85].

Identifying the specific source of the biomarker molecule or fragment can be a problem with regard to both process and tissue. An increased rate of release of a marker may occur as a result of a net increase in degradation (resulting in net loss from tissue) or as a result of an increased rate of degradation in the presence of an increased rate of synthesis. We therefore need biomarkers specific for both degradative and synthetic events in the joint. An example of the former is the cleavage of type II collagen discussed above and of the latter the synthesis of type II procollagen where the release of the C-propeptide reflects type II collagen synthesis [86, 87].

Although "snapshot" values of biomarkers are often used to compare with other outcomes, such as loss of joint cartilage by radiography, it is possible that measuring the "area under the biomarker curve" generated by several timed measurements may compare better with cumulative cartilage loss. Several lines of evidence suggest that loss of cartilage in OA may not be a linear but an episodic process. If so, then biomarker measurements coinciding with or preceding a "loss phase" may be able to predict or monitor these episodes. Some recent reports support this concept [27, 69].

Biomarker Influences from Variables Other than OA

Serum COMP levels were shown to be influenced by ethnicity and sex [71, 88]. Several other recent publications have shown that biomarker levels are influenced by factors such as body mass index, diurnal rhythm, and physical activity [85, 88–90].

Too little is yet known of the effects of these and other variables such as comorbidities, medications, or food intake and how they may influence the utility of individual OA biomarkers.

It may be concluded that an estimate of the precise degradation rate of cartilage matrix in OA, based on assay of biomarkers, is very difficult to achieve and that the changes monitored are relative at best.

Potential Uses of Current Generation of OA Biomarkers

Roles of Biomarkers Outside Formal Classification of Types 0 to II

Biomarkers may be useful beyond the formal type 0, I, and II definitions, for example in studying OA *disease dynamics and pathogenesis*. The temporal changes in joint fluid concentrations of fragments of aggrecan, COMP, type II collagen, bone sialoprotein, MMP-3, and MMP-1 after joint injury and in developing OA are consistent with the changes in metabolic rate observed for these molecules in animal models *in vivo* and in human osteoarthritic cartilage *in vitro* and with increased human subchondral bone turnover *in vivo* [25, 26, 60, 86, 87, 91, 92]. Of particular significance here are the findings of type II collagen degradation early in the disease development pointing to a potential treatment target.

Structural analysis of molecules and their fragments released from or remaining in the cartilage matrix can yield useful information on matrix turnover, the protease(s) responsible, and so help *identify molecular treatment targets*. Some results obtained with aggrecan fragments may serve as an example. The aggrecan core protein contains multiple potential proteolytic cleavage sites, and the molecular population contained in the cartilage matrix is heterogeneous with evidence of gradual C-terminal trimming of the core protein. This confounded the search for the key proteases responsible for aggrecan release from cartilage in joint disease. However, structural analysis of aggrecan fragments from human joint fluid showed that the major N-terminal sequence was consistent with activity of an aggrecanase [61, 62]. Subsequent work leading to the identification and cloning of aggrecanases (ADAMTS-4, -5) demonstrated a key role for ADAMTS-5 in a mouse model for OA and identified it as a potential treatment target in human OA and other joint disease [64, 65]. Assays specific for aggrecan proteolytic neoepitopes (see above) will be important in establishing the role of ADAMTS-5 in human OA and screening during early stages of drug development (Fig. 16.6). In this example of candidate target development and validation, biomarkers may aid in *bridging between animal models and human phase I studies*.

A marker of disease severity, reflecting underlying pathogenic mechanisms and predicting clinical outcome independent of treatment, is defined as *a type 0 biomarker*. In OA, structural disease severity (stage) is traditionally measured by the Kellgren and Lawrence grade of radiologic changes (which measures joint remodeling as well as destruction) or by the amount of cartilage loss measured at arthroscopy or by MRI. Interestingly, a recent study using MRI documented a relationship between knee cartilage damage measured by this technique and the molecular biomarkers serum COMP and a type II collagen cleavage neoepitope [93]. This is promising in terms of understanding processes leading to OA biomarker changes, but at this stage it is simply a relationship between one biomarker and another; neither of them yet representing a true surrogate OA outcome or clinical outcome.

Several assays of molecular markers developed for patients with arthritis have been promoted as *prognostic markers* and tested to see whether they predict the onset or progression of OA. For example, levels of serum hyaluronan have in some studies on patients with clinically diagnosed knee OA predicted subsequent progression of knee OA [20–23]. An increase in serum COMP has in several reports been shown to predict subsequent radiographic progression of OA [69, 70, 94]. Consistent with a relationship between serum COMP levels and synovial inflammation [24], increased serum levels of CRP were associated with OA progression [28, 95]. Plasma levels of MMP-3 predicted radiographic knee joint space narrowing over 16 months in a prospective, longitudinal OA clinical trial [27]. Finally, increased levels in urine of type II collagen C-telopeptide cross-linked peptides (CTxII) correlated with OA disease load and subsequent disease progression [54, 96]. Such biomarkers show the promise of *predicting OA progression, selecting study populations in clinical trials, and identifying those that may best benefit from treatment.*

For all currently explored OA biomarkers, a considerable overlap exists between affected and nonaffected individuals and between those with disease progress and those without. Interpretation of results is further confounded by the fact that most comparisons between groups are cross-sectional and retrospective. Results to date are best considered as hypothesis-generating and will require confirmation in large longitudinal, prospective studies such as the OsteoArthritis Initiative.

The *evaluative test*, on the other hand, focuses on the ability of a marker to monitor change over time in the individual patient, often expressed as sensitivity to change or effect size. The effect size is dependent on the amount of change for the test, divided by the baseline variation in the test. Knowledge of longitudinal, within-patient variability and correlations with other measures of disease activity is thus important, although there are only few published studies [97]. Molecular markers that can *monitor a response to therapy in OA* may be valuable as sensitive surrogate measures of outcome in therapeutic trials, in the ideal case providing "early warning" and indications of clinical outcome. Before then we need to learn more about disease mechanisms and the release of molecular markers at the tissue level from cartilage and other joint tissues. The current lack of disease-modifying treatments in OA is a major barrier to marker validation and new randomized, controlled clinical trials will provide important opportunities.

Given that markers reflect the dynamic state of cartilage or bone metabolism, it is likely that markers will be used clinically to evaluate the dynamic changes in disease, as prognostic tools to identify those at high risk of rapid progression, or as measures of response to treatment, to identify the responders and assess the degree of response. Other potential uses of markers (e.g., as diagnostic tests) seem less likely.

Bone Biomarkers and Osteoporosis Drug Development: A Role Model for Osteoarthritis?

Approved commercial assays for biochemical markers of bone formation and bone resorption in serum and urine have been widely used to assess disease activity and responses to therapy in osteoporosis (OP), particularly in drug trials. They represent indices of bone turnover rate and the dynamic balance between resorption and formation of bone matrix, which is also altered in OA. Comparisons of different assays that superficially measure the same type of bone activity such as resorption reveal consistent differences in responsiveness, and hence discriminant validity, dependent on the clinical condition. Some markers are measured with more precision than others; others may be more specific for bone of a particular quality and yet others may have variable rates of metabolism by liver and other organs and therefore not always accurately reflect bone turnover. Despite these limitations, bone marker studies have been used to identify women with and at risk for OP, to detect high bone turnover states, and to follow treatment, especially with antiresorptive therapy [98].

In transferring the concepts of osteoporosis to OA, several issues need to be considered: (a) Alterations in subchondral bone turnover in OA, though not necessarily systemic as in osteoporosis, can be measured in serum and urine [99–101]. Cartilage turnover in a single joint may not be easily detected in serum and may require synovial fluid sampling (see discussion above). (b) Variations in clearance from synovial fluid caused by varying degrees of inflammation is a concern. (c) As discussed in other sections of this chapter, practical barriers will make it harder to validate the clinical usefulness of markers in OA compared with osteoporosis. Obtaining synovial fluid is more difficult, and having access to control subjects to assess normal levels of markers in synovial fluid in nondiseased joints is difficult. Serum levels would be much easier to determine in normal subjects, but results on serum may be harder to interpret. An example is the reduction in serum levels of the C-propeptide of type II collagen in patients with OA, despite the elevations seen in OA cartilage [87]. (d) Precise and accurate bone mineral density assessments in osteoporosis that provide a well-defined end point have provided a consensus gold standard used in patient diagnosis, management, and drug development as well as biomarker evaluation. Similar quantitative measures of disease status in an OA joint are not yet possible. Markers may therefore be more difficult to validate and use clinically in OA than they have been in osteoporosis. (e) A further obvious hindrance in OA is the lack of agents that can predictably and reproducibly alter the metabolism of joint cartilage, whereas parathyroid hormone (PTH) and other hormones, steroids, and bisphosphonates can produce clear changes in bone turnover that can be used to explore the utility of bone biomarkers.

Barriers to Validating OA Biomarkers as Surrogate End Points

Validating biomarkers as surrogate end points is a demanding process, as discussed in previous reviews [14, 15]. Aspects of a prognostic OA marker (type 0) are discussed here as an example. First, a prognostic marker should have a biological rationale. The marker should be identifiable in and highly specific for the target tissue such as cartilage or bone or be a protease, cytokine, or growth factor or some other such molecule. The role of the marker in the pathogenic pathway should be understood. Second, a prognostic marker measured at baseline in a body fluid should correlate with later patient-relevant changes. If the level of a marker is abnormal at baseline, then the risk of subsequent joint deterioration may be magnified. The course of OA should be evaluated by accepted measures that are independent from the marker. Third, the marker should be detectable in all OA patients and should correlate with appropriate measures of disease dynamics if these are available. Fourth, the validation process needs to include samples from patients with a spectrum of OA severity and range of potentially interacting variables. Fifth, any biomarker, surrogate or not, needs to be measured by reliable methods described in sufficient detail to be replicable by others. This latter issue is discussed in detail in recent guidelines on standards of diagnostic accuracy and reporting [102, 103]. It is possible that a combination of markers, or marker ratios, will prove to be more useful than a single marker [104–108].

Validating a biomarker as a surrogate end point/measure is complex. In addition to testing how well a putative surrogate end point reflects patient preference and quality of life, how well the marker responds to adverse effects that may overshadow the apparent benefit is equally important. Further, even if a surrogate end point/measure is identified and validated, beneficial effects may occur via pathways that do not include the surrogate.

For all marker applications, but in particular in monitoring treatment response, it is essential to establish the variability over time and between individuals in representative and stable cohorts of appropriate size [97]. Such data can be used in power analyses to calculate the required number of patients and the required response to treatment in a clinical trial setting.

The Promise That Broad Screens Can Identify New OA Biomarkers

Most of the OA-related work on biomarkers has thus far taken the "candidate protein" approach of exploring changes in body fluids of proteins or protein fragments with a known or suspected function in joint cartilage. Although several promising candidate markers have thus been identified, this approach has its limitations. It may be argued that the search for OA biomarkers needs to expand to be genome-, transcriptome-, proteome-, and metabolome-wide and accelerated by large-scale screening techniques as used in proteomic and gene-expression profiling, using joint tissues and circulating blood cells. For continued biomarker research using either traditional or newer approaches, access to large biological specimen repositories linked to high-quality longitudinal clinical data is critical. This may, in the face of the slow natural history progress of OA, be the most difficult limiting factor.

As an example of a broad screening approach, high-resolution nuclear magnetic resonance (NMR) spectroscopy tuned to examine body fluids for differences in low-molecular-weight metabolites revealed evidence that markers of lipid metabolism are consistently altered in animals with OA [109, 110]. Another example of a related methodology is the use of ^{1}H-NMR serum spectroscopy and multivariate statistics to detect epithelial ovarian cancer with 100% sensitivity and specificity [111]. Such technology combined with access to large, well-characterized sample collections as generated in the OsteoArthritis Initiative may improve the odds of success in the search for OA biomarkers.

References

1. Kaplan W, Laing R. Priority Medicines for Europe and the World. World Health Organization, Geneva, 2004.
2. Dieppe PA, Lohmander LS. Pathogenesis and management of pain in osteoarthritis. Lancet 2005, 365:965–973.
3. Lohmander LS, Felson D. Can we identify a "high risk" patient profile to determine who will experience rapid progression of osteoarthritis? Osteoarthritis Cartilage 2004, 12(Suppl A):S49–52.
4. OsteoArthritis Initiative (OAI). National Institute of Arthritis and Musculoskeletal and Skin Diseases. Available at: http://www.niams.nih.gov/ne/oi/index.htm. Accessed April 2005.
5. Bellamy N, Buchanan WW, Goldsmith CH et al. Validation study of WOMAC: A health status instrument for measuring clinically important patient relevant outcomes to antirheumatic drug therapy in patients with osteoarthritis of the hip or knee. J Rheumatol 1988, 15: 1833–40.
6. Roos EM, Lohmander LS. The Knee injury and Osteoarthritis Outcome Score (KOOS) – a review. Health and Quality of Life Outcomes 2003, 1:64.
7. Bischoff HA, Roos EM, Liang MH. Outcome assessment in osteoarthritis: a guide for research and clinical practice. In Osteoarthritis, 2nd ed.. Edited by Brandt KD, Doherty M, Lohmander LS. Oxford University Press, Oxford, 2003, pp. 381–390.
8. Buckland-Wright CJ. Protocols for radiography. In Osteoarthritis, 2nd ed.. Edited by Brandt KD, Doherty M, Lohmander LS. Oxford University Press, Oxford, 2003, pp. 497–500.
9. Peterfy CG. Magnetic resonance imaging. In Osteoarthritis, 2nd ed. Edited by Brandt KD, Doherty M, Lohmander LS. Oxford University Press, Oxford, 2003, pp. 433–451.
10. Ayral X. Arthroscopic evaluation of knee articular cartilage. In Osteoarthritis, 2nd ed. Edited by Brandt KD, Doherty M, Lohmander LS. Oxford University Press, Oxford, 2003, pp. 451–6.
11. Myers SL. Ultrasonography. In Osteoarthritis, 2nd ed. Edited by Brandt KD, Doherty M, Lohmander LS. Oxford University Press, Oxford, 2003, pp. 462–468.
12. NIH Workshop. Biomarkers and surrogate endpoints: preferred definitions and conceptual framework. Clin Pharmacol Ther 2001, 69:89–95.
13. Illei GG, Tackey E, Lapteva L et al. Biomarkers in systemic lupus erythematosus. I. General overview of biomarkers and their applicability. Arthritis Rheum 2004, 50:1709–20.
14. Mildvan D, Landay A, De Gruttola V et al. An approach to the validation of markers for use in AIDS clinical trials. Clin Inf Dis 1997, 24:764–74.
15. De Gruttola V, Fleming TR, Lin DY et al. Perspective: validating surrogate markers – are we being naïve? J Infect Dis 1997, 175:237–46.
16. Simkin PA, Bassett JE. Cartilage matrix molecules in serum and synovial fluid. Curr Opin Rheumatol 1995, 7:346–51.

17. Tiderius CJ, Olsson LE, Nyquist F et al. Cartilage glycosaminoglycan loss in the acute phase after an anterior cruciate ligament injury: delayed gadolinium-enhanced magnetic resonance imaging of cartilage and synovial fluid analysis. Arthritis Rheum 2005, 52:120–7.

18. Atencia LJ, McDevitt CA, Nile WB et al. Cartilage content of an immature dog. Connect Tissue Res 1989, 18:235–42.

19. Eckstein F, Reiser M, Englmeier KH et al. In vivo morphometry and functional analysis of human articular cartilage with quantitative magnetic resonance imaging–from image to data, from data to theory. Anat Embryol (Berl) 2001, 203:147–73.

20. Sharma L, Hurwitz DE, Thonar EJ et al. Knee adduction moment, serum hyaluronan level, and disease severity in medial tibiofemoral osteoarthritis. Arthritis Rheum 1998, 41:1233–40.

21. Sharif M, George E, Shepstone L et al. Serum hyaluronic acid level as a predictor of disease progression in osteoarthritis of the knee. Arthritis Rheum 1995, 38:760–7.

22. Pavelka K, Forejtova S, Olejarova M et al. Hyaluronic acid levels may have predictive value for the progression of knee osteoarthritis. Osteoarthritis Cartilage 2004, 12:277–83.

23. Elliott AL, Kraus VB, Luta G et al. Serum hyaluronan levels and radiographic knee and hip osteoarthritis in African Americans and Caucasians in the Johnston County Osteoarthritis Project. Arthritis Rheum 2005, 52:105–11.

24. Vilim V, Vytasek R, Olejarova M et al. Serum cartilage oligomeric matrix protein reflects the presence of clinically diagnosed synovitis in patients with knee osteoarthritis. Osteoarthritis Cartilage 2001, 9:612–8.

25. Lohmander LS, Hoerrner LA, Lark MW. Metalloproteinases, tissue inhibitor and proteoglycan fragments in knee synovial fluid in human osteoarthritis. Arthritis Rheum 1993, 36: 181–9.

26. Lohmander LS, Hoerrner LA, Dahlberg L et al. Stromelysin, tissue inhibitor and proteoglycan fragments in human knee joint fluid after injury. J Rheumatol 1993, 20:1362–8.

27. Lohmander LS, Brandt KD, Mazzuca SA et al. Utility of the plasma Stromelysin (MMP-3) concentration in reflecting progression of knee osteoarthritis. Arthritis Rheum 2005, 52:3160–7.

28. Sharif M, Shepstone L, Elson CJ et al. Increased serum C reactive protein may reflect events that precede radiographic progression in osteoarthritis of the knee. Ann Rheum Dis 2000, 59:71–4.

29. Sturmer T, Brenner H, Koenig W et al. Severity and extent of osteoarthritis and low grade systemic inflammation as assessed by high sensitivity C reactive protein. Ann Rheum Dis 2004, 63:200–5.

30. Sowers M, Lachance L, Jamadar D et al. The associations of bone mineral density and bone turnover markers with osteoarthritis of the hand and knee in pre- and perimenopausal women. Arthritis Rheum 1999, 42:483–9.

31. Saxne T, Lindell M, Månsson B et al. Inflammation is a feature of the disease process in early knee joint osteoarthritis. Rheumatology 2003, 42:903–4.

32. Hsu YH, Hsieh MS, Liang YC et al. Production of the chemokine eotaxin-1 in osteoarthritis and its role in cartilage degradation. J Cell Biochem 2004, 93:929–39.

33. McNearney T, Baethge BA, Cao S et al. Excitatory amino acids, TNF-alpha, and chemokine levels in synovial fluids of patients with active arthropathies. Clin Exp Immunol 2004, 137: 621–7.

34. Pelletier JP, Martel-Pelletier J, Abramson SB. Osteoarthritis, an inflammatory disease: potential implication for the selection of new therapeutic targets. Arthritis Rheum 2001, 44: 1237–47.

35. Benito MJ, Veale DJ, Fitzgerald O et al. Synovial tissue inflammation in early and late osteoarthritis. Ann Rheum Dis 2005;64:1263–7.

36. Goldring SR, Goldring MB. The role of cytokines in cartilage matrix degeneration in osteoarthritis. Clin Orthop Rel Res 2004, 427(Suppl):S27–36.

37. Fosang AJ, Stanton H, Little CB et al. Neoepitopes as biomarkers of cartilage catabolism. Inflamm Res 2003, 5:277–82.

38. Hanson DA, Weis MAE, Bollen A-M et al. A specific immunoassay for monitoring human bone resorption: Quantitation of type I collagen cross-linked N-telopeptides in urine. J Bone Min Res 1992, 7:1251–8.

39. Risteli J, Elomaa I, Niemi S et al. Radioimmunoassay for the pyridinoline cross-linked carboxy-terminal telopeptide of type I collagen: a new serum marker of bone collagen degradation. Clin Chem 1993, 39:635–40.

40. Eyre DR. The specificity of collagen cross-links as markers of bone and connective tissue degradation. Acta Orthop Scand 1995, 266(Suppl):166–70.

41. Eyre D, Shao P, Weis MA et al. The kyphoscoliotic type of Ehlers-Danlos syndrome (type VI): differential effects on the hydroxylation of lysine in collagens I and II revealed by analysis of cross-linked telopeptides from urine. Mol Genet Metab 2002, 76:211–6.

42. Apone S, Lee MY, Eyre DR. Osteoclasts generate cross-linked collagen N-telopeptides (NTx) but not free pyridinolines when cultured on human bone. Bone 1997, 21:129–36.

43. Atley LM, Mort JS, Lalumiere M et al. Proteolysis of human bone collagen by cathepsin K: characterization of the cleavage sites generating by cross-linked N-telopeptide neoepitope. Bone 2000, 26:241–7.

44. Eyre DR, Atley LM, Wu J-J. Collagen Cross-links as markers of bone and cartilage degradation. In: The Many Faces of Osteoarthritis. Edited by Hascall VC, Kuettner KE. Birkhäuser Verlag, Basel, Switzerland, 2002, pp. 275–84.

45. Eyre DR. US Patent No. 5,140,103. Peptide fragments containing HP and LP cross-links. 1992.

46. Eyre DR, Atley LA, Vosberg-Smith K et al. Biochemical markers of bone and cartilage collagen degradation. In: Chemistry and Biology of Mineralized Tissues. Edited by Goldberg M, Boskey A, Robinson C. AAOS, Rosemont, 2000, pp. 347–50.

47. Atley L, DeLustro B, Eugui E et al. RS-130830, a selective inhibitor of collagenase-3 blocks the release of hydroxyproline and metalloproteinase specific neoepitope, COL II CTx, from bovine cartilage exposed to IL-1. Arthritis Rheum 1997, 40(9S):584.

48. Atley LM, Sharma L, Clemens JD et al. The collagen II CTx degradation marker is generated by collagenase 3 and in urine reflects disease burden in knee OA patients. Trans Orthop Res Soc 2000, 25:168.

49. Lohmander LS, Atley LM, Pietka TA et al. The release of cross-linked peptides from type II collagen into human joint fluid is increased early after joint insult and in osteoarthritis. Arthritis Rheum 2003, 48:3130–9.

50. Matyas JR, Atley L, Ionescu M et al. Analysis of cartilage biomarkers in the early phases of canine experimental osteoarthritis. Arthritis Rheum 2004, 50:543–52.

51. Lindhorst E, Wachsmuth L, Kimmig N et al. Increase in degraded collagen type II in synovial fluid early in the rabbit meniscectomy model of osteoarthritis. Osteoarthritis Cartilage 2005, 13:139–45.

52. Nishi Y, Atley L, Eyre DE et al. Determination of bone markers in pycnodysostosis: Effects of cathepsin K deficiency on bone matrix degradation. J Bone Mineral Res 1999, 14:1902–8.

53. Everts V, Hou WS, Rialland X et al. Cathepsin K deficiency in pycnodysostosis results in accumulation of non-digested phagocytosed collagen in fibroblasts. Calcif Tissue Int 2003, 73:380–6.

54. Reijman M, Hazes JM, Bierma-Zeinstra SM et al. A new marker for osteoarthritis: cross-sectional and longitudinal approach. Arthritis Rheum 2004, 50:2471–8.

55. Bingham CO 3rd, Buckland-Wright JC, Garnero P, et al. Risedronate decreases biochemical markers of cartilage degradation but does not decrease symptoms or slow radiographic progression in patients with medial compartment osteoarthritis of the knee: results of the two-year multinational knee osteoarthritis structural arthritis study. Arthritis Rheum 2006;54:3494–507.

56. Norlund LL, Shao P, Yoshihara P et al. Markers of bone type I and cartilage type II collagen degradation in the Hartley guinea pig model of osteoarthritis. Trans Orthop Res Soc 1997, 22:313.

57. Pratta MA, Yao W, Decicco C et al. Aggrecan protects cartilage collagen from proteolytic cleavage. J Biol Chem 2003, 278:45539–45.
58. Heinegard D, Inerot S, Wieslander J et al. A method for the quantification of cartilage proteo-glycan structures liberated to the synovial fluid during developing degenerative joint disease. Scand J Clin Lab Invest 1985, 45:421–7.
59. Møller HJ, Larsen FS, Ingemann-Hansen T et al. ELISA for the core protein of the cartilage large aggregating proteoglycan, aggrecan: comparison with the concentrations of immuno-genic keratan sulphate in synovial fluid, serum and urine. Clin Chim Acta 1994, 225:43–55.
60. Lohmander LS, Ionescu M, Jugessur H et al. Changes in joint cartilage aggrecan after knee injury and in osteoarthritis. Arthritis Rheum 1999, 42:534–44.
61. Sandy JD, Flannery CR, Neame PJ et al. The structure of aggrecan fragments in human synovial fluid. Evidence for the involvement in osteoarthritis of a novel proteinase which cleaves the Glu 373-Ala 374 bond of the interglobular domain. J Clin Invest 1992, 89: 1512–6.
62. Lohmander LS, Neame PJ, Sandy JD. The structure of aggrecan fragments in human synovial fluid: evidence that aggrecanase mediates cartilage degradation in inflammatory joint disease, joint injury and osteoarthritis. Arthritis Rheum 1993, 36:1214–22.
63. Malfait A-M, Liu R-Q, Ijiri K et al. Inhibition of ADAM-TS4 and ADAM-TS5 Prevents Aggrecan Degradation in Osteoarthritic Cartilage. J Biol Chem 2002, 277:22201–8.
64. Stanton H, Rogerson FM, East CJ et al. ADAMTS5 is the major aggrecanase in mouse car-tilage in vivo and in vitro. Nature 2005, 434:648–52.
65. Glasson SS, Askew R, Sheppard B et al. Deletion of active ADAMTS5 prevents cartilage degradation in a murine model of osteoarthritis. Nature 2005, 434:644–8.
66. Lark MW, Bayne EK, Flanagan J et al. Aggrecan degradation in human cartilage. Evidence for both aggrecanase and matrix metalloproteinase activity in normal, osteoarthritic and rheumatoid joints. J Clin Invest 1997, 100:93–106.
67. Dickinson SC, Vankemmelbeke MN, Buttle DJ et al. Cleavage of cartilage oligomeric matrix protein (thrombospondin-5) by matrix metalloproteinases and a disintegrin and metallopro-teinase with thrombospondin motifs. Matrix Biol 2003, 22:267–78.
68. Vilim V, Voburka Z, Vytasek R et al. Monoclonal antibodies to human cartilage oligomeric matrix protein: epitope mapping and characterization of sandwich ELISA. Clin Chim Acta 2003, 328:59–69.
69. Sharif M, Kirwan JR, Elson CJ et al. Suggestion of nonlinear or phasic progression of knee osteoarthritis based on measurements of serum cartilage oligomeric matrix protein levels over five years. Arthritis Rheum 2004, 50:2479–88.
70. Petersson IF, Boegard T, Svensson B et al. Changes in cartilage and bone metabolism iden-tified by serum markers in early osteoarthritis of the knee joint. Br J Rheumatol 1998, 37: 46–50.
71. Jordan JM, Luta G, Stabler T et al. Ethnic and sex differences in serum levels of cartilage oligomeric matrix protein: the Johnston County Osteoarthritis Project. Arthritis Rheum 2003, 48:675–81.
72. Dragomir AD, Kraus VB, Renner JB et al. Serum cartilage oligomeric matrix protein and clinical signs and symptoms of potential pre-radiographic hip and knee pathology. Osteoarthritis Cartilage 2002, 10:687–91.
73. Clark AG, Jordan JM, Vilim V et al. Serum cartilage oligomeric matrix protein reflects osteoarthritis presence and severity: the Johnston County Osteoarthritis Project. Arthritis Rheum 1999, 42:2356–64.
74. Lorenzo P, Bayliss MT, Heinegard D. Altered patterns and synthesis of extracellular matrix macromolecules in early osteoarthritis. Matrix Biol 2004, 23:381–91.
75. Hauser N, Geiss J, Neidhart M et al. Distribution of CMP and COMP in human cartilage. Acta Orthop Scand 1995, 66(Suppl 266):72–3.
76. DiCesare P, Hauser N, Lehman D et al. Cartilage oligomeric matrix protein (COMP) is an abundant component of tendon. FEBS Lett 1994, 354:237–40.

77. DiCesare PE, Carlson CS, Stolerman ES et al. Increased degradation and altered tissue distribution of cartilage oligomeric protein in human rheumatoid and osteoarthritic cartilage. J Orthop Res 1996, 14:946–55.
78. Poole AR. Cartilage in health and disease. In Arthritis and Allied Conditions. A Textbook of Rheumatology, 14th ed. Edited by Koopman W. Lippincott Williams & Wilkins, Philadelphia, 2000, pp. 226–84.
79. Downs JT, Lane CL, Nestor NB et al. Analysis of collagenase-cleavage of type II collagen using a neoepitope ELISA. J Immunol Methods 2001, 247:25–34.
80. Wu W, Billinghurst RC, Pidoux I et al. Sites of collagenase cleavage and denaturation of type II collagen in aging and osteoarthritic articular cartilage and their relationship to the distribution of matrix metalloproteinase 1 and matrix metalloproteinase 13. Arthritis Rheum 2002, 46:2087–94.
81. Poole AR, Ionescu M, Fitzcharles MA et al. The assessment of cartilage degradation in vivo: development of an immunoassay for the measurement in body fluids of type II collagen cleaved by collagenases. J Immunol Methods 2004, 294:145–53.
82. Billinghurst RC, Mwale F, Hollander A et al. Immunoassays for collagens in chondrocyte and cartilage explant cultures. Methods Mol Med 2004, 100:251–74.
83. Deberg M, Labasse A, Christgau S et al. New serum biochemical markers (Coll 2-1 and Coll 2-1 NO2) for studying oxidative-related type II collagen network degradation in patients with osteoarthritis and rheumatoid arthritis. Osteoarthritis Cartilage 2005, 13:258–65.
84. Poole AR, Ionescu M, Swan A et al. Changes in cartilage metabolism in arthritis are reflected by altered serum and synovial fluid levels of the cartilage proteoglycan aggrecan - implications for pathogenesis. J Clin Invest 1994, 94:25–33.
85. Kobayashi T, Yoshihara Y, Samura A et al. Synovial fluid concentrations of the C-propeptide of type II collagen correlate with body mass index in primary knee osteoarthritis. Ann Rheum Dis 1997, 56:500–3.
86. Lohmander LS, Yoshihara Y, Roos H et al. Procollagen II C-propeptide in joint fluid. Changes in concentrations with age, time after joint injury and osteoarthritis. J Rheumatol 1996, 23:1765–9.
87. Nelson F, Dahlberg L, Reiner A et al. Evidence for altered synthesis of type II collagen in patients with osteoarthritis. J Clin Invest 1998, 102:2115–25.
88. Mundermann A, Dyrby CO, Andriacchi TP et al. Serum concentration of cartilage oligomeric matrix protein (COMP) is sensitive to physiological cyclic loading in healthy adults. Osteoarthritis Cartilage 2005, 13:34–8.
89. Roos H, Dahlberg L, Hoerrner LA et al. Markers of cartilage matrix metabolism in human joint fluid and serum: the effect of exercise. Osteoarthritis Cartilage 1995, 3:7–14.
90. Manicourt DH, Poilvache P, Nzeusseu A et al. Serum levels of hyaluronan, antigenic keratan sulfate, matrix metalloproteinase 3, and tissue inhibitor of metalloproteinases 1 change predictably in rheumatoid arthritis patients who have begun activity after a night of bed rest. Arthritis Rheum 1999, 42:1861–9.
91. Lohmander LS, Saxne T, Heinegård D. Increased concentrations of bone sialoprotein in joint fluid after knee injury. Ann Rheum Dis 1996, 55:622–6.
92. Lohmander LS, Poole AR. Defining and validating the clinical role of molecular markers in osteoarthritis. In Osteoarthritis, 2nd ed. Edited by Brandt KD, Doherty M, Lohmander LS. Oxford University Press, Oxford, 2003, pp. 468–77.
93. King KB, Lindsey CT, Dunn TC et al. A study of the relationship between molecular biomarkers of joint degeneration and the magnetic resonance-measured characteristics of cartilage in 16 symptomatic knees. Magn Reson Imaging 2004;22:1117–23.
94. Sharif M, Saxne T, Shepstone L et al. Relationship between serum cartilage oligomeric matrix protein levels and disease progression in osteoarthritis of the knee joint. Br J Rheum 1995, 34:306–10.
95. Spector TD, Hart DJ, Nandra D et al. Low-level increases in serum C-reactive protein are present in early osteoarthritis of the knee and predict progressive disease. Arthritis Rheum 1997, 40:723–7.

96. Garnero P, Ayral X, Rousseau JC et al. Uncoupling of type II collagen synthesis and degradation predicts progression of joint damage in patients with knee osteoarthritis. Arthritis Rheum 2002, 46:2613–24.
97. Lohmander LS, Dahlberg L, Eyre D et al. Longitudinal and cross-sectional variability in markers of joint metabolism in patients with knee pain and articular cartilage abnormalities. Osteoarthritis Cartilage 1998, 6:351–61.
98. Delmas P, Hardy P, Garnero P et al. Monitoring individual responses to hormone replacement therapy with bone markers. Bone 2000, 26:553–60.
99. Astbury C, Bird HA, McLaren AM et al. Urinary excretion of pyridinium crosslinks of collagen correlated with joint damage in arthritis. Br J Rheum 1994, 33:11–5.
100. Thompson PW, Spector TD, James IT et al. Urinary collagen crosslinks reflect the radiographic severity of knee osteoarthritis. Br J Rheum 1992, 31:759–61.
101. Sowers M, Jannausch M, Stein E et al. C-reactive protein as a biomarker of emergent osteoarthritis. Osteoarthritis Cartilage 2002, 10:595–601.
102. Bossuyt PM, Reitsma JB, Bruns DE et al. Standards for Reporting of Diagnostic Accuracy. The STARD statement for reporting studies of diagnostic accuracy: explanation and elaboration. Clin Chem 2003, 49:7–18.
103. Bossuyt PM, Reitsma JB, Bruns DE et al. Standards for Reporting of Diagnostic Accuracy. Towards complete and accurate reporting of studies of diagnostic accuracy: the STARD initiative. Standards for Reporting of Diagnostic Accuracy. Clin Chem 2003, 49:1–6.
104. Otterness IG, Weiner E, Swindell AC et al. An analysis of 14 molecular markers for monitoring osteoarthritis. Relationship of the markers to clinical end-points. Osteoarthritis Cartilage 2001, 9:224–31.
105. Otterness IG, Zimmerer RO, Swindell AC et al. Analysis of 14 molecular markers for monitoring osteoarthritis. Segregation of the markers into clusters and distinguishing osteoarthritis at baseline. Osteoarthritis Cartilage 2001, 8:180–5.
106. Garnero P, Piperno M, Gineyts E et al. Cross sectional evaluation of biochemical markers of bone, cartilage, and synovial tissue metabolism in patients with knee osteoarthritis: relations with disease activity and joint damage. Ann Rheum Dis 2001, 60:619–26.
107. Bruyere O, Collette JH, Ethgen O et al. Biochemical markers of bone and cartilage remodeling in prediction of longterm progression of knee osteoarthritis. J Rheumatol 2003, 30: 1043–50.
108. Garnero P, Mazieres B, Gueguen A et al. Cross-sectional association of 10 molecular markers of bone, cartilage, and synovium with disease activity and radiological joint damage in patients with hip osteoarthritis: The ECHODIAH Cohort. J Rheumatol 2005, 32:697–703.
109. Damyanovich AZ, Staples JR, Chan AD et al. Comparative study of normal and osteoarthritic canine synovial fluid using 500 MHz 1H magnetic resonance spectroscopy. J Orthop Res 1999, 17:223–31.
110. Damyanovich AZ, Staples JR, Marshall KW. 1H NMR investigation of changes in the metabolic profile of synovial fluid in bilateral canine osteoarthritis with unilateral joint denervation. Osteoarthritis Cartilage 1999, 7:165–72.
111. Odunsi K, Wollman RM, Ambrosone CB et al. Detection of epithelial ovarian cancer using 1H-NMR-based metabonomics. Int J Cancer 2005, 113:782–8.
112. O'Kane JW, Hutchinson E, Atley LM, Eyre DR. Sport-related differences in biomarkers of bone resorption and cartilage degradation in endurance athletes. Osteoathritis Cartilage 2006;14:71–6.

Chapter 17
Role of Genetics and Genomics in Clinical Trials in Osteoarthritis and Rheumatoid Arthritis

Stuart H. Ralston

Introduction

Identifying the genetic variants that contribute to the pathogenesis of common diseases and the variation in therapeutic response to drugs is an important goal of biomedical research. With completion of the Human Genome Project, researchers have open access to high-quality databases that contain extensive information on gene structure and on polymorphic variation within genes. Other developments such as the Haplotype Mapping Project provide powerful tools for rapid identification of informative variants in candidate genes without the need for extensive resequencing. These developments are likely to make a major impact on all common diseases but are particularly relevant to conditions such as osteoarthritis (OA) and rheumatoid arthritis (RA), which have a strong genetic component. The application of genetics and genomics to clinical trials in arthritis has so far been limited, but this is certain to change in the future as our knowledge about the molecular-genetic basis of these conditions increases and new drugs are developed that target specific molecular pathways.

This chapter will review some basic principles relevant to the genetic dissection of complex traits; briefly review the role of genetic factors in the pathogenesis of OA and RA, and discuss the current status of genetics and pharmacogenetics as applied to these diseases with particular emphasis on the potential application to clinical trials.

Approaches to the Identification of Complex Disease Genes

The approaches that have been used to identify genes that predispose to common diseases are illustrated in Figure 17.1 and are discussed in detail below.

S.H. Ralston
Head of School of Molecular and Clinical Medicine & arc Professor of Rheumatology, Molecular Medicine Centre, University of Edinburgh, Edinburgh UK

D.M. Reid, C.G. Miller (eds.), *Clinical Trials in Rheumatoid Arthritis and Osteoarthritis*,
© Springer-Verlag London Limited 2008

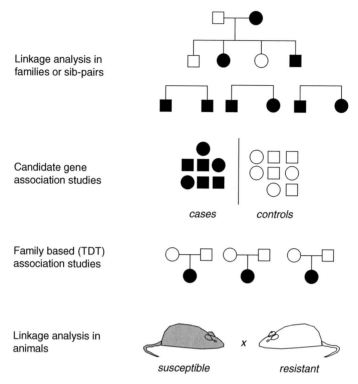

Linkage analysis in
families or sib-pairs

Candidate gene
association studies

cases   *controls*

Family based (TDT)
association studies

Linkage analysis in
animals

susceptible   *resistant*

Fig. 17.1 The figure illustrates the four main approaches used in the identification of genes for complex diseases. See the text for more details of each approach

Linkage Analysis

The classic approach used for gene identification is linkage analysis in families. This involves identifying a model of inheritance for the disease (e.g., autosomal dominant) and looking for evidence of segregation of the disease within a family according to that model, in relation to the inheritance of a panel of genetic markers. If specific genetic markers are inherited by individuals within a family who have the disease, but not by unaffected individuals, this provides evidence of *linkage*. Because the chromosomal location of genetic markers is known, successful linkage studies can localize susceptibility genes to a specific chromosomal region, allowing positional candidate genes to be screened for disease-causing mutations. The results of linkage analysis are reported in *lodscore* units. The lodscore is defined as the logarithm of the odds that the disease and the genetic marker are inherited together within a family (linked) compared with being inherited independently (unlinked). By convention, linkage is considered significant when the lodscore exceeds about +3.0, whereas linkage is considered suggestive when the lodscore exceeds +1.9. Conversely, linkage can be excluded by the finding of a lodscore below −2.0. Linkage studies are usually performed on a genome-wide basis, with a panel of 300 to

400 markers spaced approximately 8 to 10 centimorgans (cM) apart, but they also can be conducted in relation to a specific locus or gene. Linkage analysis has been spectacularly successful in identifying genes for monogenic diseases but with a few exceptions [1] has been little applied to complex diseases such as OA or RA because of uncertainty about the mode of inheritance and the difficulties that are involved in collecting families that are large enough to be informative.

Nonparametric Linkage Analysis

The technique of *nonparametric* linkage analysis is also based on looking for evidence of segregation of a disease (or a quantitative trait) within a family in relation to the inheritance of a panel of genetic markers. In this case, however, no model of inheritance is assumed, but rather, the hypothesis to be tested is that relatives who are affected by a disease should inherit alleles that predispose to that disease more commonly than would be expected by chance. This allows one to localize regions of the genome that predispose to the disease and ultimately to identify the causal gene. As in the case of classic linkage, statistical significance is measured in lodscore units, but the threshold values are between +0.5 and +1.3 units higher than with classic linkage methods, depending on which statistical program is used to analyze the data [2]. The advantages of nonparametric over classic linkage analysis in complex disease is that sib-pairs or multiple small families can be used and that the mode of disease inheritance need not be known. Nonparametric linkage studies have yielded less clear-cut results in complex diseases than those of classic linkage analysis in monogenic diseases. Advances have been made in many disease areas, however, including rheumatology, where several genomic regions that show probable or definite linkage to OA and RA have been identified [3–6].

Association Studies

Association studies involve selecting a candidate gene that is considered to play a role in the disease of interest from a knowledge of cell biology or physiology; searching for potentially functional polymorphisms in that candidate gene; and comparing the frequency of these polymorphisms in subjects with the disease compared with controls. Candidate gene association studies can also be used to study quantitative traits in populations by comparing the average values of the trait under investigation in different genotype groups. Association studies are statistically powerful in that they can detect genetic associations where the effect size is modest, but a potential pitfall is that spurious results may arise as the result of population stratification. This is especially likely if the sample size is small and when insufficient care has been paid to the methods of recruitment, in terms of matching for ethnic group and other confounding factors. These problems can be partly circumvented by careful study design and by genotyping cases and controls with a series of unassociated markers [7]. False-negative results can also occur in association studies, in cases where true genetic susceptibility is masked by polymorphic variation in other candidate genes that also influence disease susceptibility. This problem can theoretically be addressed by stratification for genes that are known to predispose to the disease (e.g., HLA in RA) [8]. The problem is that only a small fraction of susceptibility alleles have been discovered for complex diseases.

Association studies have traditionally focused on polymorphisms in known candidate genes, but over recent years, interest has focused on using genome-wide association to discover new genes that predispose to common diseases [9]. This approach involves genotyping a large number of single-nucleotide polymorphisms spread across the genome to find regions of association and following this up with mutation screening of candidate genes within the associated interval to identify causal polymorphisms and mutations. The number of informative, validated, and suitably spaced single-nucleotide polymorphisms (SNPs) that have currently been identified is considered insufficient to permit this approach, but it is likely that a set of informative SNPs will soon be available for genome-wide mapping. Initiatives such as the Haplotype Mapping Project [10] will greatly facilitate the success of genome-wide association studies by allowing researchers to genotype a series of so called tagSNPs [11] that identify alleles in common haplotype blocks in genes of interest, without the need for resequencing.

Transmission Disequilibrium Test

The transmission disequilibrium test (TDT) is a family-based association study that is a test of association in the presence of linkage [12]. The TDT examines the observed frequency with which an affected individual inherits a "risk" allele from a heterozygous parent in relation to the expected frequency. Because the noninherited allele acts as the control, the TDT is unaffected by confounding due to population stratification. As originally described, the TDT requires a single affected offspring and both parents, but several variations have been devised, allowing TDT to be applied to quantitative traits; employed in sib-pairs without parents and on relatives other than sib-pairs within extended families [13, 14]. Disadvantages of the TDT include the fact that only heterozygous individuals are informative, and this limits statistical power when polymorphisms are being tested that have limited heterozygosity.

Animal Linkage Studies

Linkage studies in animals provide an additional method of identifying genes responsible for human disease, based on the assumption that key regulatory genes will be shared across species [15]. These studies involve setting up an experimental cross of animals from a strain that shows increased susceptibility to disease, with a strain of animals that are nonsusceptible. Brother-sister mating is carried out using the offspring from the first generation (F1 generation) to produce a second generation (F2) in which susceptibility alleles have segregated, allowing one to perform a genome-wide search to localize the genes responsible. Many diseases and quantitative traits have been mapped using this approach, and of relevance to this review, Barton and colleagues identified a susceptibility locus for human RA based on the fact that it showed synteny (i.e., homology) with a locus identified by linkage in an animal model of inflammatory arthritis [16].

Pharmacogenetics

Pharmacogenetic studies seek to identify the genetic determinants of drug response. Most pharmacogenetic studies involve genotyping individuals for polymorphisms in candidate genes that are thought to influence response and relating these polymorphisms to therapeutic response or adverse effects (Fig. 17.2). The best characterized examples are genetic polymorphisms in enzymes that affect drug metabolism such as thiopurine methyl transferase [17] and members of the cytochrome P450 family of enzymes that are responsible for drug metabolism [18]. For the most part, polymorphisms in these enzyme systems are inherited as simple monogenic traits that have high penetrance with clearly defined phenotypes when carriers are exposed to the drug. For many drugs, however, genetic variation in responsiveness and liability to adverse effects is determined by polygenic influences that are more difficult to identify and characterize.

Pharmacogenetic studies of drug responsiveness are potentially prone to false-positive results because of factors such as population admixture in the target population, uncertainty about compliance with treatment, and small sample sizes. False-negative results may also occur because the effects of functional polymorphisms in one component of a metabolic pathway for drug response or metabolism might be counterbalanced by the effects of polymorphisms in a different part of the metabolic pathway. Because of this, pharmacogenetics is best performed by examining the effects of polymorphisms in all known genes that affect the distribution and metabolism of a drug, rather than a single gene [17]. Large-scale randomized controlled trials (RCTs) probably represent the optimal vehicle to define the pharmacogenetic determinants of drug response, but so far, relatively few RCTs have included DNA sampling and pharmacogenetic analysis as part of the study protocol.

Microarrays and Proteomics

Microarrays and proteomic analyses are increasingly being used in both genetics and pharmacogenetics to facilitate the discovery of genes that predispose to disease and to identify predictors of drug response. This approach involves a systematic interrogation of RNA or protein expression in a diseased tissue (e.g., tumor tissue)

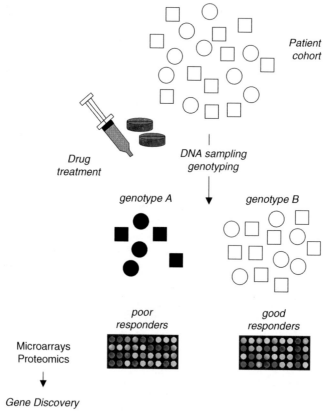

Fig. 17.2 Pharmacogenetic studies seek to identify the genetic basis of drug response and adverse effects by analyzing genetic polymorphism cohorts of patients exposed to drug treatments and relating genotype to therapeutic response. Also, tissue samples in responders and nonresponders can now be used to interrogate patterns of gene expression that correlate with response and thereby identify new molecular targets for drug design

in order to characterize the patterns of gene or protein expression that are associated with clinical response. These types of approach have been most used in the field of oncology where progress has been made to identify patterns of gene expression that are associated with prognosis [19, 20]. Microarrays have also been employed as a tool to identify new molecular targets for drug design. For example, Stegmaier and colleagues [21] were able to identify mRNA signatures that were typical of differentiated myeloid cells (compared with myeloid leukemia cells) and used this as a screening assay to identify compounds that might be able to induce differentiation in myeloid leukemia cells. Another application of this approach is to identify the signatures of gene and protein expression that are associated with adverse effects and/or therapeutic response in cells or tissue samples from patients who are treated with a therapeutic drug (Fig. 17.2).

Genetic Determinants in OA

OA is by far the most common form of arthritis. The incidence of OA increases markedly with increasing age, and it is a major cause of pain and disability in the elderly. It has been estimated that 80% of people will have some radiographic evidence of OA by the age of 65 years, although only 25% to 30% will have symptoms. The knee and hip are the most important joints affected and the principal sites of disability. Pathologically, OA is characterized focal loss of articular cartilage and proliferation and remodeling of bone around the joint to form osteophytes. Inflammation can be a feature of OA, although it is less prominent than in RA.

Environmental and genetic factors are both recognized to contribute significantly to the pathogenesis of OA. Support for the importance of genetic factors comes from twin and family studies that have shown that OA is a highly heritable condition. This is especially marked in hand OA but also holds true for hip and knee OA [22]. Several genome-wide searches have now been conducted to try and identify the genes responsible for OA and have resulted in the identification of multiple loci that influence diseases susceptibility [3–5]. The message that has emerged from these studies is that susceptibility to knee, hip, and hand OA is probably determined by different genes in different chromosomal regions and that the predisposing genes may differ in men and women [22].

Analysis of positional candidate genes within the linkage regions identified so far has revealed some interesting results. For example, polymorphic variation within the interleukin-1(IL-1) gene cluster on chromosome 2q13 has been found to predispose to knee OA in two studies [23, 24]. A missense polymorphism affecting the matrillin-3 gene has been reported to account for the linkage signal to hand OA identified on chromosome 2p24 in Icelanders [25], and a haplotype carried by individuals that consists of two coding polymorphisms of the *FRZB* gene has been shown to account for most of the linkage signal with hip OA identified on chromosome 2q32 by the Oxford group [26]. Finally, polymorphisms in the IL-4 receptor on chromosome 16p12 have been shown to confer increased susceptibility to hip OA but these do not account for the whole linkage signal in this region indicating that there may be other candidate genes within this region that remain to be discovered [27].

Many candidate gene association studies have also been performed in OA, although only a few associations have been replicated in more than one study. Some of the more notable findings that have been described come from the large, population-based Rotterdam study. These include an association between polymorphisms in the 3' flank of the vitamin D receptor gene and osteophyte formation in knee osteoarthritis [28], whereas in the same population, an association was observed between a microsatellite polymorphism close to the COL2AI gene and joint space narrowing in OA [29]. Haplotypes defined by two common polymorphisms in the 5' region of the estrogen receptor alpha gene have also been associated with osteophyte formation in OA in this population [30].

Although the emphasis in this article is upon genetics, there is a substantial body of evidence to suggest that environmental factors also play a key role in OA. Trauma is an important predisposing factor, and reflecting this fact, several occupations have been identified that are associated with an increased risk of OA include farming, mining, and professional football [31, 32]. There is also a strong association between OA and obesity. Traditionally, this has been attributed to increased mechanical loading of the joints, although it has recently been hypothesized that instead, this might reflect an intrinsic disorder of mesenchymal cell differentiation [33].

Genetic Determinants in RA

RA is the most common form of inflammatory arthritis. It is typically a symmetrical form of arthritis that affects both small and large joints that is often associated with systemic disturbance and extra-articular disease features. The clinical course is one of exacerbations and remissions although it is unusual for established disease to remit completely. RA occurs in all ethnic groups and has a prevalence in Caucasians of around 1.5% with a female-to-male ratio of 3:1. The prevalence increases with age, such that about 5% of women and 2% of men more than 55 years are affected by the condition.

Genetic factors play an important role in RA, reflected by the fact that there is a higher concordance of the disease in monozygotic (12% to 15%) compared with dizygotic (3%) twins and an increased frequency of disease in first-degree relatives of patients. Genome-wide searches have revealed that the most important susceptibility locus for the disease lies on chromosome 6p in the human leukocyte antigen (HLA) region, and about 50% of the genetic contribution to RA is thought to be accounted for by allelic variation in genes within this region. This association appears to be primarily driven by carriage of a "shared epitope" of specific amino acids in the hypervariable region of the HLA-DR β1 chain between amino acid residues 67 and 74 [34]. It is currently unclear how exactly this predisposes to RA, but possibilities include the fact that this region of HLA class II acts as a receptor for an arthritogenic agent or peptide; that there is molecular mimicry between the shared epitope and an infectious agent that triggers RA; or that the shared epitope may influence the T-cell repertoire to favor an arthritogenic response.

Many candidate genes other than HLA-DR have also been implicated in the pathogenesis of RA, with most attention focusing on genes that regulate the inflammatory response such as immune-related cytokines and their receptors. For example, several functional polymorphisms have been identified in the promoter and 5' untranslated region of the tumor necrosis factor (TNF) gene that affect TNF expression, and these have been associated with increased susceptibility to RA and with progression of erosions in some studies [8, 35]. A nonsynonymous coding polymorphism in exon 6 of the p75 TNF receptor has also been identified that is associated with RA [36]. Polymorphisms in many other cytokine genes have been associated with RA in various studies, including the IL-1 gene cluster, IL-3, IL-4, IL-10, and interferon-γ [37–39]. The identification of genetic variations in cytokine genes as possible genetic determinants of RA is of interest therapeutically, in view of the fact that biological agents that block the TNF and IL-1 signaling pathways are now being used to treat RA [40, 41].

Role of Pharmacogenetics in the Management of Arthritis

In an ideal world, the drugs that are used for the treatment of diseases such as OA and RA would be completely effective in all patients and would be free of side effects. Unfortunately, none of the medications currently available meet these expectations. Advances in genetics and pharmacogenomics offers the prospect that medicines of the present and future could be tailored to the needs of individual patients, based on their genetic makeup or disease subtype as defined by expression profiling, or proteomics. The application of pharmacogenomics to the clinical management of arthritis is in its infancy, but some studies have been conducted that have identified genetic markers of treatment response and of adverse effects.

Thiopurine Methyl Transferase and Azathioprine

Thiopurine methyl transferase (TPMT) plays a critical role in metabolizing aza-thioprine to inactive metabolites, and polymorphisms have been described in the TPMT gene that encode a variant of the enzyme with much reduced activity [42]. Black and colleagues [43] studied the relationship between TPMT polymorphisms and clinical response to azathioprine therapy in 67 patients who were prescribed this drug as a second-line antirheumatic therapy. Six of 67 (9%) patients were het-erozygous for mutant thiopurine methyltransferase alleles, and five of these patients had to discontinue therapy within 1 month of starting treatment because of leukope-nia, demonstrating that analysis of thiopurine methyltransferase genotype can be used to identify patients at risk for acute toxicity from azathioprine. Although poly-morphisms of TPMT are a very strong predictor of azathioprine toxicity, uptake of genetic testing has been limited in clinical practice, despite the evidence that it could be cost-effective in many health care settings [44].

Cytokine Gene Polymorphisms and Anti-TNF Therapy

TNF plays a pivotal role in regulating expression of other proinflammatory cytokines in RA [45], and anti-TNF therapy has emerged as an important treatment modality in patients with severe RA. Because the therapeutic response to anti-TNF therapy in RA is highly variable, interest has focused on the possibility that genetic testing could be employed to identify good and poor responders to anti-TNF treatment. In a study of 123 patients with active RA that were treated with anti-TNF antibodies, Padyukov studied the relationship between treatment response and a number of known polymorphisms in candidate genes including TNF, IL-1RN (IL-1 receptor), IL-10, and transforming growth factor (TGF)-β1 [46]. There was no significant association between polymorphisms of individual genes and the response, but on subset analysis, a combination of alleles in the IL1RN and TGF-β1 gene did influence response. This association should probably be considered provisional until it is repeated in other studies.

Application of Genetics and Pharmacogenetics in Clinical Trials

The application of genomics and genetics to clinical medicine opens up incredible opportunities for improvements in health care, and this is especially true in the clinical trials arena. Despite this, the pharmaceutical industry has been slow to incorporate genomic, genetic, and pharmacogenetic approaches into clinical trials of new drugs. Although regulatory agencies are aware of the fact that treatment responses and adverse effects are subject to genetic influences, no examples exist where genetic profiling has been successfully used to inform the risk-benefit analysis of a new drug for licensing and registration process. For this to be done, one would not only have to collect and analyze DNA samples from all participants of clinical trials included in the registration package, but one would also need to have identified a robust genetic marker for treatment response and adverse effects that could be included in the regulatory submission. It has been argued that this approach could "save" drugs that might otherwise fail to gain regulatory approval, or get withdrawn from the market, because of uncommon side effects in a genetically predisposed subgroup [47]. Under these circumstances, genetic profiling would allow one to explain the molecular basis of the adverse effect and potentially avoid exposing susceptible individuals to the drug in question.

Unfortunately, a common perspective in the pharmaceutical industry is that genetic profiling might simply hinder drug development. Specifically, there is a concern that the introduction of DNA collections as a routine component of clinical trials might delay ethical approval and adversely affect recruitment, due to concerns about confidentiality and implications for health insurance. In fact, these concerns are largely unfounded, as participants of clinical trials who consent to provide DNA samples as part of a research project or a drug development program are not considered to have undergone genetic testing for insurance purposes. Similarly, the issues of confidentiality with DNA sampling are no different from the general principles of confidentiality regarding other biological samples and clinical information collected during the course of clinical trials.

A second concern is that the introduction of genetic profiling as part and parcel of the drug development process might limit market penetration. For example, if the beneficial effects of a drug were seen to be restricted to a specific, genetically defined subgroup of patients, then there is concern that regulatory agencies might limit the therapeutic indication to patients who have a specific genetic makeup, thus reducing market share. Incorporation of genetic analysis into studies that are conducted after regulatory approval also raises the concern that if one were to identify poor responders as defined by a genetic test, then this might be used by competitors as a negative factor in their attempts to market alternative products. The upside of identifying genetic predictors of response and adverse effects is that there is the potential to develop safer medicines that are individually tailored to a specific patient, resulting in greater efficacy and better tolerability. One of the most common questions raised by patients when discussing whether or not to commence a new treatment is whether side effects will occur. This is a common problem, and in a recent study, adverse drug reactions were estimated to account for about 6.5% of emergency hospital admissions [48]. Even if some of these adverse drug reactions could be predicted by genetic testing of a simple blood sample, this would be seen as a major bonus to most patients. How this might work in clinical practice was elegantly outlined by Bentley in a recent review on the application of genomics to clinical medicine [49].

At the end of the day, the most important drivers toward translating the advances in genetics and genomics into clinical trials and clinical practice will be a consumer-led demand for individualized medicines. For that demand to be fulfilled, regulatory agencies will have to insist that genetic profiling is included as an integral part of the registration process for new drugs. Other requirements will be the identification and validation of genetic predictors of drug response in large, properly powered, randomized controlled studies; retooling routine diagnostic laboratories with necessary equipment to undertake this diagnostic testing; educating health care professionals about how to use and apply these tests, and implementing the results in clinical practice. This is a tall order, given the financial constraints on most health care systems, but is a worthwhile goal if the promise of genetics for improvement of health is to be realized.

References

1. Leppavuori J, Kujala U, Kinnunen J et al. Genome scan for predisposing loci for distal interphalangeal joint osteoarthritis: evidence for a locus on 2q. Am J Hum Genet 1999, 65: 1060–1067.
2. Nyholt DR. All LODs are not created equal. Am J Hum Genet 2000, 67:282–288.
3. Chapman K, Mustafa Z, Irven C et al. Osteoarthritis-susceptibility locus on chromosome 11q, detected by linkage. Am J Hum Genet 1999, 65:167–174.
4. Ingvarsson T, Stefansson SE, Gulcher JR et al. A large Icelandic family with early osteoarthritis of the hip associated with a susceptibility locus on chromosome 16p. Arthritis Rheum 2001, 44:2548–2555.
5. Demissie S, Cupples LA, Myers R et al. Genome scan for quantity of hand osteoarthritis: the Framingham Study. Arthritis Rheum 2002, 46:946–952.
6. MacKay K, Eyre S, Myerscough A et al. Whole-genome linkage analysis of rheumatoid arthritis susceptibility loci in 252 affected sibling pairs in the United Kingdom. Arthritis Rheum 2002, 46:632–639.
7. Bacanu SA, Devlin B, Roeder K. Association studies for quantitative traits in structured populations. Genet Epidemiol 2002, 22:78–93.
8. Newton J, Brown MA, Milicic A et al. The effect of HLA-DR on susceptibility to rheumatoid arthritis is influenced by the associated lymphotoxin alpha-tumor necrosis factor haplotype. Arthritis Rheum 2003, 48:90–96.

9. Carlson CS, Eberle MA, Kruglyak L et al. Mapping complex disease loci in whole-genome association studies. Nature 2004, 429:446–452.
10. The International HapMap Project. Nature 2003, 426:789–796.
11. Carlson CS, Eberle MA, Rieder MJ et al. Selecting a maximally informative set of single-nucleotide polymorphisms for association analyses using linkage disequilibrium. Am J Hum Genet 2004, 74:106–120.
12. Ewens WJ, Spielman RS. The transmission/disequilibrium test: history, subdivision, and admixture. Am J Hum Genet 1995, 57:455–464.
13. Abecasis GR, Cardon LR, Cookson WO. A general test of association for quantitative traits in nuclear families. Am J Hum Genet 2000, 66:279–292.
14. Abecasis GR, Cookson WO, Cardon LR. Pedigree tests of transmission disequilibrium. Eur J Hum Genet 2000, 8:545–551.
15. Nadeau JH, Singer JB, Matin A et al. Analysing complex genetic traits with chromosome substitution strains. Nat Genet 2000, 24:221–225.
16. Barton A, Eyre S, Myerscough A et al. High resolution linkage and association mapping identifies a novel rheumatoid arthritis susceptibility locus homologous to one linked to two rat models of inflammatory arthritis. Hum Mol Genet 2001, 10:1901–1906.
17. Evans WE, Relling MV. Moving towards individualized medicine with pharmacogenomics. Nature 2004, 429:464–468.
18. Ingelman-Sundberg M. Human drug metabolising cytochrome P450 enzymes: properties and polymorphisms. Naunyn Schmiedebergs Arch Pharmacol 2004, 369:89–104.
19. Sotiriou C, Neo SY, McShane LM et al. Breast cancer classification and prognosis based on gene expression profiles from a population-based study. Proc Natl Acad Sci U S A 2003, 100:10393–10398.
20. Cheok MH, Yang W, Pui CH et al. Treatment-specific changes in gene expression discriminate in vivo drug response in human leukemia cells. Nat Genet 2003, 34:85–90.
21. Stegmaier K, Ross KN, Colavito SA et al. Gene expression-based high-throughput screening(GE-HTS) and application to leukemia differentiation. Nat Genet 2004, 36:257–263.
22. Loughlin J. Genetic epidemiology of primary osteoarthritis. Curr Opin Rheumatol 2001, 13:111–116.
23. Smith AJ, Keen LJ, Billingham MJ et al. Extended haplotypes and linkage disequilibrium in the IL1R1-IL1A-IL1B-IL1RN gene cluster: association with knee osteoarthritis. Genes Immun 2004;5:451–460.
24. Loughlin J, Dowling B, Mustafa Z et al. Association of the interleukin-1 gene cluster on chromosome 2q13 with knee osteoarthritis. Arthritis Rheum 2002, 46:1519–1527.
25. Stefansson SE, Jonsson H, Ingvarsson T et al. Genomewide scan for hand osteoarthritis: a novel mutation in matrilin-3. Am J Hum Genet 2003, 72:1448–1459.
26. Loughlin J, Dowling B, Chapman K et al. Functional variants within the secreted frizzled-related protein 3 gene are associated with hip osteoarthritis in females. Proc Natl Acad Sci U S A 2004, 101:9757–9762.
27. Forster T, Chapman K, Loughlin J. Common variants within the interleukin 4 receptor alpha gene (IL4R) are associated with susceptibility to osteoarthritis. Hum Genet 2004, 114: 391–395.
28. Uitterlinden AG, Burger H, Huang Q et al. Vitamin D receptor genotype is associated with radiographic osteoarthritis at the knee. J Clin Invest 1997, 100:259–263.
29. Uitterlinden AG, Burger H, van Duijn CM et al. Adjacent genes, for COL2A1 and the vitamin D receptor, are associated with separate features of radiographic osteoarthritis of the knee. Arthritis Rheum 2000, 43:1456–1464.
30. Bergink AP, van Meurs JB, Loughlin J et al. Estrogen receptor alpha gene haplotype is associated with radiographic osteoarthritis of the knee in elderly men and women. Arthritis Rheum 2003, 48:1913–1922.
31. Cooper C, Inskip H, Croft P et al. Individual risk factors for hip osteoarthritis: obesity, hip injury, and physical activity. Am J Epidemiol 1998, 147:516–522.

32. Croft P, Coggon D, Cruddas M et al. Osteoarthritis of the hip: an occupational disease in farmers. Br Med J 1992, 304:1269–1272.
33. Aspden RM, Scheven BA, Hutchison JD. Osteoarthritis as a systemic disorder including stromal cell differentiation and lipid metabolism. Lancet 2001, 357:1118–1120.
34. Wordsworth BP, Lanchbury JS, Sakkas LI et al. HLA-DR4 subtype frequencies in rheumatoid arthritis indicate that DRB1 is the major susceptibility locus within the HLA class II region. Proc Natl Acad Sci U S A 1989, 86:10049–10053.
35. Mulcahy B, Waldron-Lynch F, McDermott MF et al. Genetic variability in the tumor necrosis factor-lymphotoxin region influences susceptibility to rheumatoid arthritis. Am J Hum Genet 1996, 59:676–683.
36. Barton A, John S, Ollier WE et al. Association between rheumatoid arthritis and polymorphism of tumor necrosis factor receptor II, but not tumor necrosis factor receptor I, in Caucasians. Arthritis Rheum 2001, 44:61–65.
37. Yamada R, Tanaka T, Unoki M et al. Association between a single-nucleotide polymorphism in the promoter of the human interleukin-3 gene and rheumatoid arthritis in Japanese patients, and maximum-likelihood estimation of combinatorial effect that two genetic loci have on susceptibility to the disease. Am J Hum Genet 2001, 68:674–685.
38. Eskdale J, McNicholl J, Wordsworth P et al. Interleukin-10 microsatellite polymorphisms and IL-10 locus alleles in rheumatoid arthritis susceptibility. Lancet 1998, 352:1282–1283.
39. Buchs N, Silvestri T, Di Giovine FS et al. IL-4 VNTR gene polymorphism in chronic polyarthritis. The rare allele is associated with protection against destruction. Rheumatology (Oxford) 2000, 39:1126–1131.
40. Elliott MJ, Maini RN, Feldmann M et al. Treatment of rheumatoid arthritis with chimeric monoclonal antibodies to tumor necrosis factor alpha. Arthritis Rheum 1993, 36:1681–1690.
41. Bresnihan B, Alvaro-Gracia JM, Cobby M et al. Treatment of rheumatoid arthritis with recombinant human interleukin-1 receptor antagonist. Arthritis Rheum 1998, 41:2196–2204.
42. Yates CR, Krynetski EY, Loennechen T et al. Molecular diagnosis of thiopurine S-methyltransferase deficiency: genetic basis for azathioprine and mercaptopurine intolerance. Ann Intern Med 1997, 126:608–614.
43. Black AJ, McLeod HL, Capell HA et al. Thiopurine methyltransferase genotype predicts therapy-limiting severe toxicity from azathioprine. Ann Intern Med 1998, 129:716–718.
44. Marra CA, Esdaile JM, Anis AH. Practical pharmacogenetics: the cost effectiveness of screening for thiopurine s-methyltransferase polymorphisms in patients with rheumatological conditions treated with azathioprine. J Rheumatol 2002, 29:2507–2512.
45. Brennan F, Chantry D, Jackson A et al. Inhibitory effect of TNF alpha antibodies on synovial cell interleukin-1 production in rheumatoid arthritis. Lancet 1989, ii:244–247.
46. Padyukov L, Lampa J, Heimburger M et al. Genetic markers for the efficacy of tumour necrosis factor blocking therapy in rheumatoid arthritis. Ann Rheum Dis 2003, 62:526–529.
47. Roses AD. Pharmacogenetics and the practice of medicine. Nature 2000, 405:857–865.
48. Pirmohamed M, James S, Meakin S et al. Adverse drug reactions as cause of admission to hospital: prospective analysis of 18 820 patients. Br Med J 2004, 329:15–19.
49. Bentley DR. Genomes for medicine. Nature 2004, 429:440–445.

Chapter 18
Cost-Effectiveness of New Biologics for Rheumatoid Arthritis and Osteoarthritis

Yolanda Bravo Vergel and David Torgerson

Introduction

Rheumatoid arthritis (RA) and osteoarthritis (OA), the most common forms of rheumatic diseases, are significant causes of morbidity, mortality, and cost to society. The costs to society associated with these disorders are substantial, and given its progressive nature, if the onset of disease takes place relatively early in life, this will lead to a considerable social and economic impact. In the particular case of RA, it has been estimated that half of patients will be work-disabled within 10 years after disease onset [1–3], making productivity losses the predominant economic burden of the disease [4, 5]. Moreover, the economic costs of RA rise with both age and disease severity [6, 7].

Indirect costs incurred by patients and their caregivers are those related to reduced productivity and losses attributable to the disease preventing individuals from taking better-paying or full-time jobs. In studies that analyze the indirect costs of RA, in general, these are higher than direct costs, largely as a consequence of extensive work disability [7]. In the United Kingdom, direct health care costs have been shown to represent about one fourth of all costs, and these are dominated by inpatient and community day care [8]. One recent study reports that in the United Kingdom, drugs currently represent a minor cost: 3% to 4% of total costs and 13% to 15% of direct costs [9]. However, the introduction of new and costly biological response modifiers can alter the distribution of costs associated with arthritis.

Nonsteroidal anti-inflammatory drugs (NSAIDs) are useful in controlling inflammation, but most patients will require early therapy with disease-modifying antirheumatic drugs (DMARDs) to control disease progression. However, traditional DMARDs are associated with several problems, including a slow onset of action and the requirement for close patient monitoring because of toxicity (including renal disease, hepatotoxicity, and hypertension).

Numerous chemokines and cytokines are believed to play an important role in triggering cell proliferation and sustaining joint inflammation in arthritis disorders.

Y. Bravo Vergel
Research Fellow, Centre for Health Economics, University of York, York, UK

D.M. Reid, C.G. Miller (eds.), *Clinical Trials in Rheumatoid Arthritis and Osteoarthritis*,   289
© Springer-Verlag London Limited 2008

Cytokines stimulate inflammatory processes that result in the migration and activation of T cells that then release tumor necrosis factor-α (TNF-α). TNF-α, one of several proinflammatory cytokines, has been found to play a central role in the pathogenesis of RA and has therefore been the focus of research for novel therapies.

Prasad and Gladman [10] classify the new biological response modifier therapies into TNF-α antagonists (etanercept, infliximab, and adalimumab) and T-cell–targeted therapies (alefacept and efalizumab). The latter are currently used only for the treatment of psoriasis and not psoriatic arthritis. Etanercept, infliximab, and adalimumab are anti-TNF-α agents able to alter the immune function and in particular to inhibit inflammatory response. Leflunomide and azathioprine are also used in the treatment of rheumatoid diseases, leflunomide in particular interferes with T-cell production of cytokines, but both belong to the group of medicines known as immunosuppressive agents and are classified as systemic drugs by the British National Formulary (BNF). In Tables 18.1 and 18.2 we summarize the characteristics of anti-TNF-α agents and when they have been licensed in the U.S. and the European markets for the treatment of arthritis diseases. Hereafter, we will refer to them as new biologic agents.

Etanercept, infliximab, and adalimumab are licensed for moderate to severe active RA when response to other DMARDs has been inadequate.

Etanercept is also licensed in Europe for the treatment of active and progressive psoriatic arthritis in adults not responding adequately to other DMARDs and for juvenile chronic arthritis in children aged 4 to 17 years not responding adequately to conventional therapy. Infliximab is also licensed for the treatment of ankylosing spondylitis, in patients with severe axial symptoms who have not responded adequately to conventional therapy, and it is currently awaiting a final European Agency for the Evaluation of Medicinal Products (EMEA) decision on psoriatic arthritis.

The aim of this chapter is to provide a systematic review of all the economic evaluations that have been undertaken on these new biologic agents. However, before we do so, we describe, in the next section, some of the basic health economic methods and concepts in order to facilitate interpretation of the identified studies.

Background: The Role of Health Economics

Health economics is about making choices in the use of scarce health care resources. Whenever we use a resource in one way there is an *opportunity cost*, which means

Table 18.1 Classification of new biologic agents

Anti-TNF agents*	Description
Infliximab	Anti-TNF antibodies
Adalimumab	
Etanercept	Fusion protein of the p75 TNF receptor

Source: http://www.bnf.org/bnf/bnf/current/openat/index.htm (accessed 25 October 2004).
*Inhibit the activity of TNF.

Table 18.2 Licensed new biologic agents for rheumatoid diseases

Generic name	Brand name	Manufacturer	Status EMEA	FDA
Etanercept	Enbrel	Wyeth Europe Ltd.	JCA (1999) RA (2000) PsA (2003)	PsA (2002) AS (2003)
Infliximab	Remicade	Schering-Plough	RA (1999) AS (2002) PsA (2004)	RA (1998)
Adalimumab	Humira	Abbott Laboratories Ltd.	RA (2003)	RA (2002)

Source: http://www.emea.eu.int/htms/human/epar/a-zepar.htm (accessed 25 October 2004); http://www.fda.gov/cber/index.html (accessed 25 October 2004).
EMEA, European Agency for the Evaluation of Medicinal Products; FDA, U.S. Food and Drug Administration; PsA, psoriatic arthritis; RA, rheumatoid arthritis; JCA, juvenile chronic arthritis; AS, ankylosing spondylitis.

we forego a benefit of not using that resource in an alternative manner. It is generally accepted (by health economists at least) that health care decision making will be more efficient if the costs and benefits of any change in clinical policy are explicitly measured. In this way, we can see the extra benefit that any extra spending incurs and balance this against the loss of not allocating these resources elsewhere. In this section, we will briefly describe the main economic evaluation methodologies, discuss the relationship between clinical trials and economic modeling, and provide a further insight into the particular challenges of modelling chronic diseases.

Cost-Benefit Analysis

Cost benefit analysis (CBA) is the oldest and theoretically the best evaluative method to use in economics. It was developed in the early part of the 20th century to evaluate increased government expenditure on social programs. Its distinguishing feature is that as well as measuring costs in monetary values it also monetarizes benefits. Placing a monetary value on benefits can be difficult even in non–health areas, but in health care it is fraught with difficulty. Attempting to place a monetary value on increases in quality of life has not been satisfactorily resolved. Therefore, most economic evaluations in health care use cost-effectiveness analyses.

Cost-Effectiveness Analysis

Cost-effectiveness analysis (CEA) avoids the problem of monetarizing health benefits by measuring them in their natural units. These "clinical" benefits are then set against costs and informs decision making. For example, we might consider a cost per disability avoided or cost per life saved or life year gained. Although this approach makes it relatively easier for the economist to undertake an evaluation compared with CBA, this simplification loses an important aspect of CBA. CEA cannot be used to make purchasing decisions across different disease areas. Also, the end points might not capture all of the benefits of treatment. To address these weaknesses, health economists have developed a version of CEA known as cost-utility analysis.

Cost-Utility Analysis

Cost-utility analysis (CUA) measures health care benefit in terms of utility, which can be thought of as a measure of overall well-being. Patients' quality of life is measured and converted usually into quality-adjusted life-years (QALY). A QALY basically weights a person's life expectancy by some adjustment for quality of life. For example, if a person is expected to live for 10 years but their quality of life is only 50% of perfect health, they would have 5 QALYs. A CUA, therefore, addresses the weaknesses of CEA and allows the study results to be compared with health economic evaluations of quite different treatments. Nevertheless, a CUA is not without its problems. Measurment of participants' quality of life that will enable capture of all the relevant attributes that are important to a patient in a single scale is difficult. The results of a CUA are expressed in a cost per QALY. There is a debate about what cost per QALY is worthwhile. In the United Kingdom, the National Institute for Clinical Excellence (NICE) tends to approve treatments within the range of £ 20,000 to £ 30,000 per QALY.

Clinical Trials and Economic Evaluations

The most robust method of collecting data for an economic evaluation is usually through the use of a randomized trial. Economic evaluations alongside randomized controlled trials (RCTs) are increasingly common; however, the majority of pharmaceutical trials do not undertake contemporaneous economic evaluations. They often rely on evaluations being conducted after a trial has been completed, which means that often cost data cannot be directly estimated from trial participants, and economic models need to be constructed to estimate all the likely costs and benefits of treatment. Nevertheless, even when there are high-quality trials available with concurrent economic evaluation, there is still a role for economic modeling.

Economic Modeling

Economic evaluations based only on clinical trials can be of limited value for decisions about allocating resources to new treatments in chronic progressive diseases. Clinical trials are generally short in comparison with the duration of the disease and health benefits that can affect the progression of the disease. Together with the potential economic impact of treatments, health benefits will be more evident in the long-term [11]. If we want the results of the economic analysis to be of any use for decision making, the time horizon of the model should be based on the natural history of the disease and not limited to the time frame of the clinical data available.

In this sense, the economic question posed by the new biologic therapies is a good example of the relevance of long-term implications. If the progression of functional disability is delayed with the use of biologics, the resource consumption of patients can be expected to be lower, especially in the long-term (e.g., joint replacement). Also, their ability to work is maintained longer and, consequently, their quality of life increased. The initial response to therapy is still crucial, but the long-term progression for responders and nonresponders to therapy has also a decisive impact on the final cost-effectiveness results. If overall costs increase, the relevant question is whether there is an associated gain in health and whether, from a societal or health management perspective, this gain justifies the additional expenditure.

Ideal data on this would consist of a long-term RCT or, failing this, data from a good quality observational study of disability progression, but in the absence of it, an evidence synthesis of published literature is required. Thus we require a baseline against which we can evaluate new treatments within a time frame that exceeds that of the clinical trials and that incorporates good epidemiologic data; detailed resource consumption for patients at all levels of disease severity; and an effectiveness measure clinically relevant that can be expressed with one generic quality of life measure. Only a decision model will allow us to extrapolate all these costs and effectiveness parameters beyond the data observed in a clinical trial.

Modeling Methods

Markov models have traditionally been used to evaluate the cost-effectiveness of competing technologies for chronic diseases given the ability of these models to reflect patient pathways over extended time horizons [11–13]. Recently, patient-level simulation models are being used for the same purpose. Results from the two modeling techniques have been shown to be very similar in one case study [14].

Both Markov models (i.e., cohort simulation) and patient-level models are forms of simulations. In cohort simulations, the probabilities of a patient following a variety of different treatment pathways are simultaneously estimated to obtain estimates of expected costs and effects, working in terms of identifying the proportion of the total number of patients in particular states (e.g., well, symptomatic, ill, dead) at fixed periods of time (i.e., cycles). In a patient-level simulation, the progress of a patient down various individual clinical pathways is repeatedly simulated to obtain estimates of expected costs and effects.

The general limitations inherent in Markov models are, basically, the need to operate with regular cycles of fixed time length and the fact that transition probabilities between health states depend only on the state in which the patient is at the start of the cycle, with no memory of the patient's previous history before entering that state (homogeneity assumption).

Patient-level simulation models are presented as a more flexible model structure in the sense of allowing a more complicated representation of the clinical pathways being modeled [14]. But it is also a more computationally complicated decision-modeling technique, so its advantages over the more traditionally used cohort simulation should be carefully considered for each case, depending on whether outcomes are believed to be a non-linear function of different variables and whether the interaction between individuals is important (e.g., infectious diseases).

In the next section, we review the economic literature on the use of new biologic agents for the treatment of arthritis.

Critical Appraisal of Economic Evaluations of New Biologics

We have undertaken a systematic review. A systematic review differs from the *traditional* or *narrative* review in that it seeks to identify all the relevant studies within a given field. A key feature of a systematic review is its use of transparent search and inclusion criteria [15]. Non–systematic reviews may be selective in their choice of evidence to present to the reader. In addition, systematic reviews are exhaustive in their search for as many relevant studies as possible.

The study inclusion criteria specified cost-utility analysis of anti-TNF-α therapies compared with DMARDs for the treatment of the most common forms of arthritis.

Search Strategy

The aim of the search was to identify cost-effectiveness studies on new biologics for the treatment of the most common forms of arthritis. Searches were undertaken on the following databases to identify relevant cost-effectiveness literature: MEDLINE, EMBASE, CINAHL, NHS Economic Evaluation Database, EconLit, OHE Health Economic Evaluations Database, HMIC (King's Fund database, HELMIS, DH-Data), Cochrane Controlled Trials Register, SIGLE (System for Information on Grey Literature in Europe), Science Citation Index, and Scientific and Technical Proceedings. The search was dated 25 March 2004.

All databases were searched from date of inception, so there was no limit by date. Given the novelty of biologic drugs, no limit by language was imposed either, in order to make the search as comprehensive as possible. The terms for the search strategies were identified through discussion between an information officer and the research team, by scanning the background literature, and by browsing the Medline Thesaurus (MeSH).

After deduplication, a total of 1521 records were retrieved. Fifty-five economic evaluations of treatments for different forms of arthritis were identified, as well as a number of relevant systematic reviews of economic evaluations published in the field of rheumatology [16–18]. The majority of cost-effectiveness analyses were on the two most common forms of arthritis, OA and RA.

Only 12 cost-effectiveness studies on new anti-TNF-α therapies compared with DMARDs for the treatment of arthritis were found, all of them for adults with RA (Table 18.3). Their main limitations relate to the use of short-term costs and benefits while ignoring long-term impact on disease progression, cost-offsets, and mortality [19], lack of explicit modeling of response versus nonresponse [20, 21], and lack of the generic QALY as the main outcome measure [22, 23]. Two economic evaluations comparing etanercept versus infliximab were also identified [21, 27] (see Table 18.3 for further details).

After exclusion of conference abstracts, seven key published evaluations of new biologics on RA were identified: two of these analyze the cost effectiveness of infliximab [24, 25], three analyze etanercept [22, 23, 26], and the last two compare results for both etanercept and infliximab against a sequence of DMARDs [21, 27]. Two economic evaluations were excluded because they used a clinical surrogate end point (ACR) in estimating their cost-effectiveness ratio [22, 23], and so their results were not comparable with the rest of the studies. The Birmingham Rheumatoid Arthritis Model (BRAM) [27], recently published as a Health Technology Assessment report, is a revised and extended version of the Birmingham Preliminary Model (BPM) [21], so only the first is analyzed.

Summary Characteristics and Quality Assessment

Table 18.3 shows the main characteristics of the four economic evaluations selected. All four studies model the cost-effectiveness of biologic therapies in adults with RA from a health care perspective, using QALYs as their main outcome measure. Two of the studies were set within the National Health Service (NHS) in the United Kingdom [26, 27], and the remaining two were set in the United Kingdom and Sweden [24] and the United States [25]. Kobelt et al. [24] and Wong et al. [25] were analyzed from a societal as well as from a health service perspective.

None were undertaken alongside a randomized controlled trial. The studies used different modeling methods for their analyses. Like the BPM [21], the BRAM study [27] operates as a patient-level simulation model. Brennan et al. [26] is also a patient-level simulation model, whereas the other two are Markov models [24, 25]. All studies assume independence of individuals within the model and allow for an extrapolation of costs and benefits beyond trial evidence into different health states (i.e., HAQ levels and death). Three studies model the relevant costs and QALYs gained over a lifetime perspective [25–27], whereas Kobelt et al. [24] present a 10-year time framework. In the BRAM study [27], toxicity is explicitly modeled for methotrexate and ciclosporin, but none of these studies factor in toxicity or adverse events related to the use of anti-TNF-α agents (i.e., potential harmful effects on the immune system).

Table 18.3 Cost-effectiveness studies on licensed biologic agents for the treatment of RA

Study	Intervention and comparator/s	Primary outcome measure	Decision model	Perspective of the study	Setting, year
Bansback et al.*	Adalimumab vs. DMARDs, infliximab and etanercept	QALYs	IPL simulation	Swedish health service	Sweden, 2003
Bansback et al.*	Adalimumab vs. sequence DMARDs	ACR50	IPL simulation	U.S. health service	USA, 2003
Barton et al.	Infliximab and etanercept vs. DMARDs	QALYs	IPL simulation	U.K. NHS	UK, 2004
Brennan et al.*	Etanercept vs. sequence DMARDs	QALYs	IPL simulation	U.K. NHS	UK, 2001
Brennan et al.	Etanercept vs. sequence DMARDs	QALYs	IPL simulation	U.K. NHS	UK, 2004
Choi et al.	Etanercept vs. sequence DMARDs	ACR20, ACR70	Decision tree	Societal & health service	USA, 2000
Choi et al.	Etanercept vs. sequence DMARDs	ACR20, ACR70	Decision tree	Societal & health service	USA, 2002
Jobanputra et al.	Infliximab and etanercept vs. DMARDs	QALYs	Markov model	U.K. NHS	UK, 2002
Kavanaugh et al.	Hypothetical BIO vs. MTX and IMG	Response	Decision tree	Societal & health service	USA, 1996
Kobelt et al.	Infliximab plus MTX vs. MTX	QALYs	Markov model	Societal & health service	Sweden, UK, 2003
Wong et al.*	Infliximab vs. sequences of DMARDs	QALYs	Markov model	Societal & health service	USA, 2001
	Infliximab vs. sequences of DMARDs	QALYs	Markov model	Societal & health service	USA, 2002

Note: Underlined studies are those reported and compared in Tables 18.4 and 18.5.

DMARDs, disease-modifying antirheumatic drugs; BIO, novel biologic agent; MTX, methotrexate; IMG, intramuscular gold; QALY, quality-adjusted life-year; IPL model, individual patient-level simulation model; ACR20, American College of Rheumatology 20% response criteria; ACR70, American College of Rheumatology 70% response criteria.

* Conference abstract.

All studies used the Health Assessment Questionnaire (HAQ) scores to predict QALYs gained using either a published regression of HAQ versus EuroQol [24, 26], researchers' own HAQ versus EuroQol regression based on published data set [27], or self-reported visual analog scale (VAS) based on the Anti-TNF Therapy in RA with Concomitant Therapy (ATTRACT) study or the Arthritis, Rheumatism, and Aging Medical Information System (ARAMIS) cohort [25]. Direct costs were linked to HAQ scores using published data.

Brennan et al. [26] justify their modeling approach as technically required to model HAQ progression as a function of time-dependent variables (e.g., response rate, withdrawal rate, and mortality rate). The intention behind the model structure of the Brennan et al. [26] and BRAM study [27] is to produce a realistic set of virtual patient histories, replicating patient variability at all relevant points in the model.

In contrast, Kobelt et al. [24] and Wong et al. [25] assume withdrawal at 1 or 2 years based on trial evidence, representing the development of the disease by the movement of proportions of patients between health states over time (i.e., severity states based on functional disability measured by the HAQ plus a death state). Changes due to the treatment effect are calculated as the changes in the transition probabilities between health states.

In the Brennan et al. study [26], initial response to therapy (measured by the ACR20 at 6 months) and initial HAQ score improvement for ACR20 responders was based on phase III study of etanecept versus placebo. Both Kobelt et al. [24] and the Wong study [25] were based on the ATTRACT trial, a 12-month international placebo-controlled RCT of infliximab and concomitant methotrexate.

All studies required a baseline against which they could evaluate treatment effect within a time frame that exceeds that of the clinical trials. Two studies used a U.K. cohort study (ERAS) [24, 26], Wong et al. [25] used a U.S. cohort study (ARAMIS), and the BRAM study [27] used the Norfolk Arthritis Register (U.K.) and estimation of times on each DMARD based on published literature.

In all four studies, a number of assumptions including response to treatment and maintenance of efficacy beyond the clinical trial had to be made. Making assumptions in modeling studies is unavoidable, and for this very reason assumptions should be made explicit, realistic, and even conservative toward the intervention evaluated. In this sense, investigating uncertainty using univariate or probabilistic sensitivity analysis is essential to study the robustness of the findings.

Assumptions present in all four studies and with a decisive impact on the incremental cost-effectiveness ratio (ICER) are the following:

1. The positioning of biologics in the sequence.
   The models assume that the populations concerned have already failed at least two DMARDs in three of the four studies [24–26]. The BRAM study [27] presents a different approach: the aim of this study was to test the effect on the analysis results of using the DMARDs sequence that represents current U.K. practice, in order to avoid the incremental cost-effectiveness of new biologics appearing lower than they really are when inappropriate comparators are used. To ensure that the model truly reflected modern clinical practice, a postal survey

of current U.K. rheumatologic practice was undertaken, as well as a systemaric review of drug use in the treatment of RA.

2. Annual withdrawal rate.

   If patients on biologic treatment withdraw for lack of response, they will still incur large annual costs. So a high rate of treatment continuation can have a large impact on the incremental cost-effectiveness ratios (ICERs). In the study by Brennan et al. [26], the annual withdrawal rate reported for etanercept is 8.3% compared with a much higher dropout for DMARDs (between 10.6% and 25.3%).

   Both Wong et al. [25] and Kobelt et al. [24] assumed that infliximab would be discontinued after 54 weeks and that patients would then receive methotrexate and be at increased risk of flaring.

   The BRAM study [27] uses a completely different approach. The length of time a patient will spend on treatment is estimated from published literature, and withdrawal can be caused by any of four events: death, need for joint replacement, HAQ increase, or quitting the drug. The time to be spent on any treatment is sampled from a Weibull[1] distribution with parameters appropriate to the particular drug. This is added to the patient's current age to give the age at which the drug will be quit; risk of joint replacement, HAQ increase, and death are set as appropriate.

3. Annual disease progression while on treatment.

   There are also huge cost implications if continued treatment does not provide enough and sustained health benefits to compensate annual fixed costs.

   Etanercept is assumed to almost halt progression in responders in the Brennan study [26]. Based on evidence from a systematic review, the Brennan model [26] assumes a slight progression of disability over time even while patients are responding to DMARDs (annual HAQ progression rate of 0.017). HAQ progression for responders to biologics was based on evidence from the long-term open-label study of etanercept, where the initial HAQ improvement is maintained for at least 4 years. For periods of nonresponse to treatment, the average patient's HAQ progression is based on the mean annual HAQ progression rate for patients who were functional grade III+IV in the Early Rheumatoid Arthritis Study (ERAS) cohort.

   As already mentioned, both Wong et al. [25] and Kobelt et al. [24] assumed that after infliximab discontinuation, patients would receive methotrexate and be at increased risk of disability progression. The Kobelt et al. model [24] provides an element of originality. Using a subsample of patients from the ERAS cohort, transition probabilities between HAQ severity states beyond trial data (1 year) were estimated using an ordered probit regression[2] that generated transition

---

[1] Sometimes we want to fit a regression-type model to survival data. The Weibull distribution is commonly used to formulate a parametric proportional hazards model.

[2] Ordered probit regression models are widely used for analyzing outcome variables with an ordinal nature.

probabilities for a cohort that will match the patient characteristics (age, gender, time onset RA) included in the ATTRACT trial.

For all patients with RA, the BRAM study [27] assumes that the average time interval to see an 0.125 increase in the HAQ score was 4 years, based on estimates published in the literature. HAQ improvements on different biologic drugs and DMARDs were also estimated based on published trials, including the ATTRACT study for infliximab and several placebo-controlled studies on etanercept (24- and 52-week data).

4. Rebound after treatment.

For the base-case analysis of the Brennan model [26], after withdrawal the HAQ score would immediately worsen by an exactly equivalent amount to the initial improvement (i.e., rebound is equal to the health benefit gained while on treatment).

In Both Wong et al. [25] and Kobelt et al. [24], health benefits in terms of initial HAQ improvement are maintained beyond the first year (i.e., assumption of no relapse after being off biologics treatment). In other words, new biologics are assumed to slow down the curve of progression. If the HAQ progression after coming off treatment was equivalent to the natural history of RA patients, then the effect of biologics would be assumed to be merely that of symptomatic relief. In the BRAM study [27], once the time to switch treatment has been determined, if the next event is not death or joint replacement, then the HAQ is increased by the fixed quantity of 0.125, independent of the type of biologic or DMARD therapy and the amount of health benefit gained while on treatment.

All the above assumptions will have a decisive impact on the differences in the results reported in the next section. (See the main features of the modeling studies described in more detail in Table 18.4.)

Summary of Cost-Effectiveness of New Biologics in RA

For the Brennan study, the etanercept strategy provides a gain of 1.66 QALYs, resulting in a central estimate cost per QALY gained of £16,330 (lifetime perspective). Drug costs were estimated to be £30,395 higher in the etanercept sequence. These results suggest that etanercept is cost-effective after the failure of two DMARDs in the Brennan model [26]. The impact on results of alternative scenarios for the key parameters is investigated using one-way sensitivity analysis. Univariate sensitivity analyses (£7800 to £42,000) showed long-term HAQ progression on etanercept as the most sensitive variable. Even in the best scenario of including nursing home costs and productivity costs, the net cost difference is still £12,733 against etanercept.

In the Kobelt model [24], The central estimate cost per QALY gained is £25,700 (1-year treatment, only direct costs). Including effect loss at discontinuation, the ICER is reduced to £21,100 per QALY. These results are counterintuitive, as one will expect the ICER to increase when including effect loss after being off treatment

Table 18.4 Main characteristics of economic evaluations of anti-TNF-α drugs

Study	Brennan et al. [26]	Kobelt et al. [24]†	Wong et al. [25]	Barton et al. [27] (BRAM)
Modeling approach	Individual patient-level simulation	Markov model	Markov model	Individual patient-level simulation
Currency (year)*	GBP (2000/2001)	GBP (1999/2000)	$ (1998)	GBP (2000/2001)
Perspective used	UK NHS	Societal & UK NHS	Societal & US health service	UK NHS
Time frame	Lifetime	10 years	Lifetime	Lifetime
Comparators	Sequence with etanercept monotherapy third-line and traditional DMARDs afterwards vs. a sequence of traditional DMARDs only (for patients who had already failed at least two DMARDs, i.e., MTX and SSZ).	Infliximab+MTX vs. MTX alone (for patients who had already failed a mean of 2.5 to 2.8 DMARDs).	Infliximab+MTX vs. MTX only, NSAIDs, DMARDs, MTX+DMARDs (for patients who had already failed a mean of 2.5 to 2.8 DMARDs).	Two analysis were run: (1) Biologics vs. placebo; (2) sequence using biologics vs. two sequences that represent current practice in the UK.
Main source of effectiveness data	Initial response (ACR20) at 3 and 6 months obtained from patient-level trial data for etanercept (Moreland et al.) and from published literature for DMARDs. Mean HAQ progression for nonresponders (baseline) estimated from a UK cohort study (ERAS).	ATTRACT trial (UK, 54 weeks), comparing infliximab+MTX vs. MTX in 428 patients with advanced RA. For the following years, in order to estimate the transition probabilities, they use a UK cohort (ERAS).	ATTRACT trial (UK, 54 weeks). After 1 year of treatment, patients are discontinued and the projection of natural progression based on the ARAMIS cohort study (US).	HAQ improvements on different biologic drugs and DMARDs were also estimated based on published trials, including the ATTRACT study for infliximab and several placebo-controlled studies on etanercept (24 and 52 week data).

Table 18.4 (continued)

Study	Brennan et al. [26]	Kobelt et al. [24]†	Wong et al. [25]	Barton et al. [27] (BRAM)
Main source of resource use data	BSR guidelines (drug & monitoring costs). Direct health care costs estimated using published regression of HAQ scores against health care costs (Kobelt et al. [9]).	ERAS cohort study. Cross-sectional subsample of patients in the ERAS cohort study.	ATTRACT trial, ARAMIS cohort study (US). Indirect costs beyond the first year were estimated as 1 or 3 times the direct costs.	Norfolk Arthritis Register (UK). Published literature.
Main source of unit cost data	MIMS, PSSRU, Health Services Cost Index.	PSSRU, BNF, hospital accounting data.	PSSRU, Health Services Cost Index, BNF.	PSSRU, BNF, Trust Finance Department, published literature.

GBP, Great Britain pounds; DMARDs, disease-modifying antirheumatic drugs; NSAIDs, nonsteroidal anti-inflammatory drugs; MTX, methotrexate; SSZ, sulfasalazine; ACR20, American College of Rheumatology score; HAQ, Health Assessment Questionnaire; ERAS, Early Rheumatoid Arthritis Study; BSR, British Society of Rheumatology; MIMS, Monthly Index of Medical Specialities; ATTRACT, Anti-TNF Therapy in Rheumatoid Arthritis with Concomitant Therapy study; ARAMIS, Arthritis, Rheumatism, and Aging Medical Information System; PSSRU, Personal Social Services Research Unit; BNF, British National Formulary; BRAM, The Birmingham Rheumatoid Arthritis Model.

* Year to which costs apply.

† Details of the Swedish case and results for the Swedish NHS not reported.

from infliximab. In the base-case analysis when indirect costs are also included, the cost per QALY gained was £21,600. When infliximab was given for 2 years and health benefits also maintained at treatment discontinuation, the cost per QALY gained increased to £29,900. These results suggest that maintenance of health benefits after withdrawal and direct cost savings after 2 years of treatment with infliximab are not enough to offset the fixed drug costs. If continued treatment with infliximab were extended to a 3-year scenario, we could predict that results would not be cost-effective.

For the base-case scenario of the Wong model [25], the ICER of infliximab is $30,500 (1-year treatment, only direct costs). These results could remain within the usual range of treatments to be recommended in the United Kingdom. In the absence of maintenance infliximab, the clinical benefit diminished over time as disease progressed, so that one third of the clinical benefit fom infliximab was lost by 2 years and all by 10 years. If that loss of clinical benefit is accelerated to 5 years, the cost-effectiveness of infliximab rises to $47,000 per discounted QALY gained. The univariate sensitivity analysis shows that infliximab with concomitant methotrexate was relatively more cost-effective in patients who weighed less or who had more rapidly progressive RA. As reported earlier, assumptions in both Markov models [24–25] are very similar.

Not surprisingly, the BRAM study [27] reports that when placebo is used as comparator, results are consistently lower than in the base case where apropriate comparator drugs are used, as defined by a survey of current U.K. rheumatologic practice. For the base-case scenario against placebo, the ICER of etanercept is £42,289 and for infliximab £55,988. In contrast, base-case results when appropriate comparator drugs are used are both beyond the £50,000 cost per QALY gained. In any case, these results are well beyond the cost-effectiveness threshold for health technologies to be recommended in the U.K. NHS. Regarding the comparative analysis of biologics, etanercept seems to be more effective (the incremental QALY difference of both treatments compared with placebo is 0.306) but also more expensive (£7736 extra cost per patient). However, even under best scenario circumstances when only biologics can delay HAQ progression, the ICER for etanercept is.£30,141 and for infliximab £39,566.

Both costs and QALYs have been discounted in the above results, although at different discounting rates. (For a summary of the main results, see Table 18.5.)

Discussion

We have identified seven key recent published relevant studies estimating the cost-effectiveness of new biologics compared with standard therapy for RA patients. All of the economic evaluations we found were modeling studies; none had been conducted alongside clinical trials. As noted previously, modeling studies offer a number of advantages over trial-based evaluations, particularly being able to extrapolate costs and health benefits beyond the time frame of clinical trials.

Table 18.5 Economic evaluation results

Study	Brennan et al. [26]	Kobelt et al. [24]*	Wong et al. [25]	Barton et al. [27] (BRAM)
Summary of effectiveness results	Etanercept strategy provides a gain of 1.66 QALYs (lifetime perspective).	Infliximab provides a QALY gain of 0.298 for 1 year of treatment. Including effect loss at discontinuation, the QALY gain is reduced to 0.259 (10 years time horizon, only direct costs included)	Infliximab plus MTX led to a mean lfe expectancy of 0.34 QALY when compared with MTX alone (lifetime perspective).	Results for comparison of anti-TNF-α drugs against placebo show a 0.687 QALY gain for etanercept, and 0.381 for infliximab (lifetime perspective).
Summary of cost results	Drug costs estimated to be £ 30,395 higher in the etanercept sequence, although these are partially offset by cost savings as a result of reduced levels of disability and monitoring costs.	Incremental costs for 10 years are £ 7660 (1-year treatment, only direct costs); including indirect costs the difference is reduced but these will not offset the drug costs (incremental cost £ 6440).	First-year costs with infliximab plus MTX were $10,500 higher and lifetime costs $9000 than with MTX alone.	Etanercept direct costs are estimated to be £ 29,066 higher for etanercept and £ 21,330 for infliximab, both compared with the placebo option.
Summary of cost-effectiveness results	The central estimate cost per QALY gained is £ 16,330.	The central estimate cost per QALY gained is £ 25,700 (1-year treatment, only direct costs). Including effect loss at discontinuation, the ICER is reduced to £ 21,100 per QALY.	For the base-case scenario, the ICER of infliximab is $30,500 (1-year treatment, only direct costs).	For the base-case scenario against placebo, the ICER of etanercept is £ 42,289 and for infliximab £ 55,988.

(continued)

Table 18.5 (continued)

Study	Brennan et al. [26]	Kobelt et al. [24]*	Wong et al. [25]	Barton et al. [27] (BRAM)
Sensitivity analysis	Univariate sensitivity analyses (£ 7800 to £ 42,000) showed long-term HAQ progression ono etanercept as the most sensitive variable.	Including indirect costs, the cost per QALY gained is reduced to £ 21,600 for 1-year treatment.	Infliximab+MTX was relatively more cost-effective in patients who weighed less or who had more rapidly progressive RA. When including productivity costs, the ICER drops to $9100.	The ICERs shown when biologics are compared with current UK practice on DMARD use are consistently higher than when placebo is used. Under the best scenario when only biologics can delay HAQ progression, the ICER for etanercept is.£ 30,141 and for infliximab £ 39,566.
Main conclusions	Results suggest that etanercept is cost-effective after the failure of two DMARDs. However, even in the best scenario of including nursing home costs and productivity costs, the net cost difference is still £ 12,733 against etanercept.	For patients who have already failed two DMARDs, results for infliximab remain within the usual range of treatments to be recommended (£ 20,000 to £ 30,000 per QALY). Although 1 to 2 years of treatment will lead to savings in both direct & indirect costs, these will not offset drug cost.	For 1-year treatment with infliximab and for patients who have already failed two DMARDs, results for infliximab could remain within the usual range of treatments to be recommended in the UK.	Even under best scenario circumstances, results for both etanercept and infliximab are not within the usual range of treatments to be recommended in the UK.

HAQ, Health Assessment Questionnaire; DMARDs, disease-modifying antirheumatic drugs; ICER, incremental cost-effectiveness ratio; QALYs, quality-adjusted life-years; MTX, methotrexate; BRAM, The Birmingham Rheumatoid Arthritis Model.
* Results for the Swedish NHS not reported.

Most of the effectiveness data used to populate the models identified come from short-term RCTs, with 54 weeks being the longest study period. Ideally, longer-term RCTs are required to estimate health benefits, costs, and adverse events during long-term administration of these treatments. Failing the establishment of appropriate RCTs, carefully planned prospective observational studies that include an economic element ought to be undertaken.

This review suggests that new biologics cannot be regarded as cost-effective compared with standard therapy for first-line treatment based on current evidence. Only after the failure of the most effective DMARDs and under best scenario circumstances (i.e., inclusion of indirect costs, maintenance of the treatment effect of biologics after withdrawal, etc.) can results remain within the usual range of treatments to be recommended in the United Kingdom. All the key assumptions with an important impact on the cost-effectiveness of biologics have been reviewed in the above sections. The only study that provides a direct comparison of etanercept and infliximab against current U.K. practice shows that none of them are cost-effective, even under best scenario circumstances (i.e., when only biologics can delay HAQ progression).

However, there remains substantial uncertainty surrounding any decision about the use of these therapies. Additional research could focus on medium and long-term withdrawal rates due to lack of efficacy or adverse events and on maintenance of benefits for responders.

In accordance with the importance of indirect costs as part of the economic burden of RA, when indirect costs are included in the sensitivity analysis, results show an improvement in terms of a reduction of the cost per QALY to be paid. Clearly the results of these analyses are very susceptible to the fixed cost of the biologic drugs, and should these fall substantially, the results would need to be revised.

What is certain is that all new biologic agents are substantially more expensive than current standard treatment (i.e., approximately £ 10,000 per patient per year). In comparison, the cost of the common disease-modifying agent, leflunomide, also licensed in Europe for the treatment of adult patients with active RA, is approximately £ 1200 per patient per year for a standard daily dosage of 20 mg. Both figures include administration and monitoring costs. A careful consideration of the U.K. NHS priorities is needed to guarantee an efficient use of scarce resources. Only economic evaluations that present their results in terms of cost per QALY gained can enable comparability of health care technologies across different diseases.

In March 2002, NICE recommended the use of either etanercept or infliximab for highly active RA in adults who have failed to respond to at least two DMARDs, including methotrexate. NICE also recommended the use of etanercept in children aged 4 to 17 years with active polyarticular course juvenile idiopathic arthritis. The guidance pays attention to the possibility of drug-related toxicity with anti-TNFs. It recommends consultant rheumatologists to register patients with the appropriate biologics registry and forward information on dosage, outcome, and toxicity on a quarterly basis. Treatment should be withdrawn in the event of severe drug-related toxicity or lack of response at 3 months in adults and 6 months in children [28].

We can expect that the use of new biologics will require further clinical and cost-effectiveness research in the near future for the treatment of other immune-mediated chronic diseases such as ankylosing spondylitis, psoriatic arthritis, psoriasis, and Crohn's disease.

The conclusions drawn here are predominately based on the U.K. health system and costs, and so they may not be generalizable to an international context. For other health care systems with different cost profiles, the results may differ. Ideally, economic evaluations ought to be undertaken using country-specific data on costs before a decision is made on implementation of these new treatments.

References

1. Barrett E, Scott D, Wiles N, Symmons DP. The impact of rheumatoid arthritis on employment status in the early years of disease: a UK community-based study. Rheumatology 2000(39):1403–1409.
2. Young A, Dixey J, Kulinskaya E, et al. Which patients stop working because of rheumatoid arthritis? Results of 5 years follow-up in 732 patients from the Early RA Study (ERAS). Ann Rheum Dis 2002;61:859.
3. Fex E, Larsson BM, Nived K, Eberhardt K. Impact of rheumatoid arthritis on work status and social and leisure time activities in patients followed 8 years from onset. J Rheumatol 1997(25):44–50.
4. Jonsson B, Kaarela K, Kobelt G. Economic Consequences of the Progression of Rheumatoid Arthritis. A Markov Model. Stockholm School of Economics: Stockholm, 1997.
5. Kobelt G, Eberhardt K, Jönsson L, Jönsson B. Economic consequences of the progression of rheumatoid arthritis in Sweden. Arthritis Rheum 1999(42):347–356.
6. Jonsson B, Rehnberg C, Borgquist L, Larsson SE. Locomotion status and costs in destructive rheumatoid arthritis. A comprehensive study of 82 patients from a population of 13,000. Acta Orthop Scand 1992;63(2):207–212.
7. Kvien T. Epidemiology and burden of illness of rheumatoid arthritis. Pharmacoeconomics 2004;22(Suppl 1):1–12.
8. McIntosh E. Clinical audit: The cost of rheumatoid arthritis. Br J Rheumatol 1996;35: 781–790.
9. Kobelt G, Jönsson L. Lindgren P. Young A, Eberhardt K. Modeling the progression of rheumatoid arthritis: A two-country model to estimate costs and consequences of rheumatoid arthritis. Arthritis Rheum 2002;46(9):2310–2319.
10. Prasad R, Gladman D. Current and investigational treatment of psoriatic arthritis. Expert Opin Investig Drugs 2004;13(2):139–150.
11. Kobelt G, ed. Health Economic Assessment of Medical Technology in Chronic Progressive Diseases. Multiple Sclerosis and Rheumatoid Arthritis. Karolinska Institute: Stockholm, 2003.
12. Parmigiani G. Modeling in Medical Decision Making. A Bayesian Approach. John Wiley & Sons, Ltd.: Hoboken, NJ, 2002.
13. Barton P, Bryan S, Robinson S. Modelling in the economic evaluation of health care: selecting the appropriate approach. J Health Services Res Policy 2004;9(2):110–118.
14. Karnon J. Alternative decision modelling techniques for the evaluation of health care technologies: Markov processes versus discrete event simulation. Health Economics 2003;12:837–848.
15. Torgerson C. Systematic Reviews Continuum. Research Methods Series. London, 2003.
16. Emery P. Review of health economics modelling in rheumatoid arthritis. Pharmacoeconomics 2004;22(2):55–69.
17. Tella MN, Feinglass J, Chang RW. Cost-effectiveness, cost-utility, and cost-benefit studies in rheumatology: a review of the literature, 2001-2002. Curr Opin Rheumatol 2003;15(2): 127–131.

18. Maetzel A, Ferraz MB, Bombardier C. A review of cost effectiveness analyses in rheumatology and related disciplines. Curr Opin Rheumatol 1998;10(2):136–140.

19. Kavanaugh A, Heudebert G, Cush J, Jain R. Cost evaluation of novel therapeutics in rheumatoid arthritis (CENTRA): a decision analysis model. Semin Arthritis Rheum 1996;25(5): 297–307.

20. Maetzel A, Wong JB. Estimating the cost-effectiveness of lifelong infliximab for patients with rheumatoid arthritis (RA) in Canada. J Rheumatol 2003;30(8):1863–1883.

21. Jobanputra P, Bartan P, Bryan S, Burls A. The effectiveness of infliximab and etanercept for the treatment of rheumatoid arthritis: a systematic review and economic evaluation. Health Technology Assessment 2002;6(21):1–110.

22. Choi HK, Seeger JD, Kuntz KM. A cost-effectiveness analysis of treatment options for patients with methotrexate-resistant rheumatoid arthritis. Arthritis Rheum 2000;43(10):2316–2327.

23. Choi HK, Seeger JD, Kuntz KM. A cost effectiveness analysis of treatment options for methotrexate-naive rheumatoid arthritis. J Rheumatol 2002;29(6):1156–1165.

24. Kobelt G, Jönsson L, Young A, Eberhardt K. The cost-effectiveness of infliximab (Remicade) in the treatment of rheumatoid arthritis in Sweden and the United Kingdom based on the ATTRACT study. Rheumatology 2003;42(2):326–335.

25. Wong JB, Singh G, Kavanaugh A. Estimating the cost-effectiveness of 54 weeks of infliximab for rheumatoid arthritis. Am J Med 2002;113(5):400–408.

26. Brennan A, Bansback N, Reynolds A, Conway P. Modelling the cost-effectiveness of etanercept in adults with rheumatoid arthritis in the UK. Rheumatology 2004;43(1):62–72.

27. Barton P, Jobanputra P, Wilson J, Bryan S, Burls A. The use of modelling to evaluate new drugs for patients with a chronic condition: the case of antibodies against tumour necrosis factor in rheumatoid arthritis. Health Technology Assessment 2004;8(11).

28. NICE. Clearance for new arthritis drugs. Pharm J 2002;268(7191):419–425.

Abbreviations

AP	Anteroposterior
AS	Ankylosing spondylitis
ASAS	Assessment in ankylosing spondylitis
BASDAI	Bath Ankylosing Spondylitis Disease Activity Index
BASFI	Bath Ankylosing Functional Index
BASRI	Bath Ankylosing Spondylitis Radiology Index
CRP	C-reactive protein
DC-ART	Disease-controlling antirheumatic therapy
DMARD	Disease-modifying antirheumatic drug
ESR	Erythrocyte sedimentation rate
FDA	Food and Drug Administration
HLA-B27	Human leukocyte antigen B27
ICL	Imaging core laboratory
IND	Investigational New Drug
ITT	Intention to treat
LDAS	Low disease activity state
LOCF	Last observation carried forward
MCID	Minimal clinical important difference
MRI	Magnetic resonance imaging
NDA	New Drug Application
NME	New molecular entity
NRS	Numeric rating scale
NSAID	Nonsteroidal anti-inflammatory drug
OA	Osteoarthritis
RA	Rheumatoid arthritis
RCT	Randomized controlled trial
SAARD	Slow-acting antirheumatic drug
SASSS	Stoke's Ankylosing Spondylitis Spinal Score
SD	Standard deviation
SMARD	Symptom-modifying antirheumatic drug
TNF	Tumor necrosis factor
VAS	Visual analog scale

Index